Medication Errors:
Causes and Prevention

Medication Errors:
Causes and Prevention

NEIL M. DAVIS, M.S., PHARM.D.
Professor of Pharmacy, Temple University School
of Pharmacy, Philadelphia, PA, Editor-in-Chief,
Hospital Pharmacy

MICHAEL R. COHEN, B.S.
Assistant Director of Pharmacy Service, Temple University
Hospital, Philadelphia, PA, Assistant Clinical Professor,
Temple University School of Pharmacy, Assistant Editor,
Hospital Pharmacy, Editor, "Medication Errors," *Nursing '81*,
Intermed Communications

With contributions by
RUTH BUDD JACOBSEN, R.N., B.S., M.A.
Nursing Consultant, Eastern Division, Hospital Affiliates International,
Tampa, Florida

CHARLES J. MILAZZO
Loss Control Manager, Alexis Risk Management Services, Inc.,
Chicago, Illinois

George F. Stickley Company
210 West Washington Square
Philadelphia, PA 19106

iv

Contents

Acknowledgement

We thank the many dedicated health professionals who contributed their experiences or knowledge of actual medication errors by sending them to us for publication. Because of their thoughtfulness and efforts they no doubt have helped other health professionals prevent countless incidents of injury and death to patients. In our opinion, an important way of preventing errors is by learning from the mistakes of others. We will continue to serve as a clearing house for information on medication errors and disseminate this information to readers of *Hospital Pharmacy* and *Nursing '81*. We look forward to the continued support of our readers.

We offer special thanks to Frank F. Williams, Pharm.D., Salvatore J. Turco, Pharm.D., Lawrence Wolfe, B.S. Pharm., and Hedy Cohen, R.N., for serving as resource people on technical matters and for their valuable suggestions; Robin Davis for her editorial assistance, and Julie Davis and Hedy Cohen for their support and understanding.

Last, but not least, to William and Mollie Davis and Elinore and Victor Cohen, our parents, we give thanks for their encouragement.

Preface

The purpose of this book is to document the problem of medication errors, to discuss the reasons for these errors, and to suggest methods to prevent them from occurring.

The health care system has many checks and balances built in to prevent errors from reaching the patient. Errors that do reach the patient usually result from more than one breakdown or weakness in the system. This book deals with the contributions of the physician, nurse, pharmacist, and their assistants and students in causing and preventing errors. The roles of the patient and Pharmaceutical Industry in contributing to and preventing errors also are discussed.

In 1975 the journal, *Hospital Pharmacy*, solicited readers to publish anonymously errors that had occurred at their health care facility. Although medication errors are common, they are rarely publicized and it is our belief that publicizing errors will help to sensitize health professionals and administrators to this problem and serve as an educational tool. The errors have since been published on a monthly basis. Throughout our professional careers we have been interested in preventing medication errors. The publication of such errors for the past five years has heightened our knowledge and interest in the subject. This book results from these interests and our desire to make drug therapy safer and more effective by reducing the incidence of medication errors.

1

General Information

Medication Errors

How bad is the medication error problem in hospitals? The medication error studies in chapter two, in non-unit dose hospitals, found error rates of 16.6%, 13%, 7.7%, 8.3%, 9.9%, 11.4%, 20.6% and 5.3%. These rates do not include wrong time errors. This is a range of 5.3% to 20.6%, with an average of 11.6%. If we project a 12% medication error rate for a hospital with a daily census of 300 patients, the following could be expected:

300 patients x 365 days = 109,500 patient days—Each patient receives about 10 doses a day of medication—1,095,000 doses of medication are administered annually—131,400 medication errors are committed annually—360 medication errors are committed daily—

Many hospital personnel are skeptical of the validity of these studies and minimize the clinical importance of the errors they reflect. What is the true error rate in hospitals? For the disbelievers let us select an arbitrary figure of 1%, a much lower figure than any reported by studies in non-unit dose hospitals. Such an error rate would mean 10,950 medication errors annually, 30 medication errors daily. Clearly, even with a low medication error figure, the number of errors is alarming.

Many of these errors have no clinical significance and do not adversely affect the patients or extend their hospital stay, although they do affect the patient's confidence in the quality of the health care system and its personnel. But some errors do affect the patient's health. In the pages that follow, medication errors which had serious, and sometimes fatal effects on patients, are cited. If health professionals and administrators treat errors lightly simply because no harm was done to the patient, a serious error that will cause injury or death will be inevitable.

1

Obviously, when each patient is given 10 daily doses of medication ordered by physicians, dispensed by pharmacists and administered by nurses, errors will occur even in the best of hospitals; and it should be pointed out that the medication error rate in long term care facilities probably equals that found in the hospital studies. While human error is inescapable, a zero error rate must be the goal of all concerned.

The Plan of This Book

The purpose of this book is to document the problem of medication errors, to explore the causes of such errors and to suggest remedies to help in their prevention. Scientific studies and brief cases are cited to illustrate the scope and severity of the problem.

If you have worked in a hospital, long term care facility, physician's office, pharmacy, have been a patient, or have had a relative or friend who has been a patient, you are aware of the problem of medication errors. However, until studies began in 1962, the problem had never been accurately assessed (see Chapter 2).

In March 1975, *Hospital Pharmacy* began publishing a medication error report feature consisting of error reports submitted by readers and errors brought to the attention of the authors in their seminars on the subject. The reports are published anonymously. Where possible, methods of prevention were suggested. It was hoped to alert health professionals to errors that occurred elsewhere, since such errors were likely to be repeated. The first 150 errors published in *Hospital Pharmacy* appear in the appendix of this book, and are referred to by number in the body of the text.

The term *error* is used throughout this book. The classification and definition of errors used in medication error studies are discussed in Chapters 2 and 17. However, some of the incidents described below go beyond these classifications and definitions and thus are not true errors. For instance, in error #25 the patient refused to take an oral dose of paraldehyde when he noted that the medicine was dissolving a styrofoam cup. In another situation an adult patient refused Lugol's solution when he observed the word "poison" which the pharmacist placed on the label (see error #26). Neither of these incidents is an error, but if our goal is to see that the right patient receives the right drug, in its active form, in the proper amount, via the right route of administration, at the right time, such incidents are appropriate for discussion in addition to the errors that fit the classical definition.

Errors are caused by physicians in hospitals, long term care facilities and office practice, residents, interns, medical students, physician assistants, registered nurses, student nurses, licensed practical (vocational) nurses, ward clerks, pharmacists, pharmacy residents, pharmacy students, pharmacy supportive personnel, administrators, pharmaceutical manufacturers, patients and patients' visitors. Errors are common among American-trained personnel and foreign-trained personnel. They are caused by the young and the old, the experienced and the inexperienced.

Errors occur because of a lack of knowledge, substandard performance or because of defects in systems. Any individual may lack knowledge or be guilty of poor performance. Nurses are often implicated in health care facility medication errors since they are the personnel at the interface of medication and the patient. However, the nurse who administers the drug often is not responsible for the error.

An examination of poor systems which lead to errors and recommendations for improving these systems are major features of this book. Our discussion will cover personnel selection, training and supervision; written and verbal communications; after hour rounds by physicians; transcribing physician orders; reduction or elimination of non-emergency drug stocks on nursing units; adequate pharmacy hours, unit dose dispensing systems, and pharmacy I.V. admixture services.

The pharmaceutical manufacturer's selection of brand names, poor label design, and package size often contribute to the potential for errors. These problems and recommendations for correction will be found in Chapter 15.

The reasons some patients allow errors to be perpetrated on them is discussed in Chapter 13. This chapter also explores methods of educating the public to assume more responsibility for preventing errors.

Medication errors are not usually publicized within the hospital.* Some reasons for this are medical-legal implications, protection of hospital reputation, and consideration for an individual's feelings. Also, every group of professionals and every department is vulnerable, and those who are inclined to point the finger at other professionals may later find themselves involved in errors.

It should be kept in mind that avoidance of error is everyone's concern. Errors must be fully investigated to determine whether new procedures should be formulated to prevent recurrence. Once formulated, these procedures must be publicized and followed. Methods must be instituted to inform health professionals when errors occur. If, for instance, health professionals are informed about errors caused by illegible handwriting whenever one occurred, perhaps the source of error would no longer be treated as a joke.

The reporting of medication errors is presented in Chapter 17. Reporting forms, protocols, error tabulation, committee action and follow up are also discussed.

---

*Wherever used here, the term "hospital" should be understood to include long term care facilities.

The American Society of Hospital Pharmacists Guidelines on Hospital Drug Distribution and Control is an authoritative document which should be of great value in hospitals and long term care facilities in designing safe drug distribution systems. It will be found in the appendix.

An additional appendix, Hazard Warnings, was originally published in *Hospital Pharmacy*. Hazard Warnings were intended to alert health professionals to specific error-causing situations, such as poorly conceived drug names and drug product labels. Some of the Hazard Warnings resulted from errors that were reported to us; others were based on our assessment of the potential for error of new products or labels.

Halfway measures are never satisfactory. Part time supervision, programs that are not constantly monitored, poorly conceived unit dose systems, etc., eventually show their weaknesses. They slowly deteriorate to the level of safety that preceded them. Adequate programs are needed from the outset — monitored to insure that the desired level of performance and service is maintained. It is easier to start a program than to maintain one at the desired level of performance.

Unit Dose Drug Distribution Systems

Unit Dose Distribution is referred to throughout this book. A compilation of published articles describing unit dose systems is available.[1] Published medication error rate studies (see Chapter 2) show approximately 80% fewer medication errors in hospitals using a unit dose dispensing system compared to hospitals using a traditional drug distribution system. Other benefits of properly designed and controlled unit dose systems are drug control, increased accountability for doses of drugs dispensed, economy and the freeing of nursing time.

Though the unit dose system may differ in form depending on the specific needs, resources and characteristics of each institution, four elements are common to all:[2]

1. medications are contained in, and administered from, single-unit or unit dose packages;
2. medications are dispensed in ready-to-administer form, to the extent possible;
3. for most medications, not more than a 24-hour supply of doses is provided or available at the patient care area at any time, and a patient medication profile is concurrently maintained in the pharmacy for each patient.

   In a unit dose system, floor stocks of drugs are minimized and limited to drugs for emergency use, and routinely used "safe" items such as mouthwash, antiseptic solutions and other nursing necessities. The more comprehensive the system, the less need for floor stock.

For long term care facilities, some pharmacies provide a unit dose system such as we have described. Some provide what is termed a "modified" unit dose system, where more than a 24-hour supply of unit dose medication is dispensed. Others modify the system by providing medication on 30-day punch cards. These variations are improvements which offer major advantages over the traditional method of supplying medication, but are not as effective as a true unit dose system.

A flow chart diagraming the typical unit dose process is shown in Figure 1-1. Variations and more complete explanations of some of the numbered steps are as follows:

Step 1   The physician's order may be written, verbal, or computer entered.

Step 2A   Before this process is initiated, the nurse also goes through the processes described in steps 6 and 6A. Communication with the pharmacist is also part of this process. When necessary, nurses prepare stat doses which are obtained from emergency floor stock drug supplies.

Step 6   The pharmacist also assesses whether there is an indication for the drug prescribed. To calculate or verify some drug doses the pharmacist must obtain patient data such as age, weight and degree of kidney function. Also, cancer chemotherapy protocols must be available.

Step 6C   In those rare instances where there is a significant unresolved conflict concerning drug therapy further steps must be taken as described in the literature.[3] A review of this process is described in Chapter 4.

Step 6D   Physicians may write new orders or verbally modify the order to the pharmacist. Pharmacists may enter this verbal order onto the chart to be countersigned by the physician and/or may prepare a form notifying the nurse of the order change, for inclusion in the chart.

Step 9B   All drugs, with the exception of topical medications
and 10   and other drugs which do not lend themselves to unit dose packaging, are dispensed in properly labeled unit dose packages. Such packages may be for oral solid dosage forms, liquids, injections or I.V. admixtures. These products are purchased already packaged from the pharmaceutical manufacturers or are prepared by the pharmacy.

Step 11   The pharmacy maintains a set of patient labeled bins (drawers). These are filled in the pharmacy while another separate set of drawers are in the nursing unit.

6

Figure 1-1. FLOW CHART FOR A UNIT DOSE SYSTEM. (Carts = carts or cassettes, MAR = Medication Administration Record)

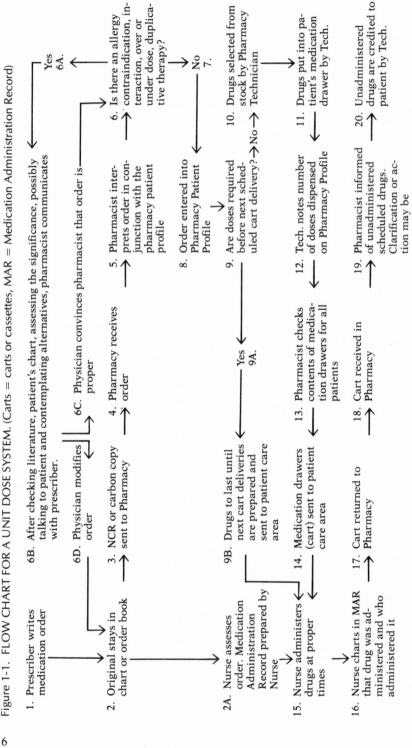

Step 14   Some systems use a drug cart with a patient labeled drawer for each patient from which drugs are administered, while others use a locked medication drawer in each patient's room. In either case labeled unit dose packages are placed in patient labeled drawers.

Step 15   The nurse first determines from the patient's MAR what drug(s) is to be administered and then finds the drug(s) in the patient's drawer.
If a scheduled drug is not administered or rescheduled the nurse completes a 'drug not administered' form (see Chapter 7) and leaves the form and the medication in the patient's drawer.

Step 17   Carts, cassettes, bins are exchanged when the medication is delivered for the next time period in Step 14.

References

1. Sourcebook on Unit Dose Drug Distribution 1978 Edition, published by the American Society of Hospital Pharmacists, 4630 Montgomery Ave., Washington, D.C. 20014.
2. ASHP Guidelines on Hospital Drug Distribution & Control, reprinted in the appendix.
3. Davis, NM. Physician-pharmacist conflict over drug therapy: a pharmacy policy statement. Hosp Pharm 1976; 11:134.

2

Published Medication Error Studies

Understanding the various medication error studies requires careful reading of all the published material on this subject. Occasionally, it is necessary to go over the study with the investigator personally to grasp some of the subtleties, for the subject is a complex one which requires detailed descriptions. The most scholarly work in the field *A Study of Medication Errors in A Hospital*, by Barker et al.[1] (1966) may be found in pharmacy school libraries.

A comparison of medication error studies is difficult because investigators measured different things in different ways at different times. Some of the variables are as follows:

1. Administration of a dose after an automatic stop order expiration date in some studies was counted as an extra dose error while other studies did not count this as an error.
2. Some studies counted wrong time errors, others did not.
3. Some studies in the 1960's counted administering a wrong brand as an unordered drug given and an omission, while other studies did not count this as an error.
4. Some studies did not count an error if observers did not see the patient take the drug, others considered as given everything that the nurse took into the patient's room and charted.
5. Some studies noted that medications administered by student nurses, private duty nurses and physicians were not counted, while others made no mention of this.
6. Some studies had a review process to verify observers' judgment.
7. Observers included specially trained pharmacy students, pharmacists, medical students, or specially trained nurses.
8. The number of observations in various studies range from 607 to 75,463.

9. Wrong dose was defined as ± 5%, ± 17% or not studied.
10. Difficulties were encountered in defining the meaning of "going to surgery" as a determinate for stopping drug orders. Was going to surgery to have a cast removed considered "going to surgery"? One study said no, while it is not known how others treated such questions.
11. Most investigators did not observe the night shift.
12. One study indicated that if the review panel found a physician's order too confusing, all doses associated with such an order were excluded from the study. Other studies made no mention of such a practice.
13. One study stated that no attempt was made to determine if the right patient received the medication. This point is not clear in other studies.
14. Difficulty was encountered in identifying the medication administered in the traditional system to determine if an error had been made, while in the unit dose system, the use of labeled unit packages aided in identifying errors of this nature.
15. One study[2] apparently tabulated errors and discrepancies that reached the patient as well as procedural errors which really are not medication errors (see Chapter 17). This study counted the incomplete entry of an order for a PRN medication onto a pharmacy patient profile which was handled as floor stock by the nurses in their tabulation of discrepancies.

While these variables do not invalidate the studies, they make comparisons difficult in that the magnitude of the occurrence of medication errors may be understated or overstated.

A valid study must report all errors known to have occurred. But because the perpetrator of an error may be unaware of his or her mistake, error studies which rely on self-reporting have been omitted from this study.

The following are major findings of the published medication error studies:

Florida Study*

In 1961 Barker and McConnell studied medication errors and the problems inherent in reporting errors at a University of Florida Teaching Hospital. The study listed thirty-one references in nursing, hospital and hospital pharmacy journals that deal with various aspects of the medication error problem, but no articles that dealt with detecting errors were included.

*Barker KN, McConnell WE. The problem of detecting medication errors in hospital. Am J Hosp Pharm 1962; 19:361.

Information about medication errors can be collected by observation, self-reporting and studying existing records. Errors may be classified as known (someone is aware of them though they may not be reported) and unknown. Thus a report covering all *known* errors may omit many errors which escaped observation.

Errors were classified as follows:

1. Omission—failure to give a dose at the time set for it.
2. Wrong dosage given (± 5%).
3. Extra dose given—Any dose given in excess of total number of doses ordered by physician.
4. Unordered drug given.
5. Wrong dosage form given—any dosage form which is not included in generally accepted interpretation of the physician's orders.
6. Wrong time—30 minutes or more before or after it was ordered, up to the time the next dose of the same medication ordered. PRN orders were not included. (In the study all wrong time errors happened to be at least one hour away from the intended time of administration.)
7. Wrong route of administration.

Observation was made with the nurses unaware of the true reason for the observer pharmacist's presence. Observation totalled 136 hours of 9 nurses administering 572 medications. Ninety-three errors were noted, resulting in an error rate of 18.4% (Table 2-1). If wrong time errors are eliminated, the error rate would be 16.6%.

Table 2-1. Frequency of Observed Medication Errors in Florida Study
(By Error Type)

Type Error	Number of Errors Observed 572 doses administered	Percentage of Total Errors
Omission	35	37
Underdose	12	13
Overdose	7	8
Extra dose	9	10
Unordered drug	17	18
Wrong dose form	4	4
Wrong time (early or late by 30 minutes)	9	10
Total	93	100%

In this study hospital in 1960, over 278,000 doses were administered, yet incident reports were submitted for only 36 errors. If the observed error rate of 18.4% were extrapolated for 1960, then 51,200 errors actually occurred. This means 1 in 1,424 errors was in fact reported. If we assume that due to the small sample size the study was inaccurate by 50%, the extrapolated errors drop to 25,600, meaning that only 1 in 712 errors was reported on an incident report.

In a questionnaire which was part of the study, nurses indicated "practical" standards of action in reporting medication errors included under reporting of errors involving drugs omitted, wrong time errors and drugs considered innocuous.

No attempt was made to determine who actually caused the detected errors, and it would be fallacious to assume that the nurses involved in the detected errors were necessarily at fault.

Arkansas Study*

This study was the result of a United States Public Health Service grant for a multidisciplinary group to study a centralized unit dose dispensing system in the 325-bed Arkansas Medical Center Hospital. The study took place in 1964 and 1965. Because of construction delays there was a shorter than anticipated break-in period for the unit dose systems. However, because the end of the funding period was approaching, the unit dose system was analyzed prematurely.

Errors were defined as deviations from physicians' orders on the patients' charts. All observers were pharmacists with special training in observational techniques. Errors were defined as:

1. Omission—failure to give a dose at the time set for it.
2. Wrong dose—any dose above or below the correct dose by 17% or more.
3. Extra Dose Given—any dose given in excess of the total number of times indicated by the physician, such as one given on the basis of an expired order.
4. Unordered drug given.
5. Wrong route.
6. Wrong time—any drug given 30 minutes or more early or late (figures are presented with and without wrong time errors).
7. Dose deteriorated.
8. Other situations judged as unwanted by physicians (administering I.V. solutions out of sequence).

Nurses were not informed that this was a medication error study. All error observations were reviewed by two additional pharmacists and a nurse before being counted as errors.

---

*Barker KN. The effects of an experimental medication system on medication errors and costs. Am J Hosp Pharm 1969; 26:325.

The results of the study are shown in Table 2-2. If wrong time errors and wrong brand errors are eliminated, the non-unit dose system had a 13% error rate, while the unit dose system had a 1.9% error rate.

Of the errors found in the non-unit dose period, a random sample of 400 errors were analyzed. In an attempt to discover the apparent origin of errors, the most outstanding characteristics of the errors are listed in Table 2-3.

Non-University Hospital Study*

A study of the nature and frequency of certain types of medication errors in a 400 bed, non-government, voluntary, general hospital was conducted. The researcher's goal was to ascertain if this type of hospital had medication errors comparable with two university hospitals that they had previously studied.

Specially trained hospital pharmacist observers were assigned to accompany 32 medication nurses (R.N.s) throughout five successive

Table 2-2. Comparison of Errors During Control and Experimental Periods with "Wrong Brand" Doses Not Counted as Errors (Arkansas Study)

| Category | Frequency | | Error Rate[a] (Percent) | |
	Control[b]	Exper.[c]	Control[b]	Exper.[c]
Omission	493	16	4.1	0.5
Wrong dose (± 17%)	534	10	5.2	0.4
Extra dose	106	2	0.9	0.1
Unordered drug	198	5	1.7	0.2
Wrong route	69	1	0.6	0.0
Wrong time (±30 min.)	1,462	340	12.9	10.1
Deteriorated	10	2	0.1	0.1
Other	48	17	0.4	0.6
Total	2,920	393	25.9	12.0
Total (wrong time not counted as error)	1,458	53	13.0	1.9

[a]Expressed as the mean of all strata (day or evening shift on any one division) means for each error type — not total errors per total opportunities-for-error.
[b]Based on sample of 11,015 opportunities-for-error observed during six month control period. Sampling unit for study was one eight-hour work shift. For the control period, 12 such units were drawn at random from each stratum.
[c]Based on sample of 3,043 opportunities-for-error observed during two month experimental period. Four sampling units were drawn at random from each stratum for the experimental period.

*Barker, KN, Kimbrough WW, Heller WM. A Study of Medication Errors in a Hospital, 1966, published by Univ. of Arkansas, Fayetteville, Ark.

work days. Errors were deviations from the physician's order as written on the patient's chart. Errors were classified as:
1. Omissions (includes wrong brand).
2. Wrong Dose Given (± 5%).

Table 2-3. 400[a] Control Period Errors Classified by Their Most Outstanding Characteristic in Decreasing Order by Frequency of Occurrence (Wrong Time and Wrong Brand Doses Not Included)—Arkansas Study

	No.	Percent
1. Nurse mismeasured, miscalculated or miscounted	112	28.0
2. Nurse selected and used wrong drug[b]	83	20.8
3. Physician ordered doses given "q1h" or "q½h"	31	7.8
4. Nurse gave by wrong route	28	7.0
5. Confusion over automatic stop orders	15	3.8
6. Drug involved in a treatment	15	3.8
7. Nurse gave extra dose past specified limit	14	3.5
8. Initiation and/or termination of orders involved	14	3.5
9. Never any order for this or similar drug	14	3.5
10. First dose on standard schedule omitted	11	2.8
11. Multiple causes—could not be categorized	8	2.0
12. Nurse did not use medication card	6	1.5
13. Order incomplete, confusing, illegible or impossible	5	1.3
14. Nurse misled by medication card	5	1.3
15. Nurse asked (or planned to ask) physician to write covering order—one or both forgot	5	1.3
16. Nurse injected I.V. solution too fast	5	1.3
17. Nurse gave only one of two drugs ordered combined	5	1.3
18. Physician ordered an unusual regimen	4	1.0
19. Nurse misidentified patient	4	1.0
20. Nurse spilled medications during preparation	3	0.8
21. "Understood" and "routine" orders and procedures	3	0.8
22. Nurse failed to return when patient momentarily couldn't take medication	3	0.8
23. Nurse selected and used wrong dosage form	2	0.5
24. Nurse knowingly erred "for patient's benefit"	2	0.5
25. Nurse knowingly erred—accuracy inconvenient	2	0.5
26. Nurse discontinued drug without authorization or comment after patient refused a dose	1	0.3
Total	400	100.7[c]

[a] A sample from a population of the 2,920 such errors which occurred during the control period.
[b] 64 of these cases involved the three products Maalox, Amphojel and Gelusil. Some nurses used these interchangeably. One said a physician told her they were interchangeable. The other 19 cases seemed to involve confusion over drug nomenclature.
[c] Failure to total 100% due to rounding off.

Table 2-4. Distribution of Errors by Type—Non-University Hospital Study

Error Type	Frequency During 9,789 Opportunities	Per Cent of Total Errors
Omission	188	13
Wrong dose	253	17
Extra dose	113	8
Unordered drug	88	6
Wrong dosage form	11	1
Wrong time	808	,55
Total	1,461	100

3. Extra Dose Given (automatic stop order not taken into consideration).
4. Unordered Drug Given (includes wrong brand).
5. Wrong Dosage Form.
6. Wrong Time—given 30 or more minutes early or late.

The observers noted 9,789 opportunities for error. The actual error rate was 15% of this figure or 7.7% if wrong time errors were not counted (see Tables 2-4 and 2-5).

The most common actions of nurses associated with specific errors (excluding wrong time) and believed useful as clues to the cause of errors were:

Nurse miscalculated or mismeasured.
Nurse selected and used wrong drug.
Nurse gave extra dose past specified limit.

Table 2-5. Errors (By Type) Shown as a Percentage of the Total Opportunities-For-Error[a]. Non-University Hospital Study

Error Type	Frequency During 9,789 Opportunities	Per Cent of Total Opp.
Omission	188	1.9
Wrong dose	253	2.6
Extra dose	113	1.2
Unordered drug	88	0.9
Wrong dosage form	11	0.1
Wrong time	808	8.3
Total	1,461	15.0

[a]The jury of two pharmacists and a nurse failed to agree upon the proper classification of twenty-five opportunities-for-error (0.3%).

Clues to causes of errors emanating from the pharmacy were discussed but not quantified.

The investigations compared the medication error rates in this non-university hospital with the error rates at the previously studied Universities of Arkansas and Florida Hospitals and found that the errors were of the same magnitude but different in the rates of the various types of errors. If wrong time errors were eliminated from the tabulation, the non-university hospital had a lower error rate than the university hospitals.

No evidence was found to support the belief that one nurse was more "error prone" than another; however, it was found that particular nurses (related to their personalities) were prone to certain types of errors.

The Kentucky Study*

This United States Public Health Service funded study was conducted to measure the rate of occurrence of medication errors in a hospital with a unit dose dispensing system which had been operational for four years contrasted with four hospitals which did not have a unit dose dispensing system. The hospitals studied were:

Community Hospital A, (Prescription Order System, 305 beds)
Community Hospital B, (Prescription Order System, 405 beds)
University Hospital C, (Floor Stock System, 450 beds)
University Hospital D, (Prescription Order System, 483 beds)
University of Kentucky Hospital, (Unit Dose System, 365 beds)

The study did not attempt to ascertain whether the proper patient received the medication. Errors were noted by observers located in the pharmacy and in the nursing unit. The definition of errors was that of Barker, as in the Arkansas study. To validate the decision-making process of error assignment, a committee consisting of professional staff personnel and including at least one pharmacist and one nurse, reviewed all errors identified. Nursing personnel at the working level at the hospitals were told that the purpose of the observation was to prepare a systems study with guidelines for unit dose systems for the Public Health Service.

The number of administered doses observed in the four hospitals was 1,921, 788, 1,432 and 1,279 respectively. At Kentucky 6,061 doses were observed. The error rates found are shown in Table 2-6. It was observed that drugs not administered often were charted by nurses as having been administered. Wrong time errors were not counted in this

*Hynniman CE, Conrad WF, Urch WA, Rudnick BR, and Parker PF. A comparison of the medication errors under the University of Kentucky Unit Dose System and traditional drug distribution systems in four hospitals. Am J Hosp Pharm 1970; 27:803

Table 2-6. Distribution of Major Causes of Error at Hospitals Using Conventional Drug Distribution Systems in Comparison to University of Kentucky Unit Dose System

Error	Comm. Hosp. A	Comm. Hosp. B	Univ. Hosp. C	Univ. Hosp. D	Univ. of Ky. Hosp.
Omission	2.81%	8.23%	6.35%	9.07%	2.67%
Wrong Drug, Dose, Form, Route, Strength	2.76%	1.16%	3.14%	6.65%	0.59%
Administered Past ASO Date	1.15%	—	0.28%	2.42%	0.18%
Administered Past Discontinued Date	0.57%	0.13%	0.56%	1.95%	0.05%
Wrong Schedule	0.83%	0.38%	1.12%	0.47%	0.03%
Other	0.22%	—	—	—	—
Total	8.34%	9.90%	11.45%	20.56%	3.52%

study. The clinical significance of the errors was not studied, but 59% of errors in the five hospitals were with central nervous system drugs, anti-infectives, electrolytes, diuretics, cardiovascular drugs, hormones, spasmolytes, blood formation and coagulation agents. Other errors occurred with gastrointestinal drugs, cough preparations, vitamins, antihistamines, ENT preparations and miscellaneous agents.

The conclusion of the study was that the error rate in the unit dose system was significantly lower than that found in the four hospitals studied having traditional drug distribution systems. The unit dose system error rate was one-fourth of the average of the other four hospitals.

Ohio State Study*

This 1972 study at the Ohio State University Hospital compared a traditional drug distribution system using unit dose packages for 50% of their doses administered with a pharmacy coordinated unit dose-drug administration system. In this latter system the functions of transcribing, ordering, preparing, dispensing, administering, charting and charging for medication were performed by trained pharmacy technicians under direct supervision of pharmacists. Unit dose carts were checked by pharmacists and exchanged four times daily. A disguised observation technique performed by trained registered nurse researchers was utilized. The unit dose system was observed five months after it was instituted.

Errors were defined as: 1. Unordered drugs, 2. Extra doses, 3. Omitted dose, 4. Unordered route of administration, and 5. Unordered strength — any dose administered that was greater or smaller than the dose strength ordered, regardless of the percentage deviation.

---

*Shultz SM, White SJ, Latiolais CJ. Medication errors reduced by unit-dose. Hosp 47:106, (Mar 16) 1973. Table reproduced with permission from *Hospitals J.A.H.A.*, published by the Amer. Hosp. Assn.

Table 2-7. A Comparison of Medication Error Rates Between The Existing System and The Experimental System During The Study Period—Ohio State Study

Type of medication error	Control system		Experimental system		Chi-square contribution
	No. of errors	Error rate	No. of errors	Error rate	
Unordered drug	17	0.47%	15	0.43%	0.08
Unordered strength	76	2.06	3	0.09	62.83
Unordered route of administration	7	0.19	0	0.00	6.56
Omitted dose	79	2.14	3	0.09	65.68
Extra dose	17	0.47	1	0.03	12.83
Total errors	196	5.33	22	0.64	147.93
Total medication events	3,678		3,447		151.97

The results of the study revealed an error rate of 5.33% in the traditional system and 0.64% in the pharmacy coordinated unit dose-drug administration system, a statistically significant difference (Table 2-7). Wrong time errors were not counted in either system. Approximately 3,500 medication events were observed in each system.

Common errors which occurred included administering Darvon Compound 65 when Darvon 65 mg was ordered, omission of antacid doses, and the administration of one 500 mg chloral hydrate capsule when 1 g was ordered.

A follow-up study of the unit dose system was conducted 2 years later to determine whether the lower error rate might have been a result of heightened interest and performance by pharmacy personnel in demonstrating the effectiveness of their new system. A total of 3,886 medication events were observed with an error rate of 0.82%. This was not statistically different than the 0.64% found in the earlier study.

Summary

The error rates (not counting wrong time errors) in hospitals not utilizing unit dose drug distribution systems were 20.6%, 16.6%, 13%, 11.4%, 9.9%, 8.3%, 7.7% and 5.3%. In the unit dose hospitals studied the error rates were 3.5%, 1.9% and 0.64%.

It is of interest to note that general revisions have been proposed for current regulations establishing the conditions which Skilled Nursing Facilities (SNFs) and Intermediate Care Facilities (ICFs) must meet in order to participate in Medicare (Title XVIII) of the Social Security Act and Medicaid (Title XIX) of the Act. The proposed rules were published in the Federal Register, Vol. 45, No. 136, July 14, 1980. They are from the Department of Health and Human Services, Health Care Financing Administration. These proposals attempt to establish an outcome standard for drug distribution systems. In other words, they do not dictate the type of drug distribution system to be used, but rather specify what results (outcomes) may be expected. The proposal rule states: "Standard: Drug administration. The system of drug ordering, storage, distribution, and administration must ensure that the drug administration error rate does not exceed 5 percent of the total dosage units administered . . ."

From the studies discussed in this chapter it is obvious that unit dose drug distribution systems have the potential to meet this outcome standard. Whether the proposed rules will be adopted and implemented is unknown at this time. Medication error studies funded by the Federal Government have been carried out in Long Term Care Facilities, but the results have not yet been published. The stated figure of 5% in the standard may be changed when the results of the study are analyzed and/or through the natural process of change which takes place in the formalization of government regulations.

References

1. Barker KN, Kimbrough WW, Heller WM. A study of medication errors in a hospital, published by the University of Arkansas, Fayetteville, Arkansas, 1966.
2. Tester WW. A study of patient care involving a unit dose system, final report, University Hospital, University of Iowa, 1967.

3

Role of Supervision in Preventing Errors

RUTH BUDD JACOBSEN, R.N., B.S., M.A.*

Though little has been written in professional literature about medication errors and their prevention, much has been done to effect change and to reduce the incidence of error.

There are recent changes in guidelines from the JCAH and many governmental agencies and also new systems of drug distribution. In spite of these improvements, errors continue to occur, though not to the same degree as formerly. In an attempt to look at this subject carefully, we will focus on specific individuals who are responsible to one another and to the patient for maintenance of quality patient care, including safety in the administration of medications.

We also will look at the drug distribution system itself to see what can be done to provide a system in which the activities of many working together are coordinated toward the goal of accuracy. The system must be as simple as possible, because the medications we are dealing with are not. We believe that the unit dose system provides a simple, well organized procedure where professional people may function well in complementary roles to provide for patient safety.

Who is giving the patient his medication today? Things are changing rapidly, and what was common practice everywhere a short time ago is likely to be much different today, depending on location, and how many nurses are available in your area.

---

*Formerly Assistant Director of Nursing Services, Kettering Medical Center, Kettering, Ohio (1966-1972); Nursing Consultant, Eastern Division, Hospital Affiliates International, Tampa, Florida 33609

It is necessary to evaluate the roles of others who have been brought in to relieve the nurse of many responsibilities. It is also vitally important to consider the supervisor because of the strategic position this person holds in supporting staff to ensure patient safety, quality patient care, and job satisfaction. The head nurse and/or supervisor "sets the pace" for staff nurses and thereby determines the climate in which patient care will be given, including the administration of medications. This is also true of supervisors in other health professions.

Today's staff nurse

There are about 1.5 million registered nurses in the United States, with two-thirds of that number currently working. Most of those who aren't working are not seeking employment.

The nurse who plans for a hospital career today faces what some have called a "changing and turbulent environment with advanced and intensive technology." This health professional has heavy responsibilities that increase with the sophistication of medical technology. Much is expected of the nurse, and it is important for all of us to recognize that because of nursing staff shortages in hospitals, this person may be pressed into functioning in areas for which he or she is not well prepared.

While the nurse's educational background covers a wide spectrum, the complex and ever-expanding field of drugs may require her or him to seek assistance in order to function at a safe and competent level. Nonetheless, today's nurses are more independent in their attitudes and their roles within the profession. More mobile than their predecessors, nurses now put less emphasis on permanent attachment to one institution. They come expecting to work for a while, get the practice they feel they need and then move on. A nurse can choose to work for one hospital, or an agency which will allow placement in one of many hospitals on a daily, weekly, or monthly basis, as needed. Because the nurse is so badly needed, many options are open; a nurse can decide to work full time, part time, or take a leave of absence.

The nurse who seeks employment still needs certain basic knowledge in order to be a reliable practitioner: knowledge of the patient, the system, the plan of therapy, and information about the drugs to be given. It is necessary to know something about each drug, the usual range of dosage, various dosage forms, methods and techniques of administration, expected effects, and symptoms of overdose. The nurse will need to work closely with the pharmacist to be knowledgeable about incompatibilities and other pertinent data. Each hospital must insist on drug distribution system orientation time for every nurse. With agencies, nursing administration must demand this as a prerequisite for every nurse who will be administering medications while working on a temporary basis.

The nurse also needs specific information about the patient who is to receive medication. In addition to name and room number, the nurse will need to know the reason for the drug, history of previous drug reactions, allergies and idiosyncracies and any additional information the physician may have. The nurse should know what the patient has been told, and the patient's reaction to the information.

Employment and orientation

While fewer nurses are now applying for hospital employment, the demands of technologically advanced health care facilities of the 80s continue to increase. Even though the needs are great, and the applicants comparatively few, screening procedures must be carefully followed in order to maintain quality patient care. This is true for all health professions. The routine application form will contribute very little, but if used in conjunction with other screening procedures, it will yield helpful information to facilitate care in job assignment and orientation.

Effective evaluation starts when a prospective employe is interviewed. If done by a qualified person in administration, the interview can be very productive. During the interview and other screening procedures, the interviewer may look for evidences of initiative and motivation. Does the applicant have good judgment? Has he or she been taught to think and to question? Will initiative be taken to secure information on new drugs, or those the applicant is not familiar with? Lack of such knowledge led one individual to administer 25 mg of morphine instead of 25 mg of meperidine because they were thought to be the same (see error #52). In error #38, a nurse prepared 20 vials of chloramphenicol for a single dose without questioning the need for so many vials. This constituted a tenfold overdose, resulting in death. A similar incident involving 10 ampuls of colchicine, also resulting in death, is described in error #98.

Letters of reference should be used cautiously. Because of rapid turnover and the likelihood that the nurse's exposure to the supervisor has been limited, the recommending supervisor's information can be superficial and inaccurate. The applicant has lost contact with a previous supervisor, or may be reluctant to ask for a recommendation, so the individual who actually writes the letter of reference may have little direct knowledge of the applicant's ability or experience. A phone inquiry may be informative if the appropriate person can be reached.

For the nurse who is hired by an agency which places her in a hospital on a daily, weekly, or monthly basis, the same screening procedures, although done by the agency, become even more vital.

The specific job assignment is made with the involvement of the supervisor who then becomes responsible for the on-going evaluation. It is also important to have the prospective supervisor involved in the interviewing and testing in order to plan the appropriate follow-up. Thus, as the newly hired employe goes through the orientation program, orientation experiences in the assigned area can be planned to fit the specific needs brought to light through the interview, letters of reference, and/or testing.

The "right person for the job" becomes even more important when viewed in terms of cost. Nursing personnel, who comprise a large percentage of the hospital budget, need to be seen in terms of possible cost containment and cost effectiveness. Cost of inappropriate orientation and preventable turnover are two areas where this can be seen.

This book illustrates a variety of errors indicating weaknesses in basic areas of knowledge; for example Chapter 10 deals with a lack of knowledge of drugs and Chapter 16 deals with mathematical deficiencies. A medication test which reflects the potential problems of the assigned nursing unit is desirable. The test becomes a tool for planned remedial work and retesting if necessary. This is done with the cooperation of the supervisor (head nurse), for input and follow-up.

Orientation should include a sufficient period of supervised on-the-job experience until the new employe and the supervisor agree that the employe is ready to assume responsibility; certainly this should apply to procedures such as the administration of medications. Some nurses, for various reasons, prefer not to administer medications, and such reservations should be respected.

Orientation, aside from the formal classwork, should be designed to fit the needs of the individual staff nurse. This is especially true for the nurse who requires a basic understanding of a unique drug distribution system, such as unit dose. A thorough orientation should include time to work with someone who can be in a supportive role until the newcomer understands the entire system and can function well in her areas of responsibility, from the time the physician writes the order until the medication has been given and charted.

The L.P.N. and Medication Technician

The Licensed Practical Nurse also is important to the medication procedure if her preparation has been adequate.

Medication technicians are now used in some places to advantage when they have received careful screening and preparation. The medication technician usually is a nurse assistant who has been specially prepared for the responsibilities of medication administration. Here preparation must be emphasized. Job descriptions must be clearly spelled out, and good supervision provided. Programs coordinated and supervised by the pharmacy department with the cooperation of nursing are also being utilized. One such program is at Ohio State University Hospital in Columbus. *No one* should be permitted to administer medications without adequate knowledge about drugs.

Screening and orientation procedures are vital for all those admitted to the drug distribution system as new employes: the registered nurse, the licensed practical nurse, the medication technician, physicians, pharmacists and pharmacy technicians.

The Supervisor

Why do some nurses achieve high productivity while others are content with a mediocre performance? With respect to responsibility for the administration of medications, this question takes on greater significance.

At least seven different theories of motivation have been discussed often and used in nursing practice. As the supervisor works with the staff nurses and others her convictions will be influential whether she believes with Frederick Taylor that money is the primary motivating factor, with Argyris, in the theory of self-actualization and positive reinforcement, or with Skinner, who emphasizes the importance of participation. Some believe that autonomy, responsibility, achievement, recognition and variety in work are priorities, and therefore influence the climate of the nursing unit. Certainly one of the most critical aspects to be considered is the relationship between the head nurse and the staff nurse, or other individual employes, because of its importance in setting the pace for growth and success on the unit.

One of the most difficult responsibilities of the supervisor or head nurse is that of staffing: it affects the patient, the nurse, and the environment of the nursing unit. And on today's busy unit, the head nurse may be faced with new people for orientation, or temporary nurses from an agency. She will have to depend on the agency for screening and testing, and upon her own skills in working with people to make the unit run smoothly.

Some writers in nursing are saying that there is no shortage of nurses, but there is a shortage of nurse managers prepared to handle the needs of professional nurses. Must nurses then be better prepared in the care and handling of people?

Variations in staffing needs occur more often because of staff illness or vacations than as a result of a change in patient mix. The entire situation on a nursing unit should be considered when setting up criteria for staffing. For example, hospitals with a large medical staff require more nursing staff to handle physicians' orders.

Ongoing evaluation of all nursing employees by a supervisor must be a daily practice in order to be effective. Records should be spot reviewed, their "products" or services checked. This is especially true for the nurse who "floats" to a unit, or is placed by an agency as a temporary worker. Some hospitals have developed their own special float pools with their own immediate supervisor, who is responsible for testing, orientation, and ongoing evaluation. The special part-time float pools are made up of nurses with skill in specific areas, and they are not expected to float to other units. Such groups need close supervision, including their own supervisor or head nurse. Evaluation is done on a daily basis.

The ongoing evaluation of all employes is also vital for pharmacists. Staff pharmacists must be responsible for pharmacy technicians. It has been said that it is impossible for a pharmacy technician to make an error. Only a pharmacist can make an error because the pharmacist is responsible for the correctness of the final product. Yet many errors occur because the work of the pharmacy technician is not adequately supervised. In error #48, a tenfold overdose of the estrogen Premarin was given to a patient, resulting in vaginal bleeding. The dose had been prepared in error by a technician and was dispensed into a patient bin without the pharmacist's knowledge, although he was present in the pharmacy at the time. Later, checking a drug cart containing the improperly prepared drug the pharmacist failed to detect the error.

Errors #139 and #148 discuss inadequate storage of the cancer chemotherapeutic drug cisplatin, due in part to a lack of supervision of pharmacy storeroom personnel. A patient received three doses of epinephrine suspension that had the active ingredient filtered out by a pharmacy technician who prepared the doses for a nurse. The technician had been told to draw up all ampul packaged injections through a filter needle (which removes glass particles that form on opening). The technician was not under supervision when the incident occurred (error #96). A patient received iron tablets instead of birth control pills in error #41!

Technicians must be instructed that they are not permitted to judge whether a dose is correct. All work must be checked by a pharmacist who is responsible for seeing that each dose is correct.

The inexperienced pharmacist should be supervised by an experienced pharmacist. Error #99 describes a situation where a young pharmacist dispensed Zetar emulsion (30% coal tar solution) instead of the ordered Zetar shampoo (1% coal tar in a lathering shampoo) because he did not know that there was more than one Zetar product.

Physicians must also be aware of their responsibility to supervise. In error #21 an oncologist instructed his medical student to prepare orders for a patient for a cancer chemotherapy protocol. The student prepared the orders correctly but wrote them on the wrong patient's chart and the error was not discovered until two weeks later, after both patients suffered harm. The orders were never countersigned by the physician.

The System

At a time of acute staffing needs and widespread problems stemming from inadequate evaluation of inpatient nursing practice, it is most important that the drug distribution system be simplified as much as possible. This makes orientation much easier, and the evaluation more clear-cut and precise.

The trend toward unit dose systems of drug distribution in this country is encouraging to see. With the complexity of medication orders it is essential that the pharmacist and nurses work together from the physicians' orders to establish separate records for the patient which must agree at all times. There are many built-in accuracy check points in the unit dose system that can be achieved in no other way. (See Chapter 1.)

If a unit dose system is not used in your hospital, it may be desirable to give serious consideration to one, first observing a hospital using the unit dose system. By studying the procedures, forms and records, it is possible to save time which otherwise might have been spent in trial and error.

If you are using a unit dose system, it may be useful to establish an interdepartmental evaluation committee, composed of personnel from nursing and pharmacy, for periodically evaluating each step of the entire procedure to determine what changes may be necessary to improve patient safety. As medication errors are analyzed in this context, with those concerned striving toward the common goal of error prevention, much can be accomplished.

Quality Control personnel have been appointed in some institutions and are given the responsibility for ongoing evaluation of each step in the medication procedure. Should these people be nurses, or pharmacists? Probably both; good communication within nursing and between nursing and pharmacy departments is essential.

Other hospitals have appointed a liaison nurse as a designated problem-solver. This position can be a very valuable one in working through problems between departments, or between medical staff members and nursing or pharmacy. Promoting an understanding of the complexity and various facets of a problem is an effective way to assure compliance with decisions.

Not all errors are realized or reported, but a goal of the head nurse should be to encourage the reporting of all incidents occurring in her nursing unit. It is possible to create a climate where there is no stigma attached to filling out a form, where instead, staff are encouraged to fill out and file reports whenever necessary. These are essential for purposes of insurance, and also as an indication of the kinds of errors occurring, so that the appropriate measures can be taken for their prevention. (See Chapter 17.)

As nursing service takes a look at the responsibilities for administration of medications, it immediately becomes obvious that this is a many-faceted problem, requiring the understanding and cooperation of many people, from the time the nursing employe is accepted for employment, and every day thereafter. But by providing for adequate screening, preparation, and evaluation of personnel, a staff can function well for effectiveness and patient safety; and a good system can be made even better. By taking an interdisciplinary approach, measurable improvement can be effected.

Bibliography

Brown, Barbara J., Editor, *Nurse Staffing*, A Practical Guide, An Aspen Publication, reprinted from Nursing Administration Quarterly, London, England, 1980.

Dixon, Norma, *Clinical Teaching Techniques*, Ed. 3, St. Louis, C. V. Mosby Co., 1975.

Douglass, Laura Mae, *The Effective Nurse*, St. Louis, C. V. Mosby Co., 1980.

Henderson, Virginia, and Nite, Gladys, *Principles and Practices of Nursing*, Ed. 6, New York, Macmillan, 1978.

Knight, Kay, and Preston, Cynthia Ann, "Opinions" *American Operating Room Nursing Journal*, March 1980, Vol. 31, No. 4.

Kohnke, Mary, *The Case for Consultation in Nursing*, Designs for Professional Practice. New York, Wiley, 1978.

LeClear, Betty, "The Liaison Nurse," The Journal for Nursing Leadership and Management, *Supervisor Nurse*, March 1980.

Marriner, Ann, *Guide to Nursing Management*, St. Louis, C. V. Mosby Co., 1980.

Martin, Ruby M., *Nursing Implications – A Pharmacy Coordinated Unit Dose Dispensing and Drug Administration System.* Am J Hosp Pharm 1970; 27:902.

Mayers, Marlene G. (Editor) *Leadership in Nursing*, Nursing Resources, Waleford, Mass., 1979.

Shanks, Mary D., and Kennedy, Dorothy, *Administration in Nursing*, Ed. 2., New York, McGraw-Hill Book Company, 1970.

4

Physicians' Orders As A Source Of Medication Errors

Poor Handwriting

Physicians' orders which are either illegible, inaudible, ambiguous, or incomplete, are the cause or a major contributing factor in many of the errors made by nurses and pharmacists. All too often the nurse or pharmacist, who is at the interface with the patient where the error occurs, is assigned the blame and the reporting responsibility for an error which was caused by the physician's poor communication. A poorly communicated order is the seed or the fertilizer for errors — the sole cause of an error, or the stimulus for the lack of knowledge or poor performance by other health professionals which results in an error.

Where students are taught to read patients' charts, invariably one will shake his head in disbelief and ask, "With something so important, how can doctors be so sloppy with their handwriting?"

How bad is the handwriting of physicians on hospital medical records? In a study published in the *Journal of the American Medical Association*, an anonymous author studied and classified the handwriting of 47 staff physicians in a 500-bed teaching hospital.[1] The results are shown in Table 4-1. Seventeen percent of the physicians had very poor handwriting (completely illegible), and an additional 17% had poor to fair handwriting.

However, it should be noted that 47% of all physicians fall in the good to excellent classification. It is true that this group is not part of the problem and must also suffer with problems created by the 34% cited above.

All health professionals have learned to read most of what is written by physicians. However, there are occasions when one must ask for help, when an order is unreadable, when guesses are made, and times when writing is read incorrectly. Would comedians joke about physi-

Table 4-1. Classification of Physicians' Handwriting[1]

Category	No. of Physicians	%
Poor (completely illegible)	8	17
Poor to Fair	8	17
Fair to average (most can be read, but it takes extra time)	9	19
Good to very good	16	34
Excellent (can be easily read — no extra time required)	6	13
Total	47	100%

cians' handwriting if it were generally known that careless penmanship causes real harm? See errors #2, #7, #12, #14, #15, #22, #23, #39, #50, #51, #57, #70, #75, and #126 for examples of this problem. Also, see Table 4-2, which lists many similar drugs which can easily be read incorrectly on poorly written orders.

Medication errors are only one aspect of the problem. Progress notes, consultations, histories and physicals, although important enough to write, often cannot be deciphered and hence are not used. The problem certainly is not new. The blame should be placed on the medical educators, hospital administrators and health care workers who must read the writing. Health care workers such as nurses, pharmacists and physicians have not documented the problem. Errors are not reported or publicized. Sloppy writing is tolerated and accepted as an inevitable fact of life even as the air and water pollution of our mid-century.

The 1980 edition of the Accreditation Manual for Hospitals, published by the Joint Commission on Accreditation of Hospitals, includes the following:

Standard III—"Medical records shall be confidential, secure, current, authenticated, legible, and complete."

Their interpretation of this Standard includes the following comments:

". . . The quality of the medical record depends in part on the timeliness, meaningfulness, authentication, and legibility of the informational content."

Hospital administrators are not familiar with the problem or take no leadership role to correct it. They know the cost of insurance has skyrocketed, but they have not looked at physicians' handwriting as a contributing factor to hospital misadventures. Medical educators in medical schools and teaching hospitals also seem to be unwilling to attack the problem.

Table 4-2. Look-Alikes and Sound-Alikes*

A	B
Aarane .... Anturane	Bactocill .... Pathocil
Aarane .... Artane	Bactrim .... Bacitracin
Aberel .... Iberol	Banesin .... Benisone
Acetohexamide ... Acetazolamide	Banthine .... Bentyl
Achromycin ...... Aureomycin	Belladonna .... Belladenal
Adapin .... Atabrine	Benadryl .... Belladenal
Adroyd .... Android	Benadryl .... Bentyl
Aerolone .... Aralen	Benadryl .... Benylin
Aerolone .... Arlidin	Benadryl .... Caladryl
Afrin .... Afrinol	Bendopa .... Bendectin
Afrin .... Aspirin	Benemid .... Beminal
Agoral .... Argyrol	Benoxyl .... PanOxyl
Aldactone .... Aldactazide	Bentyl .... Aventyl
Aldoril .... Aldomet	Bentyl .... Bontril
Alu-Cap .... Aluscop	Benzedrex .... Benzedrine
Ambenyl .... Ambodryl	Betalin .... Benylin
Ambenyl .... Aventyl	Betapar .... Betapen
Amodrine .... Amonidrin	Bicillin .... V-Cillin
Amoxil .... Amcill	Bicillin .... Wycillin
Ananase .... Orinase	Bontril .... Vontrol
Ananase .... Tolinase	Brethine .... Banthine
Anavar .... Antepar	Brondecon .... Bronkotabs
Ancobon .... Oncovin	Butabarbital ...... Butalbital
Anturane .... Antuitrin	Butibel .... Butabell
Anturane .... Artane	Butisol .... Butabell
Anusol .... Aplisol	Butisol .... Butazolidin
Anusol .... Aquasol	
Aplisol .... Apresoline	**C**
Aplisol .... Atropisol	Calcidin .... Calcidrine
Appedrine .... Ephedrine	Calcitriol .... Calcitonin
Apresoline .... Priscoline	Capastat .... Cepastat
Aralen .... Arlidin	Catapres .... Catarase
Arfonad .... Afrin	Catapres .... Diupres
Arthralgen .... Auralgan	Cephalexin .... Cephalothin
Asminyl .... Asmolin	Cephapirin .... Cephradine
Asminyl .... Esimil	Chlorambucil ..... Chloromycetin
Asminyl .... Ismelin	Chloromycetin .... Chlor-Trimeton
Atarax .... Enarax	Chlorpromazine ... Chlorpropamide
Atarax .... Marax	Clinitest .... Citanest
Ativan .... Avitene	Clofibrate .... Clorazepate
Auralgan .... Ophthalgan	Clonidine .... Quinidine
Azathioprine ...... Azulfidine	Clonopin .... Clonidine
Azene .... Azatadine	Clonopin .... Clopane
Azolate .... Azolid	Codeine .... Coldene
Azotrex .... Azo-Stat	Codeine .... Cordran
Azotrex .... Tetrex	Coenzyme-B ...... Cotazym-B

---

*Teplitsky B., "Caution: 1000 Drugs Whose Names Look Alike or Sound Alike."
Pharmacy Times, Nov. 1979. Reprinted by permission.

Colestid . . . . Colistin
Colistin . . . . Colestipol
Combid . . . . Combex
Combipres . . . . Catapres
Compazine . . . . Compocillin
Compocillin . . . . . . Ampicillin
Consotuss . . . . Cotussis
Coramine . . . . Calamine
Cortone . . . . Cort-Dome
Cuprimine . . . . Cuprex
Cyclopar . . . . Cytosar
Cytarabine . . . . Vidarabine
Cytellin . . . . Cytoferin
Cytoxan . . . . Cytosar

D

Dalmane . . . . Demulen
Danocrine . . . . Dacriose
Dantrium . . . . Danthron
Daranide . . . . Deraprim
Daricon . . . . Darvon
Darvon-N . . . . Darvocet-N
Decadron . . . . Decaderm
Decadron . . . . Percodan
Decagesic . . . . Duragesic
Decholin . . . . Daxolin
Delalutin . . . . Deladumone
Delta-Dome . . . . . . Deltasone
Demerol . . . . Demulen
Demerol . . . . Dicumarol
Demerol . . . . Dymelor
Demerol . . . . Pamelor
Deprol . . . . Demerol
Desferal . . . . Disophrol
Desipramine . . . . . . Deserpidine
Desoximetasone . . . Dexamethasone
Desoxyn . . . . Digitoxin
Dexameth . . . . Dexamyl
Dextran . . . . Dexedrine
Diabinese . . . . Dianabol
Diafen . . . . Delfen
Dialog . . . . Halog
Dialose . . . . Dialog
Dialume . . . . Dalmane
Dialume . . . . Dialose
Diasal . . . . Diasone
Diazepam . . . . Diazoxide
Dicarbosil . . . . Dacarbazine
Digitoxin . . . . Digoxin
Digoxin . . . . Desoxyn
Dilantin . . . . Delalutin
Dilantin . . . . Deltalin
Dilantin . . . . Phelantin
Dilaudid . . . . Dilantin

Dimacol . . . . Dimercaprol
Dimetane . . . . Dimentabs
Dipaxin . . . . Digoxin
Disipal . . . . Disophrol
Disomer . . . . Disophrol
Disophrol . . . . Isuprel
Disophrol . . . . Stilphostrol
Disopyramide . . . . . Dipyridamole
Diuril . . . . Doriden
Diutensen . . . . Salutensin
Diutensen . . . . Unitensen
Dobutamine . . . . . . Dopamine
Dolene . . . . Dilone
Dolene . . . . Dolonil
Dolonil . . . . Dilone
Donnatal . . . . Dianabol
Donnatal . . . . Donnagel
Donnazyme . . . . . . Entozyme
Dopar . . . . Dopram
Dopram . . . . Dopamine
Doriden . . . . Doxidan
Doriden . . . . Loridine
Doxan . . . . Doxidan
Doxinate . . . . Doxan
Dyazide . . . . Diasone
Dyazide . . . . Thiacide
Dyclone . . . . Dilone
Dyclonine . . . . Dicyclomine
Dyrenium . . . . Pyridium

E

Ecotrin . . . . Edecrin
Elase . . . . Alidase
Elavil . . . . Aldoril
Elavil . . . . Mellaril
Emetine . . . . Emetrol
Enarax . . . . Marax
Endecon . . . . Edecrin
Endecon . . . . Enduron
Enderin . . . . Empirin
Enduron . . . . Enderin
Enduron . . . . Eutron
Enduron . . . . Imuran
Ephedrol . . . . Tedral
Equagesic . . . . Decagesic
Esimil . . . . Estinyl
Esimil . . . . Ismelin
Eskatrol . . . . Hexadrol
Estinyl . . . . Estomul
Estomul . . . . Esimil
Estomul . . . . Ismelin
Ethabid . . . . Ethamide
Ethamide . . . . Ethionamide
Ethinamate . . . . Ethamide

Ethionamide . . . . . . Ethinamate
Eurax . . . . Urex
Euthroid . . . . Thyroid
Eutonyl . . . . Eutron

F

Felsules . . . . Feosol
Feosol . . . . Feostat
Feostat . . . . Feostim
Fer-in-Sol . . . . Feosol
Festal . . . . Feosol
Fiogesic . . . . Wygesic
Flagyl . . . . Flexical
Flexeril . . . . Flexical
Fluocinonide . . . . . Fluocinolone
Folbesyn . . . . Fulvicin
Fostex . . . . pHisoHex
Furacin . . . . Fulvicin

G

Gamastan . . . . Garamycin
Ganatrex . . . . Kantrex
Gantrisin . . . . Gantanol
Garamycin . . . . Terramycin
Gelfoam . . . . Ger-O-Foam
Geritol . . . . Cheracol
Gevral . . . . Gevrine
Glucagon . . . . Glucoron
Glutethimide . . . . . Guanethidine

H

Haldol . . . . Winstrol
Haldrone . . . . Haldol
Halodrin . . . . Haldrone
Halog . . . . Haldol
Halog . . . . Mycolog
Halotestin . . . . Halothane
Halotex . . . . Halotestin
Harmonyl . . . . Hormonin
Hexadrol . . . . Hexaderm
Hexadrol . . . . Hexalol
Hexalol . . . . Hexestrol
Hispril . . . . Hiprex
Homapin . . . . Hormonin
Hycodan . . . . Hycomine
Hycodan . . . . Vicodin
Hycomine . . . . Hycodan
Hydropres . . . . Catapres
Hydropres . . . . Diupres
Hydroxyzine . . . . . . Hydroxyurea
Hygroton . . . . Hykinone
Hypersal . . . . Hyperstat
Hyperstat . . . . Hyper-Tet

Hyperstat . . . . Nitrostat
Hytone . . . . Hytrona
Hytone . . . . Vytone

I

Ilosone . . . . Ionosol
Imipramine . . . . Imferon
Imuran . . . . Imferon
Inderal . . . . Enderin
Inderal . . . . Imuran
Inderal . . . . Isordil
Indocin . . . . Lincocin
Indocin . . . . Minocin
Intropin . . . . Ditropan
Isopto Carpine . . . . Isopto Eserine
Isordil . . . . Isuprel
Isuprel . . . . Ismelin

K

Kafocin . . . . Keflin
Kaon . . . . Kaolin
Keflex . . . . Keflin
Keflex . . . . Kelex
Kemadrin . . . . Coumadin
Ketalar . . . . Kenalog
K-Lor . . . . Kaochlor
K-Lor . . . . Klor

L

Lactinex . . . . Lactocal
Larotid . . . . Lomotil
Lasix . . . . Esidrix
Lasix . . . . Laxsil
Levophed . . . . Levoprome
Levorphanol . . . . . . Levallorphan
Lidaform . . . . Vioform
Lidex . . . . Lasix
Lidone . . . . Dilone
Lincocin . . . . Cleocin
Loridine . . . . Leritine
Luminal . . . . Tuinal
Luride . . . . Loryl

M

Maalox . . . . Camalox
Maalox . . . . Maolate
Maalox . . . . Marax
Mebaral . . . . Mellaril
Mebaral . . . . Tegretol
Medrol . . . . Mebaral
Mellaril . . . . Meltrol
Mellaril . . . . Moderil
Mephenytoin . . . . . Mesantoin
Meprobamate . . . . . Mepergan

Q

Quaalude	Quinidine
Quarzan	Questran
Quinidine	Quinine
Quintess	Quiess

R

Regroton	Hygroton
Regroton	Regonol
Reticulex	Reticulogen
Rifadin	Ritalin
Ritalin	Ismelin

S

Salrin	Saluron
Sandril	Tandearil
Sanorex	Ser-Ap-Es
Sansert	Singoserp
Santyl	Sandril
Sebical	Sebulex
Sebutone	Sebulex
Senokot	Senokap
Ser-Ap-Es	Catapres
Serax	Eurax
Serax	Psorex
Serax	Xerac
Serenium	Dyrenium
Serentil	Saronil
Serentil	Surital
Silon	Silain
Simethicone	Cimetidine
Simron	Sintrom
Sinarest	Allerest
Singoserp	Sinequan
Sinulin	Sonilyn
Sinurex	Sinarest
Somophyllin	Slo-Phyllin
Sorbitrate	Sorbutuss
Sparine	Sterane
Sporostacin	Sporicidin
Sterazolidin	Butazolidin
Sterazolidin	Stelazine
Sudafed	Sudolin
Sulfamethazine	Sulfamethizole
Sulfasalazine	Sulfathalidine
Surfak	Surbex
Synalar	Synasal

T

Tace	Tao
Taractan	Tinactin
Tedral	Teldrin
Tegopen	Tagamet
Tegopen	Tegretol
Tegopen	Tegrin
Tegretol	Tegrin
Temaril	Demerol
Tepanil	Demerol
Tepanil	Temaril
Tepanil	Terfonyl
Tepanil	Tofranil
Terfonyl	Tofranil
Testolactone	Testosterone
Theolix	Theolixir
Thiamine	Thiomerin
Thiamine	Thorazine
Thyrar	Thyrolar
Thyrar	Tryptar
Thyrolar	Theolair
Tigan	Ticar
Tobramycin	Trobicin
Tolinase	Toleron
Torecan	Toleron
Triamcinolone	Triaminicin
Triaminic	Triaminicin
Triolos	Tricon
Triconol	Tricofuron
TriHemic	Triaminic
Trophite	Troph-Iron
Tuinal	Tylenol

U

Unipen	Unicap
Unipen	Urispas
Unitensen	Salutensin
Uracel	Uracil
Uracil	Uracid
Urised	Uracel
Urised	Urestrin
Urispas	Urised
Urispas	Uristat
Uristat	Uristix

V

Valium	Nalline
Valmid	Valpin
Valmid	Velban
Valpin	Valium
Vasodilan	Vasocidin
Velban	Valpin
Versapen	Verstran
Verstran	Vastran
Vesprin	Vastran
Vicodin	Hycomine
Vigran	Wigraine
Viomycin	Vibramycin
Vitron	Viteron

Vitron-C	Vicon-C	**Z**	
Vontrol	Vastran	Zactane	Zactirin
VoSol	Vontrol	Zactirin	Zarontin
Vytone	Vitron	Zactirin	Zentron
W		Zarontin	Zaroxolyn
		Zarontin	Zentron
Wyamine	Wydase	Zentinic	Zymatinic
Wycillin	V-Cillin	Zetone	Zentron

Many of us have two handwriting levels. At one level we consciously write legibly, on the other we write with no thought given to legibility. The second level may be used when we feel we do not have time to write carefully. The second level may be used as an unconscious symbol of superiority: "My time is more valuable than yours. You can take the time to decipher what I write."

Another consideration is that the writer may have a motor coordination deficit and is unable to write legibly. In this case the writer must print, type, or have someone else write his or her orders.

When are pharmacists, nurses and physicians going to say, "We've had enough of this illegible writing. We are not going to spend time trying to decipher this scribble any longer. We refuse to go from colleague to colleague to ask for aid in reading what the prescriber did not take time to make legible. Illegible orders cannot be carried out. They will be delayed pending clarification orally or in writing by the prescriber." It may be 20 years before the computer-generated medical record is commonplace, and that's too long to wait!

When one complains to the administrator or to the facility's Pharmacy and Therapeutics Committee that nursing and pharmacy will no longer respond to illegible orders, it will be pointed out that of course no one should respond to illegible orders, and there should be no guessing. It should then be noted that time is wasted in "group deciphering" or in contacting the prescriber or in implementing orders, and that occasional guessing is a fact. The problem must be faced squarely; support for corrective action must come from the top.

Poor handwriting by nurses and pharmacists also causes errors, delays and a lack of communication.

Verbal Orders

Verbal orders which are not heard correctly are a source of error. Fourteen sounds like forty, sixteen sounds like sixty (see error #4), Mannitol sounds like Amytal (see error #97), and Pitocin sounds like Potassium.

An error was reported where a consulting physician was asked to see a patient with an unexplained purpura.[2] It was discovered that a local medical doctor, two weeks earlier, had telephoned a prescription for

Kemedrin 5 mg (an anti-parkinsonism agent) to the pharmacist. The pharmacist heard it as the anticoagulant, Coumadin 5 mg, and dispensed it as such.

Listed in Table 4-2 are 1000 drug names that either sound alike or, when handwritten, may look alike. To make matters worse, in some cases dosage ranges overlap, making error even more likely (see error #12).

In addition to errors caused because the order is not heard correctly, errors can result because, like the written orders, verbal orders can be incomplete or ambiguous (see error #87). Error #103 describes the bizarre problem of an impostor phoning a medication order which, if carried out, would have proven harmful to the patient.

Verbal orders from nursing personnel to patients can also be a problem. Errors have been reported when nursing assistants have placed a cup of Phisohex on a pre-op patient's night table and said "Here is your Phisohex." The patient drank the Phisohex that was intended to be used as a body scrub in the shower. Besides poor communication, a break in procedure occurred in this instance where the Phisohex was taken out of its original container.

The Joint Commission on the Accreditation of Hospitals (see appendix) addresses the issue of verbal orders in the Pharmaceutical Service Section, stating, "Verbal Orders for drugs may be accepted only by personnel so designated in the medical staff rules and regulations, and must be authenticated by the prescribing practitioner within the stated period of time." The Medical Staff Section states rules and regulations should "specify identity of categories of personnel who are qualified to accept and transcribe verbal orders, regardless of the mode of transmission of orders." The Medical Records Services Section states: "Verbal orders of authorized practitioners shall be accepted and transcribed by qualified personnel who shall be identified by title or category in the medical staff rules and regulations. The medical staff should define any category of diagnostic or therapeutic verbal orders associated with any potential hazard to the patient, which orders shall be authenticated by the responsible practitioner within 24 hours."

The American Society of Hospital Pharmacists Guidelines on Hospital Drug Distribution and Control System (see appendix), approved by the American Nurses Association, states: "Physician's Drug Order: Writing the Order—Medications should be given (with certain specified exceptions) only on the *written* order of a qualified physician or other authorized prescriber. Allowable exceptions to this rule (i.e., telephoned or verbal orders) should be put in written form immediately and the prescriber should countersign the nurse's or pharmacist's signed record of these orders within 48 (preferably 24) hours. Only a pharmacist or registered nurse should accept such orders.

Provision should be made to place physician's orders in the patient's chart, and a method for sending this information to the pharmacy should be developed."

It has been suggested by Anderson[3] that only the charge nurses or nursing supervisors should take verbal orders, and that difficult drug names be spelled out. Anderson also recommends that decimal designations such as 0.5 g not be used, 500 mg being preferred. This suggestion also holds true for written orders.

Verbal orders must be discouraged and limited to emergency situations where no other suitable alternative can be found for alleviating significant patient discomfort, or to correct or clarify existing orders. The physician must clearly identify himself or herself and give the full name of the patient. Orders must be dictated slowly and distinctly. As with all orders, they must be complete and unambiguous. The recipient should immediately transcribe the order and read it back to the prescriber. Particular care must be taken with prescribers and transcribers whose primary language is not English.

Ambiguous Orders

The meaning of drug orders must not be ambiguous or the intent of the physician will not be communicated.

An order written for a patient on 80 mg of prednisone daily read "decrease prednisone 5 mg daily." The order was transcribed as "prednisone 5 mg daily" (see error #89).

An order was written for "Inderal ½ tablet 40 mg qid." It was unclear whether 20 mg (½ a 40 mg tablet) or 40 mg (½ an 80 mg tablet) was desired (see error #144).

One time orders such as "Lasix 40 mg P.O. in the AM" are on occasion incorrectly interpreted as daily orders, rather than one time orders. An order intended for continuous daily administration would read "Lasix 40 mg P.O. in the AM daily." For the one time dose, it would be best to write "Lasix 40 mg P.O. in the AM on 6/17/80."

A bizarre error occurred when a one time dose for insulin was administered daily, "NPH Insulin 8 units, S.C. in AM Daily." Dr. Daly was the physician's signature, which became "AM Daily." (See error #115. Chapters 5 and 6 may also be consulted for additional comments relating to ambiguous orders.)

Once written, all orders must be carefully read by the prescriber. Is the order for the right patient? Is it legible? Is it correct? Is it complete? and is it clear in its meaning? Is it open to misinterpretation? This also holds true for nurses and pharmacists in their transcriptions on Nursing Medication Administration Records and Pharmacy Patient Profiles.

The Time of Day Orders are Written

Hospital staffing is geared toward fullest coverage during the day. While twenty-four hour pharmacy service is currently seen in many hospitals of 300 beds and over, most larger hospitals do not have 24 hour pharmacy service.[4] The ratio of nursing personnel to patients is lower on the evening and night shifts, and often part-time personnel are assigned to these unpopular shifts. Some physicians make rounds after 9 P.M. as a matter of common practice. During these rounds, orders are written which are intended for use within hours. In error #104 an order written at night resulted in an error which led to a patient's death. The medical staff and the hospital administration should not permit physicians to make routine patient rounds at night unless hospitals are staffed with the quality and quantity of personnel necessary to carry out these orders.

Lack of Understanding Medication Order Systems

Medical students, house staff and staff physicians must know how drug orders should be written and how they are processed. Health care facilities have systems to alert nursing to begin processing when an order is written. If this alerting system is poor or ignored, major delays in initiating therapy will result leading to a breakdown in the entire drug distribution system. This is a serious problem in many facilities.

The order is then transcribed by nursing on to a nursing document and an actual carbon or NCR copy of the order is sent to the pharmacy. To change an order the physician must initiate a new order modifying the initial order and must again alert the nurse to the fact that a new order has been written. Error #19 describes a physician who lowered the dose of a 0.25 mg digoxin order by inserting a 1 between the decimal point and the 2, making it 0.125 mg. The original order had been processed and the lowering of the dose was not noted. The order should have been written "Change digoxin dose to 0.125 mg P.O. daily."

If an error is made at the time of writing an order, do not erase or otherwise obliterate the entry. Simply put one line through the item and write the word "error" above the lined out area together with your signature and date. Then make the proper entries on the next line. Never obliterate or otherwise alter an order once it has been written. It is easy for an expert to spot an altered document, which can be a cause for prosecution under law.

Prescribing Errors

Physicians make mistakes in prescribing. The error may be a mistake in calculating a dose, as seen with vincristine (see error #86), or in selecting a dose, as seen with meperidine (see error #16). The physician may order a dose, intended to be given over an extended period of time, to be given over a shorter period of time, thus causing toxicity as seen with mithramycin, potassium chloride and vincristine (see errors #24, 67, 71, 86). When prescribing two drugs, the physician may transpose the doses as seen with Keflin and gentamicin when Keflin 60 mg and gentamicin 1 g were ordered and administered (see errors #91, 92). This simple mental error caused a death. The physician may write the wrong drug name as seen in error #72 when the intramuscular preparation, aqueous procaine penicillin was ordered to be given intravenously. Procaine penicillin is a suspension. The incorrect use of the word aqueous contributed to the error. An incorrect order can be written as a result of a faulty history as seen when 100 units of regular insulin were ordered (see error #7). The patient was using U-100 insulin, not taking 100 units of insulin. Prescribing from a mistaken prescription label caused 2.5 mg of digoxin to be administered (see error #49). A physician may have misunderstood what he was told by a senior staff member to order as seen when a 40% rather than ¼% acetic acid irrigating solution was ordered (see error #123). A physician may order a drug to be given by the wrong route, as was seen when vancomycin 500 mg/10 ml was ordered I.M., rather than I.V. (see error #65). A physician may order a drug to be administered in too concentrated a form, as seen with I.V. potassium chloride (see error #67). A physician may write an incomplete order, as seen when "54 units of NPH Insulin SC" was ordered in the evening instead of ordering "54 Units of NPH Insulin SC in the AM, 10/1/80" (see error #79).

These occurrences emphasize the need for physicians to review orders after they are written, and the need for good nursing and pharmacy services to stand between the physician and the patient to serve as a check.

Failure to Write Orders

Failure to order significant medications to provide continuous therapy when a patient is first admitted to an institution or when patient medication orders are resumed after surgery is a source of error. A case has been reported[5] in which a patient with a history of polycythemia vera experienced an adrenal crisis brought on by the error of omission in post-operative orders. The patient had been taking 150 mg of cortisone daily prior to surgery. When the post-operative orders were written, cortisone therapy was not re-instituted.

A timely and complete drug history must be taken on admission. When post-operative orders are written, previous medication orders must be thoroughly reviewed. Specific orders should be written. A physician's order stating, "Resume previous medications" is not ac-

ceptable. The monitoring of physicians' performance of these responsibilities by nursing and pharmacy can prevent these errors from
occurring.

Prescribing for Outpatients

In addition to points already discussed above and in the chapters
that follow, outpatient prescriptions require some additional attention. The following suggestions will aid in preventing patients from
making errors, help compliance and facilitate the obtaining of an
accurate and complete drug history.

1. The name and strength of the drug dispensed should be recorded on the prescription label by the pharmacist unless
   otherwise directed by the prescriber. Abbreviated drug names
   should not be used.
2. Whenever possible, specific times of the day for drug administration should be indicated. (For example, "Take one capsule
   at 8 am, 2 pm and 8 pm," is preferable to "Take one capsule
   three times daily." Likewise, "Take one tablet two hours after
   meals," is preferable to "Take one tablet after meals.")
3. Vague instructions such as, "Take as necessary," or "Take as
   directed," which are confusing to the patient are to be avoided.
   Such directions expose the prescriber to unnecessary liability
   if a patient does not take his/her medication properly. Specific
   directions also help prevent dispensing errors. (See error #2.)
4. If dosing at specific intervals around the clock is therapeutically important, this should be stated on the prescription by
   indicating appropriate times for drug administration.
5. The symptom, indication, or the intended effect for which the
   drug is being used should be included with instructions whenever possible. For example, "Take one tablet at 8 am and 8 pm
   for high blood pressure," or "Take one teaspoonful every 4
   hours if needed for cough."
6. The prescription order should indicate whether the prescription is to be renewed and, if so, the number of times and the
   period of time each renewal is authorized. Statements such as
   "Refill prn" or "Refill ad lib" are not acceptable.
7. When institutional prescription blanks are used, the prescriber should print his/her name, and registration number
   on the prescription blank in addition to the signature.

Unapproved Uses

When a use, dose or method of administration ordered for an already
marketed drug differs from the official product literature, the pharmacy should ask the prescriber to cite a reference which can be

checked if such a reference is not already on file in the pharmacy. Such prescribing is referred to as an "unapproved use" of a drug, and such references should be copied and kept in the pharmacy. Copies or abstracts of these references should be supplied to nurses who must administer these drugs or monitor their effects. This should be done whenever an "unapproved use" first occurs.

Physicians may deviate from an official product insert for an individual patient without the need to file a new drug application and protocol. Such a formal filing is necessary only if a physician is carrying out a study. When physicians deviate from the official literature (product insert), as they often are required to do, they should have a sound basis for doing so. All of these checks and guarantees are necessary because physicians make mistakes in prescribing, and professionals, such as pharmacists and nurses, are not carrying out their responsibilities to patients if they accept orders as being correct unless they are certain there is no error.

Procedures for handling these common situations can be formulated by the Pharmacy and Therapeutics Committee of the facility.

Conflicts Over Drug Therapy*

One of the hospital pharmacist's responsibilities is to monitor drug therapy. When a nurse is concerned that physician-ordered drug therapy may not be safe, the hospital pharmacist should be contacted. When the pharmacist suspects that drug therapy is potentially harmful, he should pursue the matter until he is satisfied that the therapy will not harm the patient, or until the physician changes the order. Confirmation of safety may come from studying the patient's chart, discussing the matter with the physician, talking to the patient, researching the matter, or consulting with other pharmacists or physicians. If the pharmacist is not satisfied that no harm will come to the patient, and the ordering physician will not change the drug order, other options are open. Each option should be weighed carefully, depending upon potential for harm, time of day, service involved, degree of certainty on the part of the pharmacist, time span before which the harmful effect may occur and so on. The ideal situation is when the pharmacist and physician resolve the problem to their mutual satisfaction on a professional-to-professional basis. If this fails, the options are:

1. Consult with the physician's chief resident, chief attending physician, head of department, patient's attending physician, or a specialist in the area of drug therapy ordered. The individ-

---

*This is a sample of one hospital's policy on handling situations where conflict over drug therapy exists between physicians and pharmacists or nurses. Each hospital should develop its own policy in conjunction with legal counsel.

ual consulted can prevail on the pharmacist to modify his opinion, or may get in touch with the ordering physician to effect an order change.

2. If time or other circumstances do not make it practicable to carry out (1), request assistance from another pharmacist (preferably the Drug Information Pharmacist or a knowledgeable supervisor).

When the Order is not Modified or Cancelled

If, after extraordinary effort, option one or two above cannot be accomplished, one of the following options is available.

1. Refuse to dispense the drug. One must be reasonably sure that a more significant morbidity would result from administering the drug than from withholding the dose or doses.

2. Request the physician administer the drug himself (not the nurse). In such a case, the physician should note and sign on the Physician's Order form that he gave the medication. The nurse would then note on the medication record, "Given by M.D." The nurse can also make this entry on the verbal acknowledgement of the physician. In this situation the pharmacist may still be held partially responsible if harm comes to the patient.

When either of the latter options is required, the standard hospital incident report should be completed by the pharmacist, citing the circumstances, stating the pharmacist's position on the matter and efforts made to resolve the situation. If the physician persists in administering the drug, a statement that this action is against the pharmacist's (and nurse's) professional judgment should be included. It should also be noted that the physician assumes all responsibility and will hold the pharmacist (and nurse) guiltless in the event of patient injury. Have the physician sign the form and allow him to make comments if desired. If the physician will not sign the form, a nurse, as a witness, should sign and date the form. The writer should keep a copy for his or her own information and see that the Director of Pharmacy (and Nursing) is given the original as soon as possible.

More on Look-alike and Sound-alike Drug Names

There have been many reports in the literature related to look-alike-sound-alike drug names; Amicar has been given instead of amikacin[6]; acetohexamide for acetazolamide[7]; aminophylline for ampicillin[8]; potassium chlorate for potassium chloride[9]; Dolophine for Demerol[10]; neostigmine for physostigmine[11]; to cite a few.

These reports involve errors caused by physicians, nurses and pharmacists. Again what is needed is careful, knowledgeable professionals operating with drug distribution systems which possess built in checks and balances.

References

1. A study of physicians' handwriting as a time waster, JAMA, 1979; 242:2429-30.
2. Whitaker RL. Confused drug names. Ann Intern Med., 1980; 93:933. Letter.
3. Anderson DR. The physician's contribution to hospital medication errors, Am J Hosp Pharm 1971, 28:18.
4. Stolar MH, National survey of hospital pharmacy service, Am J Hosp Pharm 1979, 36:316.
5. Hubay CA., Weckesser EC., Levy RP., Occult adrenal insufficiency in surgical patients. Ann Surg 1975; 181:325-32.
6. Solomon KJ, Medication errors from similar trademarks letter. JAMA 1978; 239:1130.
7. Hargett N, Ritch R, Mardtrossian J, Kass NA, Podos SM., Inadvertent substitution of acetohexamide for acetozolamide. Am J Ophthalmol 1977; 84:580-3.
8. Barter B, Roberts RJ. Unusual case of aminophylline intoxication. Pediatrics 1973; 52:608-9.
9. Vakili M. Chlorate poisoning in childhood — a case report. J Trop Pediatr 1977; 23:119.
10. Simons PS. The treatment of methadone poisoning with naloxone (Narcan). J Pediatr 1973; 83:846-7.
11. Janson PA, Watt JB, Hermos JA. Doxepin overdose. Success with physostigmine and failure with neostigmine in reversing toxicity. JAMA 1977; 237:2632-3.

5

Need for Proper Expression of Drug Names, Strengths and Other Elements of a Complete Order

In order for a drug to be administered correctly, one must know the drug to be administered, the dosage form, the route of administration, the dose to be administered and the frequency of administration. In some cases the strength, dilution, rate of administration, and time of administration must also be specified. If these essential elements are poorly written or omitted, the intention of the writer will not be achieved.

Material presented in the Dangerous Abbreviation Section (Chapter 6) also applies to this section.

Drug Names

Only the generic or trade names should be used if delays in therapy and errors are to be avoided.

The use of chemical symbols causes error (see error #70).

The use of lettered abbreviations such as CPZ, MTX and ARA-A, for drug names may cause errors (see error #34, 110, 150).

The use of research or chemical names such as 6-mercaptopurine and 6-thioguanine, in place of the official names, mercaptopurine and thioguanine, has been implicated in resulting deaths (see error #13, 104).

The use of coined names such as "Black and White," "Pink Lady," "Dynamite" and "Chicken Soup," creates problems and errors (see error #84).

Dosage Form

Expressing the dosage form desired can be an important part of the drug order. Whether a cream or an ointment is used can mean the difference between success or failure of therapy. In the rare instances where both tablets and capsules of a dosage form are available, unnecessary patient apprehension can be avoided if a specific dosage form is requested.

Route of Administration

If the route of administration is not specified, delays in initiating therapy or error can result as seen with cromolyn sodium, phenobarbital, kanamycin, Sus-phrine, Urecholine and K-Lyte (see errors #31, 42, 44, 73, 91, 108). This is a very serious problem to which prescribers must pay close attention.

Dose to be Administered

The dose to be administered must be clearly stated. Medication orders stating, "administer 1 tablet," without a specific strength, or one teaspoon or one ampul, without specifying a strength and amount cause delays in therapy and error (see errors #2, 27, 33). When a drug such as Lasix Tablets is first marketed, it is not uncommon that only one strength is available (40 mg). Eventually, a 20 mg and 80 mg tablet were placed on the market. An order written "Lasix tablet P.O. daily" would cause no problem when the drug was first marketed, but today it is incomplete and would result in a delay in instituting therapy. Hundreds of similar examples could be cited. Even if only one strength is available in a given dosage form, the strength must be specified, as chances are good that a second strength will eventually be marketed. This is important for pharmaceutical companies to remember when formulating advertising material.

Frequency of Administration

It is obvious that frequency of administration must be stated. One must be familiar with the hospital procedure for the literal meaning of a frequency designation. "Twice a day" may signify 10 A.M. and 6 P.M., whereas "every 12 hours" may mean 10 A.M. and 10 P.M. Drugs are administered at the given hour each day, for example H.S., (bedtime) may be at 10 P.M. Unless the H.S. order is written PRN (if required) it will be given every night.

Orders which are written for administration out of the normal time periods for medication administration, such as every 14 hours or every 20 hours, are more likely to result in errors than orders which adhere to established time schedules. Where possible, it is best to adjust dose rather than specify an awkward schedule (see error #51).

Expressing Weights, Volumes and Units

Never leave a decimal point naked. Always place a zero before a decimal expression less than one (see error #3).

Correct 0.5   Incorrect .5

The decimal point may not be seen if the number is written incorrectly as shown above, especially if written on lined forms, NCR forms or carbons, and a tenfold overdose occurs.

Avoid using decimal expressions where recognizable alternatives exist, as whole numbers are easier to work with.

0.5 g should be expressed as 500 mg

0.05 mg should be expressed as 50 mcg

Use the metric system exclusively. Never use grains, drams or minims (see error #74).

Never place a decimal point and zero after a whole number, as the decimal point may not be seen, resulting in a tenfold overdose (see errors #50, 98).

Correct 2 mg   Incorrect 2.0 mg

In typed or computer-generated material, leave a space between the number and its units, as it is more easily read.

Correct | Incorrect
20 mg | 20mg
200 mg | 200mg

Always spell out the word "units." The abbreviation "U" for unit can be mistaken for a zero (error #1), causing a tenfold overdose.

6

Dangerous Abbreviations

Certain abbreviations cause errors. These occur because personnel may not be familiar with the meaning of the abbreviation, the abbreviation may have several meanings, or it may be poorly written and mistaken for another abbreviation.

The use of the abbreviation q.d. to mean "every day" has caused errors because it has been read as q.i.d. (four times daily) when the hand written period after the q. is mistaken for an i (see error #112).

The abbreviation O.D., which means "right eye," has caused errors when it was intended to mean "once daily." Multi-vitamin solution has been administered in the right eye when ordered O.D. (see error #105). Potassium chloride liquid has been given in the right eye for the same reason. It has also been reported that Lugol's solution and saturated solution of potassium iodide have been administered in the right eye when O.D. administration was ordered. The belief that these drugs were meant for the eye was reinforced because the liquids are dispensed in dropper bottles. There is no safe abbreviation for "once daily"—it must be written in full.

The hand written abbreviation U, for unit, has been read as a zero, causing a tenfold overdose of insulin (see error #1). This can also cause errors with heparin doses. The abbreviation can also be misread as a four (see error #1).

Seldom used abbreviations such as AU (each ear) have been misinterpreted as "each eye" (see error #8).

The poorly written abbreviation O.J., was read as O.D., which was thought to mean right eye, resulting in a patient receiving Lugol's solution in the right eye rather than orally in orange juice (see error #15). O.J. has also been read as O.S. (left eye) (see error #69).

The abbreviation D/C was read to mean "discontinue" when it was intended to mean "discharge," thus prematurely cancelling medication orders which were intended to be discharge prescription orders (see error #143).

The poorly written and poorly conceived abbreviation QN, intended to mean "every night" was read as every hour (see error #43).

The apothecary system and its abbreviations are a source of error: mx for "minim" has been mistaken for ml, causing a sixteenfold error (see error #128). The symbol for one dram, ʒT, has been mistaken for 3T, (in cooking a capital T is a tablespoon), thus 3 tablespoons (45 ml) were administered rather than 5 ml (see error #117). The abbreviation for "grain" and "gram" can be confused (see error #116). The abbreviation gtts, for drops, has been taken to mean teaspoon (see error #69). The prescribing of fractional parts of grains, rather than milligrams or micrograms, has caused errors (see error #74).

When μg is used as the abbreviation for microgram, it can be mistaken for mg, a 1000-fold error (see error #107). The handwritten abbreviation mcg, is less likely to be confused for mg than is μg.

The use of chemical symbols causes errors when they are misinterpreted or not understood (see error #70). Such symbols as KI, KC1, HC1, CaC1$_2$, H$_2$O, etc., should not be used in order writing or on medication administration records.

Drug names should not be abbreviated (see errors #34, 110, 150). There are hundreds of three and four-letter abbreviations for drug names used in textbooks and journal articles that, when used in drug order writing, cause delays in initiating therapy and error.

The Joint Commission on the Accreditation of Hospitals requires hospitals to promulgate an approved list of abbreviations which are to be used in the hospital. Each abbreviation should have only one meaning. Such a list should be compiled with the cooperation of physicians, nurses, pharmacists and medical record administrators, and approved by the Medical Staff. Only abbreviations which have through wide use achieved 100% understanding should appear on the list. The following items should *NOT* appear on any list and a statement forbidding their use should be included.

Problem Term(s)	Reason	Suggested Term
O.D. for once daily	interpreted as right eye	write "once daily"
q.o.d.	interpreted as meaning once daily or read as q.i.d.	write "every other day"
q.d. for once daily	interpreted as q.i.d.	write "once daily"
q.n. for every night	read as every hour	write "every night or H.S."
U for Unit	read as 0 or 4	write "unit"
O.J. for orange juice	read as OD and OS	write "orange juice"
μg (microgram)	misread as mg	write "mcg"
Chemical symbols	not understood	write full name
Lettered abbreviations for drug names	not understood or misunderstood	use generic or trade name
Apothecary Symbols or terms	not understood or misunderstood	use metric system

7

Drug Distribution and Administration Systems Failure

Every institution must have detailed written procedures governing the ordering, order processing, dispensing and administration of medications. When procedures are not followed or when the normal checks and balances of a well designed drug distribution system are not used appropriately, errors occur. Elmina Price[1] has stated "a system which calls for the transcription of the order by nursing personnel in conjunction with the nurse choosing the drug from floor stocks is potentially the most dangerous system." Such a system has no checks and balances.

NCR (no carbon required) forms used by thousands of hospitals for physicians' orders, provide for an original for the patient chart and an exact copy for the pharmacist. This practice saves the time of nurses and ward clerks who formerly had to transcribe orders from the original physician order sheet to a pharmacy order slip. And the use of NCR copies helps to prevent errors. The transcription step by the nurse or ward clerk who is not as familiar as the pharmacist with the milieu of drug entities available allows misinterpretation of drug, dose, route or frequency of administration. Another problem associated with transcriptions is that an order not seen by a nurse will mean a delay in therapy. When the pharmacy receives an NCR the possibility of this kind of error is greatly reduced or eliminated. Though the use of NCR physician order copies is a significant improvement, errors associated with their use have been reported.

Errors involving NCR physician order forms have resulted from inadvertent copying of orders onto more than one form at a time. This happens when more than one form is kept in the physician order section of a patient's chart or when orders are written on the top form of several NCR forms. A copy of the original order is made not only on the top form, but also on forms beneath the top form. When these other forms are used subsequently, the pharmacist receives copies of orders, previously written for the same patient, and such orders may be hours to days old. If the forms are in a single pile, but not already identified

48

by patient name, the copies received by the pharmacist could be associated with another patient's name! Error #18 illustrates this serious error: A course of chemotherapy came to pharmacy on a copy of orders addressoplated with the name of the patient intended. At the same time, identical orders came through for a second patient. The pharmacist became suspicious, investigated, and found that the ordering physician had inadvertently kept a second order sheet under the first when the order was being written.

However, the advantages of NCR forms far outweigh their potential disadvantages. Problems can be avoided if those using the forms ascertain that no other form is underneath the one being used. In patient charts or order books, extra forms must be separated by heavy Manila, cardboard or old X-ray film. A ball point pen must always be used to insure that copies are clear and easy to read.

As part of the system, forms used in the processing of drug orders normally include space for recording allergy and diagnosis information about the patient. It is helpful if this information is included by physicians on order forms (some hospitals pre-print the words "allergy" and "diagnosis" at the top of the first physician order form). This information can help to prevent some of the more serious types of medication errors. In error #78, although nurses, physicians and pharmacists were aware and had recorded an allergy to Mandelamine (methenamine mandelate), the information was not used to prevent an allergic reaction suffered by the patient when Hiprex (methenamine hippurate) was ordered. Apparently, no thought was given to the potential cross-allergenicity. Adding medications to a patient's regimen requires thoughtful attention. Gathering and recording allergy information must be routine, with a careful review of the information whenever a new medication is added to a patient's regimen.

Diagnostic information about each patient is valuable in preventing errors. Since drug therapy must correspond to diagnosis, orders inadvertently written on the wrong patient's records may be exposed. For example, the cancer chemotherapy in error #21 was ordered for a patient who did not have cancer. Had the patient's diagnosis been obtained and/or used by nurses and pharmacists caring for the patient, the error would have been prevented. (See also errors #44, 50, 70, 106, and 146).

As well-intentioned as a pharmacist may be in using allergy, diagnostic and other information to prevent drug errors, his or her work can be bypassed and serious errors result when floor-stock systems are in use, or when drug administration personnel "borrow" doses intended for one patient to administer to another. These practices can completely neutralize the pharmacist's safety value. In serving as a check on the safety of the order, the pharmacist may wish to delay initiation of therapy until further investigation is made. A pharmacist therefore must be given the opportunity of reviewing all non-emergency orders prior to drug administration. This cannot be accomplished when borrowing exists. In error #119, the patient suffered a severe allergic reaction to carbenicillin because a nurse, wanting to initiate therapy immediately, "borrowed" a dose of carbenicillin from another patient's supply. The pharmacist was withholding therapy because he was aware that the patient had a history of penicillin allergy. Pharmacists must communicate as soon as possible with nurses and physicians to explain why the medication is being withheld. Most important, the drug distribution system must be designed to allow for a pharmacist's review and interpretation of every medication order (except emergencies) and resolution of problems or uncertainties prior to allowing a drug into the dispensing system.

The person administering medications must positively identify each patient by checking the patient's identification armband. Any other procedures used to identify patients may lead to error (see Chapter 11 on patient identification).

When medication administration is in process, the person responsible for this task must stay with the patient until the dose has been taken. Exceptions to this rule are for medications kept at bedside by physician order or with formal self-administration programs. Hoarding of doses left with the patient is well known to experienced personnel. There is danger that these doses may be held for a suicide attempt, given to another patient, or important drugs may not be taken.

Patients have been known to inadvertently drink rubbing alcohol or pHisohex placed in cups at the bedside.

In error #5, a medication nurse noted that her patient was falling out of bed. Hurrying to assist the patient, she left several medication doses intended for the patient on another patient's bedside table. After helping the falling patient, she returned to the other patient's bedside table to obtain the medications. The other patient had taken the drugs.

Whenever medications are given, the nurse should make sure the patient has taken the medication. All administered or omitted doses should be recorded in the medication administration record (MAR) immediately after administering medications to each patient and before administering to the next patient. Errors #45 and #46 discuss at length the error potential when medications are recorded in MARs before dose administration or after all medication administration for a given round has taken place. If a dose of medication is charted before it is given, the potential exists for dose omission should the person who charted it be called off the floor or otherwise distracted before dose administration. Conversely, if a dose of medication is given to a patient with the intention of charting the dose later, the potential exists for an extra dose of medication to be given to the patient. This is more often seen with medications such as insulin or warfarin, whose time of administration may be different from the usual medication administration hours.

DRUG NOT GIVEN NOTICE

Patient Name _____ Bed # _____

Date _____   Time _____

1. Notify MD when important medication(s) are missed or refused.
2. If medication is in drawer but not on medication sheet:
   Look for original order on the chart. If none is found, call pharmacy.
3. If medication is listed on medication sheet but is not in drawer:
   Look for D/C order on chart. If none is found, call pharmacy.
4. Place this form in patient's medication drawer.

Drug Not Given	Reason	Reschedule for (if indicated) Time _____	Was MD Notified? (if indicated)

_____ RN/LPN
(signature)

Figure 7-1. "Drug Not Given Notice" for Nursing to Pharmacy Communication. Left with unadministered dose(s) of medication in patient bin of unit drug cart.

In a unit dose system, medications which have been dispensed but not administered can be discovered and investigated by nursing and pharmacy. More accurate charging is then possible and errors of omission can be corrected and followed up. To do this, doses which have not been administered to the patient must remain in the patient drawer. The reason that the drug was not administered should be communicated by the nurse to the pharmacist (see figure 7-1). Only medications returned to stock in unopened, sealed packages should be reused. Error #140 demonstrates an error that occurred when the nurse removed from stock a previously unwrapped IV Solution Bag of 5% Dextrose Injection that had been replaced in stock by another nurse. Unknown to both of these nurses, a third nurse had previously added 4 ampuls of dopamine to the bag during a cardiac arrest emergency. The bag was not labeled, never used, and was returned to the nursing stock during clean-up operations after the coronary resuscitation effort.

Reference

1. Price EM. A nurse looks at hospital drug distribution systems. Am J Hosp Pharm. 1967; 24:105.

8

Reading Labels

When a mistake is made because the wrong drug or the wrong amount is administered, the error may stem from a lack of knowledge or failure to read the label.

Lack of knowledge was at fault when normal saline was requested of a part time pharmacist who dispensed a product labeled "Sodium Chloride Injection 50 mEq - 20 ml." This product, which is a concentrate used in preparing hyperalimentation solutions, is 16 times more concentrated than normal saline solution. The pharmacist was not familiar with this concentrate. It was not failure to read the label, but rather not knowing what he or she was reading (see error #63).

One must read labels with care, for reading labels mechanically can lead to serious errors, as when a nurse received an order for 10 mg of Haldol Injection. She "read" on the edge of the box, Haldol Injection 1 ml, which she erroneously interpreted as 1 mg in each 1 ml ampul. The ampuls were in fact labeled 5 mg/ml. She administered a fivefold overdose (see error #91, 92). The labeling of the ampul was difficult to read, but it was clear and it was correct.

Sometimes products look alike, and if labels are not read with care, mistakes will occur. Lasix 40 mg tablets and Phenergan 12.5 mg tablets are both packaged in unit dose silver foil packages (see error #29). Wyeth's unit dose Codeine Sulfate tablets 30 mg and phenobarbital tablets 30 mg are packaged identically (see error #29). Talwin and a generic diphenhydramine injection are available in the same size ampul, with identical red color bands and the same color ink (see error #32). Phenobarbital and Pentobarbital Tubex look alike (see error #114). Clindamycin ampuls, paraldehyde ampuls and Phenytoin ampuls were all mistakenly used as 0.9% sodium chloride injection to dissolve powder antibiotic injections (see error #20). Chloromycetin Ophthalmic Ointment was dispensed instead of Ophthcort (see error #77). A 50% Dextrose Infusion was administered instead of 5% Dextrose (see error #9, 10). In one situation, U 40-80 syringes were used rather than U-100 (see error #9, 10). In all of the situations the packages, package size and colors were the same. But the error occurred because of failure to read the label.

When pharmacists purchase drugs, labeling clarity and appearance are important determinants in brand selection. Errors can be avoided if look alike products are avoided. When the similarity of product appearance is not perceived by the pharmacist as a problem, nurses and physicians should point out the potential for error and suggest a different item be purchased. Occasionally there may be no adequate substitutes, but much of the time there are.

Some favor and some oppose color coding, while others advocate its use in problem areas only. This topic is covered in Chapter 15.

It is an old and wise maxim in nursing and pharmacy to read labels three times carefully. For instance, in drug preparation, the label should be read when the drug package is selected, when the medicine is prepared, and the partially used medication is returned to its storage area or disposed in the trash. The empty container should be held for a time in case there is a further need for checking. A used container should not be left out too long, as it may interfere with the next task. Physicians also must read labels carefully three times. In those procedures which do not afford an opportunity to read labels three times, the first reading should be done with exceptional care.

In one situation Amyl Nitrite crushable ampuls were used rather than the intended aromatic ammonia (see error #138). The amyl nitrite has a yellow netting over the label and the more frequently used aromatic ammonia has white netting. Both ampuls are the same size.

In many of the errors cited above a drug was returned to stock and placed with other drugs which appeared the same but in fact were not. When drugs were later taken from stock the misplaced drug was used in error.

In some instances an infrequently used drug was discontinued, but returned with other drugs in the nursing unit. Personnel used these "strangers" in the belief that they were the more commonly used products which they resembled. This has occurred where 50% Dextrose Injection has been used rather than 5% Dextrose. Such errors have moved the Joint Commission on Accreditation of Hospitals to require monthly nursing unit drug inspections by pharmacy and to recommend unit dose systems and pharmacy I.V. admixture programs.

Errors occur because strengths are misread. Deaths have been reported when tenfold overdoses of chloromycetin were administered. The 10 ml vial was labeled "100 mg chloramphenicol" per ml when reconstituted "-10 ml Package." It was believed that each vial contained 100 mg (see error #38). A commercial 500 ml I.V. solution container was labeled as to electrolyte content in mEq per liter. This caused a patient to receive one-half of the intended dose when this fact was not noted (see error #28). Three unit dose packages, each labeled as Quinidine Sulfate Tablets 200 mg, were administered for a 200 mg dose (see error #6). An entire 100 ml bottle of V-Cillin K oral suspension labeled 250 mg/5 ml was administered for a 250 mg dose (see error #61).

A few products are inactive diluents or flavors to be used with active ingredients and labeled as such. Care must be taken to make sure the diluent is not mistakenly used in place of the active ingredient. This happened when the diluent for Coly Mycin S Ophthalmic Solution (see error #40), Vivonex Flavor Packets (see error #68) and Normal Saline for use with Evans Blue Injection USP (see error #38) were used in place of the active ingredient.

Whenever a label is incorrect or misleading, you should consider completing an FDA-USP defect Reporting Form (see Chapter 15). If your observation is correct, the label will be changed and greater safety assured. Though such corrections are helpful, the basic problem remains persistent failure to read labels carefully and thoroughly.

The FDA and the USP are to some degree part of the problem in that they require manufacturers to place certain information on the product label and also dictate its location. This is especially troublesome when designing a label for a small package such as an ampul.

Manufacturers must be sensitive to the user's need to read essential information on a label. This is discussed in Chapter 15.

9

Errors Associated with Drug Dispensing

Medication dispensing practices are the responsibility of the pharmacy. The pharmacist must follow policies and procedures that have been developed to provide safe distribution of drugs to patients served by hospitals and other institutions. For this reason many state governmental agencies and the Joint Commission on Accreditation of Hospitals require that hospital pharmacies have updated procedure manuals.

Many of the errors reviewed in this chapter might have been prevented if specific procedures had been followed. In some cases, closer attention to the work at hand, or more concern with professional responsibility would have prevented the error. Failure to read labels is a common cause of errors by pharmacists (see Chapter 8) as well as other health professionals.

Labeling Errors

Errors associated with product labeling have caused wrong drugs to be administered, wrong route of administration to be used, drug overdoses and underdoses and much patient apprehension. The prudent pharmacist adheres to labeling guidelines such as those listed by the American Society of Hospital Pharmacists.[1] When labels are prepared by pharmacy supportive personnel, the pharmacist must insist on reviewing the product prior to dispensing. As with all endeavors associated with drug dispensing, the pharmacist must take care to assure that labeling is accurate and complete.

Examples of labeling errors and their results include a tenfold overdose of dexamethasone injection (see error #66). A pharmacy technician prepared syringes of 10 mg instead of the ordered 1 mg. The technician labeled the 10 mg syringes as 1 mg, and the pharmacist in charge failed to note the error. Errors #48 and #69 describe other drug overdoses caused by inaccurate or incomplete drug labels.

Occasionally patients have received wrong drugs. Error #41 describes a situation where a female with vaginal bleeding received iron tablets instead of Norlestrin. Both drugs were packaged in a birth control pack. A pharmacist had previously used up the Norlestrin tablets, leaving the iron tablets and returning the pack to stock. The label no longer accurately reflected the package's contents, leading to the error described.

Error #59 describes an outpatient pharmacy label mixup where a patient's eye drop medication labels were switched and placed on the wrong containers. The error occurred in a busy pharmacy where pharmacists normally worked on more than one prescription at a time. Added caution must be exercised in checking the finished product in such cases.

When a pharmacist accidently hit a wrong key on a typewriter (M instead of V) a patient received an extremely irritating 10 ml of vancomycin injection IM instead of IV. A final label check would have prevented this error.

Error #137 describes an incident where too little Kayexalate was administered to a patient because pharmacy's label did not mention what volume contained the requested dose.

The labeling on the manufacturer's container of Neutraphos, although not prominent, states that the capsules are not meant to be swallowed whole, but that their contents should be mixed with water then drunk. Because of the pharmacist's failure to put this information on the label, the patient received the concentrated product orally before dilution (error #149) with resulting severe gastrointestinal upset.

Pharmacists should use caution when clinical information about the patient appears on the prescription. In error #142, a cancer patient first learned that her condition was considered "terminal" by reading it on a pharmacy label. The pharmacist who typed "pt. has terminal Ca" on the label used poor judgment. The information was placed on the prescription by the physician for the pharmacist's use only.

Auxiliary Labels

Had a pharmacist taken the "extra step" needed to prevent others from making an error, a patient would not have received a non-sterile enteral alimentation suspension intravenously (error #147). A regular hospital I.V. label was used on the fluid container. If a different color label with an auxiliary statement such as "For Enteral Alimentation Only—Not for Injection" had been used, the error might have been avoided. In other cases, ear drops were given in the eyes (error #8), a cocaine-epinephrine solution meant for topical use in epistaxis was given orally (error #87), and Lasix oral solution was given intravenously (error #124). Each of these errors might have been prevented had pharmacists used auxiliary labeling in addition to normal labeling. Nurses and physicians who note preparations that lack such labeling should request that their pharmacists use them.

The following are examples of pharmacy auxiliary labels which could help prevent errors: not to be taken internally, shake well before using, for the eye, to be taken orally, for inhalation only, not to be taken by mouth, for external use, for the ear, not for injection, for the nose, not to be swallowed, for the throat, chew tablets before swallowing, for vaginal use only, use as a gargle, not to be swallowed, for rectal use only.

Containers and labels for prescription use only

Many hospital pharmacists have made it a practice never to allow empty prescription containers or pharmacy labels to be given to individuals or departments outside the pharmacy, because once these items leave the pharmacy, there is no control over how they will be used. How does one know that the dietary department will not use pharmacy containers and labels for packaging small amounts of insecticide? Perhaps a patient care assistant will use a vial for a urine sample. Liquid floor wax might be kept in prescription bottles by housekeeping personnel. Depending on where these items are stored, they may be confused by an employe or patient as a medicine, leading to a poisoning or other unpleasant incidents.

In error #94, a patient's husband assumed that a prescription container placed at his wife's bedside by a laboratory employe contained pain medication and administered it to his wife. The contents actually were the woman's gallstones which had just been removed.

Pharmacy containers or labels must not be used by anyone but pharmacy personnel.

Lack of Familiarity with Drug Products and Names

In error #99 a pharmacist dispensed a product without taking into account its full name. The pharmacist received a prescription for Zetar Shampoo, but the only Zetar product he was aware of was Zetar Emulsion, which he dispensed. The shampoo has 1% coal tar, while the non-lathering emulsion contains 30% coal tar. Physicians may occasionally be imprecise in writing prescriptions, but most of the time they are precise. Whenever there is doubt, one of the common references (American Drug Index, Facts and Comparisons, American Hospital Formulary Service, etc.) should be consulted to determine whether a dispensing error is possible.

In another case (error #110) a pharmacist received an order for MTX 30 mg IM. MTX is an abbreviation for methotrexate, used by some oncologists. The pharmacist interpreted it to mean mustargen, and prepared and dispensed it; the patient received 30 mg of the potentially necrotizing mustargen intramuscularly. While the abbreviation led the pharmacist to commit the error, he was not certain that MTX meant mustargen. If he had checked with a knowledgeable colleague, this serious error could have been avoided.

In error #63, a part-time weekend pharmacist dispensed a concentrated sodium chloride injection instead of 0.9% sodium chloride injection. In error #25, double the concentration of epinephrine ophthalmic drops prescribed was dispensed by a pharmacist who switched brands without realizing that each product contained different salts of epinephrine. In error #145 a pharmacist dispensed a non-sustained release theophylline product instead of the prescribed sustained release product because of a lack of knowledge concerning brand names and full generic names. None of these errors would have occurred had these pharmacists taken the time to check on names or products with which they were unfamiliar. The same holds true for nurses when required to administer a drug.

Error #129 describes an incident where a nurse mixed up Bactrim with Bactrim DS. For some time the drug Bactrim (also brand name Septra), a combination of two antimicrobials, was available in one strength only. But the adult dose had long been two tablets. Then a double strength product known as Bactrim DS (Septra DS) became available. Since the nurse was used to administering two tablets when Bactrim was ordered, she administered two double strength tablets at a time when the pharmacist began dispensing the DS product. While the pharmacist failed to inform the nurses of the change, the nurse could have prevented an error if she had inquired about the name change.

Misreading Prescriptions

The health care system evolved over many years, and various responsibilities and checks and balances have been built into the system to make it safe. When an error is investigated, it is often found that several factors were involved before the error reached the patient. This is often the case with errors involving misread prescriptions.

A case was reported[2] where a man had recurrent prolonged hypoglycemia associated with normal plasma insulin levels. The patient was admitted to the hospital in a hypoglycemic coma. It was subsequently discovered that the patient was taking chlorpropamide 250 mg (an oral hypoglycemic agent) three times daily, rather than chlorpromazine 25 mg (a major tranquilizer) which had been prescribed. The wrong drug had been dispensed. A similar mistake occurred when chlorothiazide was ordered for a patient and chlorpropamide was dispensed.

Another case reported[3] a woman who had been referred to the Mayo Clinic for further evaluation of a suspected insulinoma. It was discovered that three months earlier, Tolectin had been prescribed for her arthritis. The pharmacist mistakenly dispensed Tolinase 250 mg and labeled it Tolectin. The patient did not have an insulin secreting tumor, but had received a sulfonylurea in error. A physician has reported a similar situation where Ananase was prescribed and Orinase was dispensed.[4] Hydralazine has been dispensed for hydroxyzine, and tolbutamide has been dispensed for terbutaline.[5]

Closely related to misread prescriptions are prescriptions which are not heard correctly (see section on verbal orders in Chapter 4). A physician telephoned a prescription to a pharmacist for Kemadrin 5 mg, one tablet three times daily. It was heard as Coumadin 5 mg and dispensed as such. The error was discovered and the patient went to a consulting physician because of her unexplained purpura.[6]

Fiorinal was dispensed instead of the intended Florinef (see error #2). The female hormone Estratab was dispensed to a male patient rather than the prescribed muscle relaxant, Ethatab (see error #146).

This type of error can be prevented by certain precautions, beginning with the drug name. In Chapter 4, 1000 look-alike, sound-alike drug names are listed. Manufacturers (see Chapter 15) and the United States Adopted Name (USAN) Council must be sensitive to the problem of similar names as a cause of error.

Physicians must write legibly (see Chapter 4), and must also write complete prescriptions (see Chapter 5). In the case of the Florinef prescription above, the physician did not specify a strength. If 0.1 mg had been written, Fiorinal would not have been dispensed since this is not the strength of Fiorinal. The directions on the Florinef prescription were "Take as Directed." If the directions, "Take one daily," were written, Fiorinal would not have been dispensed, since these directions are obviously inappropriate for Fiorinal. In the case of the Ethatab, if the physician had written Ethatab 100 mg, the mistake would not have occurred since the greatest available strength of Estratab is 2.5 mg.

Pharmacists must be knowledgeable and attentive to their important reponsibility in seeing that the patient receives the intended medication. The environment in the prescription laboratory should be conducive to allowing the pharmacists and their supportive personnel to concentrate on their important work. Pharmacists must not permit themselves to be placed in a situation where the workload may prevent taking the time needed to properly dispense medication and counsel patients. The public must realize that the pharmacist should not be subjected to pressure for fast service. Thorough and complete service should be sought.

Maintaining and utilizing pharmacy patient profiles can aid the pharmacist in preventing errors. In the case of the chlorpromazine-chlorpropamide, and in the Tolectin-Tolinase mix-ups, a listing of previous prescriptions or lack of a diabetes diagnosis on the patient profile might have alerted the pharmacist that the prescription had been misread.

In the situation where the female hormone was dispensed to the male patient, the pharmacist might have acted without first considering obvious questions. What is Estratab? Is it appropriate for this male patient to receive this female hormone?

Errors can be detected in the process of the pharmacist's counseling the patient on how to take the medication. If a pharmacist had counseled the patient who received Coumadin when Kemadrin was ordered, the error probably would have been discovered during the dialogue. The counseling process provides an additional opportunity to check for correctness of the label and proper contents of the container.

The government, third party agents and the public must realize that dispensing prescriptions properly requires time and that must be paid for. Time is needed to work at a safe speed, provide a double check system, maintain and utilize pharmacy patient profiles, contact physicians concerning incomplete prescriptions, counsel patients and to keep current on drug therapy.

Dispensing after pharmacy hours

It has been the practice in many hospitals that when the pharmacy is closed, an authorized nursing supervisor, who maintains a pharmacy key, enters the pharmacy for the purpose of obtaining needed medication. This practice has led to grave errors. Only authorized pharmacy personnel should be permitted to dispense drugs. In error #104, for example, a nurse who was unfamiliar with the anti-cancer drug thioguanine, misinterpreted a physician's 9 P.M. order for 6 thioguanine and removed what proved to be a sixfold overdose for a patient from the pharmacy. The patient died after receiving the overdose.

If orders are routinely written after pharmacy hours, pharmacists and nurses should demand that provisions be made to extend pharmacy hours. When 24-hour pharmacy service is impossible or not practical, a separate stock cabinet or lockable cart located in some area other than in the pharmacy should be maintained. The cabinet or cart should be stocked with prepackaged labeled drugs in quantities sufficient for starting a patient. Unit dose medication is ideal for this purpose. Drugs should be limited to those medications which must be administered before a pharmacist arrives in the morning. For any item needed which is not present, a pharmacist should be on call to come to the hospital if required. Such a system is advocated by the Joint Commission on the Accreditation of Hospitals.[7]

This use of nursing supervisors to act as pharmacists at night or on weekends when the pharmacy is closed is no longer standard practice.

There has been an expansion from five day a week pharmacy service to seven day a week service. Pharmacies have gradually extended their hours from 5 P.M. to 7 P.M. to 9 P.M. to 11 P.M. A study by Stolar[8] reported that in 1975 hospital pharmacies were open an average of 74 hours per week, in 1977, 79 hours per week, and in 1978, 83 hours per week. Advanced pharmacy systems and services such as I.V. admixture, unit dose dispensing, monitoring drug therapy, drug information services, participation in CPR activities, are provided around the clock in many hospitals by pharmacists. In 1975 6% of hospitals had their pharmacies open 24 hours a day, in 1978 this figure had reached 12%. Twenty-four hour service was available in 40% of hospitals of 400 beds or more, 16% of the 200-399 bed hospitals, and 3% of the 6-199 bed hospitals.

Hospital Pharmacy Directors must exercise care when selecting pharmacists for night work, as an experienced, high-caliber pharmacist is needed. These pharmacists are essentially on their own, with no pharmacy director, no drug information pharmacist or colleague present to consult. In many cases no staff physician is readily available. What is often present in hospitals is a tired first, or second team of physicians who have already worked many hours, and are now writing orders for patients who may be unknown to them. Drug orders arise from emergency medicine involving night admissions or patients who "go bad." The nursing department is comparatively understaffed, often with part-time nurses.

Aside from the physician, the night pharmacist normally is the most educated person working in the hospital at night. At this time the pharmacist covers the entire patient load, so he or she cannot be as familiar with the patients as are day pharmacy personnel. The night pharmacist must also be able to quickly review a pharmacy patient profile or patient's chart, and to talk to nurses and physicians with knowledge and authority. The night pharmacist, besides providing continuity to the drug dispensing systems, is a primary source of drug information, providing much advice where needed.

Errors Peculiar to Unit Dose Systems

As the studies cited in chapter two have shown, a unit dose system reduces medication errors about 80%. However, it should be noted that when a unit dose system is instituted, the number of reported medication errors increases. At first glance it might be supposed the unit dose system is not as safe as the traditional drug distribution system it replaced. This is not the case for a well designed system monitored to assure quality. Two problems may arise. The new system may have some procedural or performance problems in the beginning which must be corrected. With good pharmacy and nursing communications these problems are quickly solved. In the long term what must be realized is that all the activities associated with a unit dose system involve labeled individual doses of medication and an effective pharmacy-nursing double check system. There is heightened interest in drug distribution and accuracy. Omitted doses are obvious since the dose or doses are left unadministered in the patients' bins. No such telltale doses are left in the traditional drug distribution system. When a dose is missing, it may be traced to a dose being administered to the wrong patient, or to a double dose being administered. These factors expose errors which may never have been observed and hence never reported under the traditional non-unit dose drug dispensing system. Much the same can be said for a pharmacy I.V. admixture program.

Unit dose dispensing systems are not error free, and in fact create unique opportunities for errors. The section following and the errors cited in the beginning of this chapter address some of these problems.

Individual doses packaged in unit dose strip packs with perforations between doses are best separated prior to storage. In error #6, a pharmacist handed a nurse a strip of four 200 mg quinidine tablets, a 24 hour supply for a new order, saying "here's the quinidine 200 mg." The nurse, used to unit dose and the one package-one dose concept, did not perceive the strip as four individual doses, although they were labeled as such. She thought the four tablets equaled one dose and administered 800 mg to the patient. When nurses become used to receiving all doses in single dose packaging, this type of error may occur. In error #11, a vial of 10 Lasix 40 mg tablets was dispensed. The label on this glass prescription vial simply stated, "Lasix 40 mg." A nurse used to the one package-one dose concept gave all 10 tablets when a 40 mg dose was requested. Error #61 demonstrates that standard multi-dose containers of antibiotic liquids of 60 ml and 100 ml have mistakenly been administered as single doses by nurses when placed in a patient's bin in a unit dose cart. Once a unit dose system of drug distribution has been introduced, it is a dangerous practice to allow non-unit dose containers to be used for normal dispensing.

Pharmacists must do everything possible to provide all products in unit dose form. For doses of more than one tablet, the multiple tablets should be placed in one package or in single packaged tablets stapled together. Strip packs should be separated into the number of tablets equaling a single dose. When the exact strength of a tablet or capsule is available, the pharmacy should purchase and supply this product, rather than two half-strength products. If it is absolutely essential to dispense a non-unit dose item, accurate, precise labeling is essential. The Lasix label above, for example, should have read "Lasix 40 mg per tablet, 10 tablets."

In this review of errors associated with unit dose, some mention should be made of reconstitution of powders in unit dose containers. When an exact volume for reconstitution is recommended and appears on the label, this volume must be used. In error #88, a pharmacist failed to pay attention to the volume requirement listed on the label. Since it was a unit dose container, he simply added enough water to fill the vial and dispensed it in this fashion. When a nurse needed 800 mg of erythromycin suspension, she used the volume listed on the label as providing 200 mg/in 5 ml to calculate an 800 mg dose. Since the volume was not accurate, the patient did not receive the required dose.

If it is not practical for the pharmacist to reconstitute the unit dose powder with exact volumes, it should be dispensed unreconstituted to the nurse.

In a unit dose system "stat" doses, starter doses, and "one time only" doses are generally dispensed alone, that is, not with other doses in the drug cart. These may be dispensed by messenger, pneumatic tube or some direct method. Doses that are returned unadministered and have potential for reissue, should not be marked with a patient name and/or bed number. In error #130 this practice caused a dose of ampicillin to be given to the wrong patient. A dose of ampicillin previously dispensed as a starter dose had a bed number written on it. The dose was not administered and was returned to pharmacy and placed in stock. The dose was later dispensed for another patient, but the old bed number had not been erased. A nurse who failed to follow normal procedure in reviewing the medication administration record before administration, gave the capsule to the patient whose bed number was printed on the label and who was the wrong patient.

When a single dose must be patient identified, it is best that it be dispensed with a tear-off label or from a labeled zip-lock plastic bag. Alternatively, a pharmacy messenger should place the dose in the patient's drawer.

The Paradox of Trusting

In order for the full benefits of a unit dose system to be realized, there must be an element of trust, but not blind trust. To begin with two conflicting truisms: everyone makes mistakes, yet must trust that what others do is correct. The reason we can live with this conflict is that we cannot do everything ourselves, and that we ourselves make mistakes. By the use of common sense and with experience, we learn what to accept with trust and what to question.

When a pharmacist talks about a unit dose program with Nursing, a nurse's reaction might be, "I would never administer an injection I didn't prepare myself." It is best for the pharmacist to agree with the nurse and say, "I wouldn't either if I were you, under the traditional drug distribution system." The nurse has learned this good rule in nursing school.

Assume you are a nurse coming on duty. The off-going nurse points to an unlabeled syringe with a liquid inside and says, "That's 1 million units of Penicillin for Mr. Smith in 425-B." Would you give the drug? No! It should be pointed out that in a unit dose dispensing system, the syringe would be prepared in the pharmacy under the laminar flow hood, be properly labeled, and the pharmacy responsible for its contents. In the past nurses have accepted without hesitation 20 white tablets of prednisone 5 mg, or 120 ml of the red liquid Phenobarbital Elixir, in labeled bottles prepared by the pharmacy. The injection would be accepted in the same way, once the similarity is properly explained. The nurse trusts the labeled product coming from the pharmacy. Now the paradox: The nurse must trust to a point, but never let her knowledge or experience be overshadowed by her trust. If the pharmacy supplies a syringe with a clear-water-white liquid labeled Vitamin B-12 1000 mcg/ml-1 ml, the nurse must question this product because she knows it should be pink. There is a natural tendency to trust the pharmacy's accuracy after several months of successful unit dose service. But nurses should not refrain from questioning whatever is different or unusual. The nurse's knowledge and experience are invaluable. These matters should be stressed in procedure and as part of inservice training.

We have cited mistakes pharmacists in unit dose systems have made in preparing and labeling syringes. Even though imperfect, the unit dose system in which injections are prepared and labeled in pharmacy offers safety advantages such as:

1. A triple-check system for pharmacy-prepared parenterals in unit dose; the checkers are the pharmacy supportive personnel, the pharmacist and the nurse. Only a single-check system would exist without pharmacy preparation. Pharmacists and nurses are human and will commit errors. The nurse may prevent errors committed by pharmacists in syringe preparation (volume, color, labeling, and route of administration may be questioned). Errors arising from syringes wrongly prepared by a nurse lack this potential for being stopped.

2. Syringes prepared by the pharmacy are fully labeled (intravenous medications also include patient name and bed number, and expiration dates). In addition, in the case of bulk syringe preparation by pharmacists, control numbers are maintained and sterility testing is accomplished.

3. To increase the likelihood of producing a sterile product, all pharmacy preparation is done under laminar flow, using acceptable sterile technique. Filtration is accomplished when necessary to decrease particulate contamination.

4. Partial doses removed from vials are best calculated by a pharmacist.

5. Experienced pharmacists are most adept at choosing appropriate diluents and volumes for parenterals requiring reconstitution. Pharmacists not having this expertise rapidly acquire it.
6. Unit dose syringes allow for accountability of each dose to be administered. Nurses and pharmacists check to ascertain why unadministered doses have been returned.
7. Since labels are attached to each syringe (including expiration date and control number, as mentioned above), unused doses can be returned for reissue at considerable cost savings to the hospital.
8. The full implementation of the unit dose system is a recommendation of the Joint Commission on the Accreditation of Hospitals (JCAH). The current standard states that "The use of floor stock medications should be minimized; the unit dose drug distribution system, which permits identification of the drug up to the point of administration, is recommended for use throughout the hospital. Individual drugs should be administered as soon as possible after the dose has been prepared, particularly medications prepared for parenteral administration, and, to the maximum extent possible, by the individual who prepared the dose, except where unit dose distribution systems are used."
9. Total parenteral nutrition solutions and enteral alimentation solutions containing electrolytes, vitamins, etc., are prepared extemporaneously and labeled by pharmacy. This is a recommendation of the National Coordinating Committee on Large Volume Parenterals and JCAH.
10. Some hospital pharmacies are using vertical laminar flow containment hoods to minimize exposure of their personnel to excessive amounts of cancer chemotherapy agents.[9]

If the expected safety is to be realized from a unit dose system, pharmacy and nursing personnel must follow established procedure. Some nursing personnel become so trusting of pharmacy that they break procedure and administer an extra dose that might have been mistakenly placed in a patient's bin, or fail to request a missing dose that was omitted from a patient's bin. The nurse should not have blind faith in what is or is not in the patient's bin. The nurse must check the patient's chart or contact the pharmacy when there is an apparent discrepancy between the medication in the patient's bin and her medication administration record.

On the other hand, the pharmacy cannot accept the nurse's word that a drug was omitted from the patient's bin. If a nurse asks for an omitted drug, the pharmacist must check his patient profile. The drug may have been discontinued and nursing did not note it. The drug may never have been ordered for the patient. The dose may have been administered by another nurse who did not chart it. A dose might have been used to start another patient on a new order. The pharmacist must check carefully before the requested dose is dispensed. Additional causes of these kinds of occurrences have been published. [10,11]

There must be mutual respect and trust between Nursing and Pharmacy. A good unit dose dispensing system has built-in procedures to minimize the possibility of human error. The better the system, the fewer mistakes, and the more chance there is to trust, rather than question. Double checks, professional experience, and common sense are not to be replaced by trust in the infallibility of a pharmacist or nurse.

References

1. ASHP guidelines on hospital drug distribution and control. (See appendix)

2. Stocks AE, Martin FI. Hypoglycemia due to erroneous drug ingestion. Med J Aust 1(24):1256-8, 10 Jun 1972.

3. Ahlquist DA, Nelson RL, Callaway CW. Pseudoinsulinoma syndrome from inadvertent tolazamide ingestion. Ann Intern Med. 1980; 93:281-2.

4. Sandor IM. Ann Intern Med. 1980; 93:933 Letter.

5. Aldrich TK. Ann Intern Med. 1980; 93:933-4. Letter.

6. Whitaker RL. Confused drug names. Ann Intern Med. 1980; 93:933. Letter.

7. Accreditation Manual for Hospitals 1980, Pharmaceutical service section, standard IV, JCAH, 875 N. Mich. Ave., Chicago, Ill. 60611. (See Appendix)

8. Stolar MH. National survey of hospital pharmacy service 1978. Am J Hosp Pharm. 1979. 36:316.

9. Hoffman DM. The handling of antineoplastic drugs in a major cancer center. Hosp Pharm 1980; 15:302.

10. Kitrenos JG, Gluck, Stotter ML. Analysis of missing medication episodes in a unit dose system. Hosp Pharm 1979; 14:642.

11. Cohen MR. Discrepancies in unit dose cart fills. Hosp Pharm 1980; 15:17.

10

Errors Associated with a Lack of Knowledge About Drugs

All health professionals occasionally show lack of knowledge about drugs. This is why it is necessary for the pharmacist to see a copy of the original physician's order before the first dose is administered, why drug floor stock should be limited as much as possible to emergency items, and why unit dose dispensing systems and pharmacy I.V. admixture systems should be used. The pharmacist is grateful when a knowledgeable nurse is the last check on his or her work prior to administration of a drug.

With thousands of drugs available and the tens of thousands of generic names, trade names, synonyms, abbreviations, strengths, dosage forms, etc., in use, there will be many incidents where health professionals are not familiar with a drug which has been ordered. When this understandable ignorance is compounded with poorly communicated physician orders (see Chapter #4), the use of improper drug names (see Chapter 5), improper abbreviations (see Chapter 6), and poorly labeled containers (see Chapter 15), the problem is vastly expanded. In these situations, the person committing the error is only partly to blame, since if the drugs were correctly ordered, and/or the container was properly labeled, the error might not have occurred.

Some of the errors cited below can only be attributed to a lack of knowledge on the part of the person who made the error. These errors reflect poor training concerning drugs and their administration, poor training in seeking reliable information when one is uninformed, poor job assignments, and poor supervision.

Medication errors stemming from a lack of knowledge may involve ignorance concerning the drug product, properties of the drug, route of administration, dose, rate of administration, indication and nomenclature. Errors concerning mathematical miscalculations are discussed in Chapter 16.

Lack of Knowledge of the Drug Product

Zetar Shampoo was ordered but Zetar Emulsion was dispensed because this was the only Zetar product the pharmacist was familiar with (error #99).

A student nurse was out of Vitamin B_{12} and wanted to know if a double dose of Vitamin B_6 could be given instead (error #17).

Tylenol #3 was ordered, 3 tylenol tablets were administered rather than Tylenol 300 mg and codeine 30 mg (error #27).

Folinic acid was not given during methotrexate rescue therapy until the following morning because the person administering the drug did not want to awaken the patient just for a "vitamin" (error #47).

Part-time pharmacy personnel receiving an order for normal saline solution vials dispensed sodium chloride 100 mEq in 40 ml. This solution is 16 times more concentrated than 0.9% sodium chloride injection and is meant to be used in a pharmacy I.V. admixture program (error #63).

Camphorated opium tincture 5 ml was ordered; 5 ml of opium tincture was administered. Opium tincture is 25 times more potent than camphorated opium tincture (paregoric) (error #100).

Lack of Knowledge Concerning Properties of Dosage Form

A pharmacy technician filtered Sus-phrine Injection when drawing up the product from an ampul into a syringe. The product is a suspension and the active ingredient was thus removed by filtration (see error #96).

A pharmacist prepared a Haldol solution by crushing tablets and dissolving them in water, using the clear solution that passed through the filter and discarding the insoluble residue on the filter paper. Haldol is not soluble in water. A subpotent preparation was dispensed (see error #75).

Lack of Knowledge Concerning Route of Administration

"Aqueous Procaine Penicillin G" was ordered I.V. This suspension is only to be administered I.M. (see error #72). The correct terminology for this drug is penicillin G procaine.

Vancomycin was ordered and administered I.M. It should only be used I.V. (see error #65).

Cocaine and epinephrine was given orally when it was intended to be used on packing in the nose (see error #87).

Lugol's solution was given in the eye (see error #15).

Cromolyn sodium capsules were given orally rather than correctly opened and the powder inhaled (see error #31).

Lack of Knowledge Concerning Proper Dose

Twenty-five grams of Amytal was going to be administered rather than mannitol (see error #97).

For a renal patient, gentamicin was given every four hours instead of every 24 hours (error #51).

A "dab" of Nitroglycerin Ointment was applied to the chest rather than a 1 inch ribbon (see error #102).

A 10 mg I.V. fatal overdose of colchicine was administered rather than 1 mg (see error #98). Ten 1 mg ampuls were administered.

A 40% Acetic solution for irrigation was ordered rather than the ¼% intended (see error #123).

Ferrous Fumerate was ordered as 200 mg. The product was labeled as to the content of elemental iron, 66 mg per tablet. Three tablets were dispensed in error when in fact 200 mg of Ferrous Fumerate = 66 mg of iron (see error #60).

A 1 g I.V. dose of gentamicin was administered when ordered (see errors #91, 92). Thirteen 1 g vials were administered.

Vincristine overdoses of 32 mg to a 13-year-old, 3.5 mg to a 5-year-old, 6.5 mg to an 8-year-old, 13.5 mg to a 7-year-old, and a 7-year-old given a monthly dose on 2 consecutive days, resulted in 3 deaths (see error #86). An 8 mg overdose of vincristine was administered (error #71). Overdoses of vincristine also appear in error #131.

A physician ordered mithramycin 3750 mg I.V. over 24-hour period rather than 1250 mg per day (see error #24).

Lack of Knowledge Concerning Rate of Administration of a Drug

A physician ordered and his order was subsequently administered for 60 mEq of Potassium Chloride in 100 ml of 5% Dextrose to be administered in one hour followed by 40 mEq of Potassium Chloride in 40 ml of 5% Dextrose. The drug was too concentrated and administered too rapidly (see error #67).

Lack of Knowledge of Indication for a Drug

The anti-cancer drug Leukeran was administered to a patient who did not have cancer when the order was written on the wrong patient's chart (see error #21).

A nurse did not want to awaken a patient to take a dose of lactulose. Lactulose is used to treat hepatic coma (see error #111).

The dose of Mucomyst 20% 3.5 g P.O. q 4 hr did not correspond with its recommended mucolytic dose. Only 3.5 ml was administered. The drug was being used as an antidote for acetaminophen overdose and 17.5 ml should have been administered (see error #134).

Lack of Knowledge of Nomenclature and Terminology

An order for a Black and White 30 ml at bedtime resulted in the dispensing of Black and White Scotch, rather than the laxative mixture of Milk of Magnesia and Aromatic Cascara Fluid Extract when this old synonym (see error #84) was used.

Three tablespoons (45 ml) of medication were administered instead of a teaspoon (5 ml) because the apothecary symbol for teaspoon was not understood (error #117).

Ten ml (160 minums) was administered because the apothecary symbol for 10 minum was not familiar to the health care worker (error #128).

A drug order using a research name Ara A was wrongly thought to be the same as cytarabine, whose research name was ARA C (error #150).

The Drug Enforcement symbol for a class IV substance was thought to connote intravenous administration when in fact the drugs were not intended for I.V. administration (errors #42 and #109).

A drug was given in both eyes (O.U.) when an order was written A.U. (both ears) (error #8).

Sixfold overdoses of 6-mercaptopurine and 6-thioguanine were administered because personnel did not know that "6" was part of the research name for the drugs mercaptopurine and thioguanine (errors #13 and #104).

Some of the problems caused by lack of education of young health professionals will fade away when the older physicians are no longer practicing medicine and the apothecary system disappears (minums and grains). The use of research names after an official name is assigned and the use of abbreviated or coined names must be abandoned by physicians and researchers. Educators in our schools and hospitals must do a more thorough job of teaching health professionals about drugs. Employers must do a better job in screening job applicants, placing applicants, post employment indoctrination and training, supervision and in inservice education. The trend towards relicensing examination and/or required continued education are positive steps to provide knowledgeable health professionals.

11

Patient Identification

Patients for whom medication is intended should be positively identified prior to drug administration. This is best accomplished by checking a patient's identification armband. Most other methods of patient identification can lead to drug administration to the wrong patient. In error #53, a nurse believed she identified a patient by the bed the patient occupied. But the former occupant had just been transferred to another room without the nurse's knowledge. A new patient was in his place and the nurse assumed it was the former patient! In other instances a nurse may be in the wrong patient room. Though it may be inconvenient to look at the armband of a patient who has supposedly been in the same bed for weeks, such inspection will prevent momentary lapses in room orientation by the medication nurse and misidentification because of last-minute patient transfers.

When armbands are removed from patients for OR procedures, tests, etc., they should be replaced before any medications are administered. Temporary armbands, which are stored and created on the nursing unit, should be used until one is obtained from the usual source.

Do not rely on a patient for his or her name. Often patients on the same floor will have identical surnames (error #56) or may have organic brain syndrome or some other deficiency such as poor hearing and be unable to respond with the correct name (error #55). Asking a patient to confirm the name you are calling him also may not work, for the same reasons. In a bizarre case, a nurse asked a patient if he was Mr. Thomas. "Wright!" he answered. Mr. Wright received Mr. Thomas's medication (error #141).

Besides medication errors, misidentification of patients has been responsible for laboratory errors, dietary errors, operating room errors and even autopsy errors.

Forms used for drug orders must be patient identified. Those who transcribe and note orders must see that complete identification is used on the form. If an addressoplate is not available, full name, bed number and patient identification number (chart number) should be used. Physicians should not write on non-patient identified order sheets. A case has been described where an order was sent to pharmacy marked only with "E. Jackson" as identification. The order, written for Edna Jackson, was mistakenly scheduled and dispensed by pharmacy to Ellen Jackson, a patient on the same floor (error #30).

Hospital admitting offices should make every effort to put patients with the same surname into different areas of the facility. Amazingly, patients with identical surnames (but not related) have been placed in the same room (error #56). This is an extremely hazardous practice.

Hospital personnel must also take time to confirm that they are documenting information on correctly identified patient records. Writing drug orders on the wrong patient's chart can have disastrous consequences (error #21). Likewise, transcription of orders on the wrong patient profile or wrong medication administration record may lead to serious error. Carelessness is usually the cause of such errors. While there is no specific system designed to prevent such errors, a physician order form-medication administration record system developed by Leiman (see error #13 for brief description) helps prevent transcribing orders on the wrong patient's medication record. Physician order forms which are addressoplated once on the front and then several times on the back side of the form (segmented second sheet) are dangerous, as the unseen imprint may be incorrect. In addition, the importance of nurses and pharmacists maintaining diagnostic information on their records cannot be overemphasized. In this way, one can at least assure that drug therapy corresponds to diagnosis. For example, one would not schedule and administer cancer chemotherapy to a patient (as was done in error #21) unless there was an indication in pharmacy and nursing records that the patient in fact had cancer. Nor would insulin be administered unless the patient for whom it was ordered had diabetes mellitus. Assuring that drug therapy corresponds to diagnosis will help to prevent errors resulting from prescribing or transcribing onto the wrong patient record.

12

Errors Associated with Medication Administration

Assurance that the right patient will receive the right drug in the right dose by the right route at the right time is the essence of preventing medication error. The following general considerations regarding the administration of medications to institutionalized patients are basic procedures which will help to prevent error.

Unless following an approved protocol, never administer any medication, including topical preparations, antacids or placebos, without a physician's order. If the order is given verbally, make sure that it is reduced to writing in accordance with procedure before the drug is administered unless an emergency exists. Verbal orders are discussed in Chapter 4.

When transcribing orders on medication administration records (MAR), be especially careful to record accurately the date, drug, dose, dosage form, route and time(s) to be administered on the correct patient's record. Also record any stop time that might have been specified in the physician's order. This information will continue to be referred to as long as the order is in effect, so it must appear correctly from the start. Some system of notation should be used to serve as a reminder to hold certain doses when a patient is scheduled for an operation or procedure that contraindicates a particular drug or route of administration (i.e., NPO for OR or laboratory procedure).

When making entries on to the MAR, legibility is an important factor in avoiding errors. In error #15 the poorly written abbreviation, O.J., was mistaken for O.D., resulting in an error. The use of unapproved abbreviations on MARs has caused errors. In error #8 the abbreviation A.U. (both ears) was interpreted as both eyes. If physicians use unapproved abbreviations in order writing, these abbreviations should not be entered on the MAR, but the meaning of the abbreviation should instead be entered in its place. The physician must then be told of the dangers inherent in the use of the unapproved abbreviations (see Chapter 6).

Timely Administration

Doses of medication should be administered within 30 minutes of the time due. The busiest medication round is usually in the morning when once, twice, three and four times daily medications are usually given at one time. If sufficient adequate nursing personnel are not available, timely medication administration may not be possible. It has been determined that it takes more time to administer digoxin than any other oral medication, since it is necessary to take an apical and radial pulse before it is administered. To lighten the workload of this busy morning medication round, some hospitals have established a procedure directing that all once-daily digoxin doses be given in the afternoon. This practice also permits physicians to delay one day's therapy of digoxin, since such a holding order written in the morning can be initiated the same day.

Timely drug administration may be delayed in the traditional drug distribution system where nurses must prepare (pour) medications. In the preparation of medications, the nurse must select the drug from the proper container, place a dose in a souffle cup, in some cases oral liquids must be poured and measured, I.V. admixtures mixed, etc. With a unit dose drug distribution system, the pharmacy is responsible for providing labeled unit dose medication in a timely fashion. When this is achieved, medication administration can also be timely and efficient.

Before drug administration in a non-unit dose system, doses must be "poured" or prepared by the person who will administer them. The label on the original container must be read three times (when taking it from the shelf or cart bin, when preparing the dose, and when returning the original container). There must be a method for identifying what doses are being prepared for what patient. Medications should never be poured in advance of drug administration time. Physician orders may subsequently be written that change or modify the original therapy.

In a unit dose system doses are prepared and labeled by pharmacy and placed in patient bins in a drug cart. Prior to drug administration, the person administering drugs simply compares the labeled doses with doses scheduled according to the medication administration record. In a unit dose system, it is necessary for the pharmacist to prepare medications in advance. The pharmacist is responsible for updating prepared doses for administration, but the person administering medications must be aware of last minute changes. The fact that each dose is labeled facilitates the implementation of last minute changes by physicians. In a unit dose system, doses of medications are prepared by the pharmacist and administered by another person. Since all doses are labeled, the system allows for a check that does not exist in a non-unit dose system, where medications are prepared and administered by the same person. Whenever discrepancies exist, a notation should be made on a separate piece of paper. After a medication round, all discrepancies are resolved with the pharmacist. Removal of doses from unit dose packages prior to actual drug administration defeats the purpose of the unit dose system. This practice is condemned.

When doses are prepared for administration or when the label of each dose is compared against the medication administration record, the expiration date on the container or unit dose package is checked and the dosage form is observed for proper color, consistency and, if a liquid, the presence of precipitation. For intravenous medications, observance for precipitates or other forms of particulate matter must occur during drug administration. Absence of such a check has had disastrous consequences, as when a precipitate formed in an IV line when cephalothin and gentamicin were administered simultaneously through the same line. The precipitate was not noticed until the patient developed acute respiratory distress and cyanosis (error #76). Cephalothin and gentamicin are incompatible and should have been administered through separate lines.

When medications are transcribed onto medication administration records or made ready for administration, the purpose and dosage range must be understood. Where unfamiliar medications are involved, time must be taken to obtain appropriate information. In all cases, drug therapy and dose must "make sense" for the patient. It is the job of physician, nurse and pharmacist to assure this! Error #21 describes a situation where an anti-cancer drug was administered to a patient who did not have a diagnosis of cancer.

To the extent possible, medications should be referred to by their generic name. When a medication is dispensed under a name different from the name prescribed (i.e., generic name on label of medication prescribed by brand name), the pharmacist must devise a system so that drug administration personnel can identify what has been dispensed. Ordinarily, the pharmacist label should include both names. Other alternatives are placement of a drug synonym list on the nursing unit, or readily available formularies listing all the names. In no case should the person administering medications give a dose without first having identified the product.

Prior to the administration of any medication, the patient must be properly identified. Each patient should have an armband (see Chapter 11 for errors related to misidentification of patients). The armband must be checked and the patient addressed by name prior to drug administration.

It is common practice for nurses to crush tablets prior to administration when patients cannot swallow or are on tube feeding. The pharmacist should be informed when this is done, for a liquid dosage form of the drug may be available from the pharmacy. Enteric coated tablets should not be crushed. In this situation the pharmacist may be able to suggest alternative therapy to the prescribing physician.

In a unit dose system, when patients are able to open the package, the labeled dose of oral medication may be handed to the patient at the time of administration. This allows the patient to serve as the final check and also is a positive step in patient education.

Observe the patient swallowing oral medications. Never leave medications at bedside for the patient to take later. In error #5, medications placed at bedside were later taken by the wrong patient. Doses may be hoarded by the patient or not taken at all if left at bedside. Exceptions are doses specifically ordered by the physician to be left at bedside for self administration by the patient. Medications such as nitroglycerin, antacids, some lotions and ointments and anticholinesterase drugs used in treatment of myasthenia gravis are often ordered in this manner. Formalized medication self-administration programs are another exception.

Immediately after drug administration has occurred, doses are recorded as given on the medication administration record. If a patient questions any dose, do not administer the drug. See Chapter 13 on the patient's responsibility in preventing medication errors. Check the original order or check with the prescriber to make sure that the medication dose is correct. If a patient refuses a dose in a unit dose system, this should be noted on the medication administration record. Make sure that both the prescriber and the pharmacist are informed (a notation system has been designed for this purpose — see Chapter 7). The dose should be left in the patient bin with the explanatory note. In a non-unit dose system, the prescriber is informed and doses unadministered should be discarded. No attempt should be made to return these non-unit dose drugs to a container or re-use any dose at a later time.

Although patient refusal is not classified as an error, the result is the same as an omitted dose. When patients refuse to take a drug because of an unpleasant taste or otherwise objectionable characteristics of a dosage form, alert the pharmacist to this fact. There may be an alternative dosage form available which would be more acceptable to the patient.

When more than one medication is ordered for a patient, the timing of doses may be important. For example, one would not schedule oral tetracycline and antacid doses to be given at the same time. A drug interaction occurs that interferes with the absorption of tetracycline. Gentamicin and cephalothin interact when placed in the same container, causing precipitation. In error #113, medication being administered through a nasogastric tube was given with tube feedings. When the patient had trouble tolerating the tube feeding, gastric contents were suctioned and along with it the medications were withdrawn from the stomach. Seizures finally occurred, since the patient was supposed to be receiving the anticonvulsants phenobarbital and phenytoin. Pharmacists should routinely observe medication administration records to help prevent drug interactions related to simultaneous administration. A general awareness of this problem by all involved with medication handling is in order.

When administering PRN medications, make sure that enough time, as specified in the physician's order, has passed since the last dose.

When a patient is having intake and output recorded, make sure that all fluid administered in conjunction with a drug dose is recorded.

Never borrow a medication intended for one patient for use with another patient. There may be a good reason why a patient's medication is missing, such as dispensing delayed by pharmacist until prescribing problem resolved, mistranscription on nursing record, or pharmacy not having received original order. Borrowing often leads to serious medication error (see error #119).

If more than one or two dosage units (tablets, capsules, vials, ampuls, etc.) are needed to prepare a single adult dose, something may be wrong! Unless you are quite familiar with this need, check with a pharmacist or knowledgeable colleague before preparing the dose. If large numbers of tablets or capsules are found to be necessary, the pharmacist might be able to prepare a dosage form that would be more convenient for the patient. Errors #13, 38, 91, 92, 98 and 104 point out situations where tragic errors were made when nurses used many dosage units to administer a single dose.

The majority of errors reported in this book relate in some way to medication administration. The vast majority of errors resulting from a breech of basic nursing procedures are so common that they are not reported to us (i.e., error resulting from nurse not checking armband, wrong time errors, not reading a label, etc.)

Errors relating to drug administration not cited above, while rare, are sure to be repeated elsewhere. We review them here to give the reader an awareness of some of the unusual errors that occur which result in patient harm. In error #93, subtherapeutic insulin doses were administered to patients because of the needle size used. The insulin was ordered to be given intramuscularly. Doses were prepared (drawn up) with an intradermal (25 g x ⅝") needle attached to the syringe. But the syringe contents were administered using a 21 g x 1½" needle. The dead space in the I.M. needle held most of the dose.

Error #124 describes administration of an oral liquid dose of Lasix via an intravenous catheter. Although the dose was prepared in an "oral syringe" with a tip that could not accommodate a needle, the syringe was held against a luer connector and injected intravenously. The person administering medications explained that she thought the syringe was designed to accommodate a needle for intravenous injection, but had a malformed tip.

Although nitroglycerin ointment is supposed to be given by squeezing out a ribbon of ointment on an applicator paper measured in inches, error #102 describes an error that occurred when a dab of ointment was placed on the paper and smeared out to the required number of inches.

Error #136 describes an error in dosing with oral pediatric antibiotic suspension that occurred because those responsible for drug administration used plastic teaspoons for "teaspoonful" doses. The teaspoons actually measured only 3 ml, rather than the intended 5 ml.

References

1. Nursing 80. Nurse's guide to drugs, 2nd ed. Horsham PA, Intermed Communications 1980.
2. Loebl S, Spratto G, Wit A, eds. The Nurse's Drug Handbook. New York: John Wiley and Sons.

13

The Patient's Contribution to Medication Errors and Their Prevention

Mauksch gives us great insight on what it is like to be a patient and why patients allow hospital personnel to commit errors without defending themselves. "A patient, like anyone in a dependent position, devotes a significant part of his energy to survival and to adaptation in the institution that holds him captive. Hospitalization is a form of captivity that makes jail rank somewhat higher on personal freedom." [1]

Mauksch describes how office patients are given prescriptions which are filled as well as labeled by pharmacists. As outpatients they are trusted to take their own medicine. Then, when the need arises, arrangements for hospitalization are made. Numerous forms are completed at the admission office. The attachment of an ID band is a symbolic communication, "You are ours now." What happens to you isn't your problem any more, it is the hospital's responsibility. You are escorted to your room and helped to undress so that the hospital can cope with you. You are ordered to bed. You are given a gown that leaves your rear end exposed. The gown is also too short. If you are not in "uniform," the hospital cannot cope with you. This is part of the "stripping" process seen in the army and in prison.

You are put in a room with a stranger. Several times during the first day personal questions are asked about your bowel habits, the state of your marriage, your sex life, your drinking habits, and so on. A thin curtain is all that shields your answers from the ear of this stranger in the next bed. The doctor then proceeds to examine your orifices.

You must surrender any drugs. Yesterday you were capable of taking your drugs, today you are not. They are no longer your responsibility. Last week your physician weighed you, took X-rays, EKGs, and made other tests. Once admitted to the hospital, patients must take the same tests again, as if the results obtained by your regular physician cannot be trusted.

Mauksch goes on to state that people who are ill tend to develop "dependence manifestation," because illness tends to create preoccupation with self. In the hospital, however, dependence manifestation is a realistic adaptation to the conditions which the individual experiences. The patient is dependent on the nurse, the maid, the physician, the intern, the dietician, and others. He or she is dependent for survival, for continuity of service, for personal consideration, for reward and for punishment. Good behavior will bring bathroom privileges! The patient views a hospital as a place where others have power over him, and therefore devotes significant energy to gaining good will, exploring his rights and obligations and finding out what will achieve favorable acceptance. Only by this means can he earn what he seeks: safe, effective, personalized care.

In these circumstances it is no wonder that the patient who has been receiving ear drops for several days when instructed by a nurse to "put your head back, I have your eye drops," obediently lets the nurse make a mistake (see error #8). Similarly, a patient did not question the administration of an unordered Lugols Solution into his eye when there was nothing wrong with the eye (see error #15).

There are, of course, valid reasons for hospital policies and procedures which tend to make patients dependent and to inhibit behavior which they believe might prejudice hospital personnel against them. Consumers must be educated to question what is happening to them and to protest, I am not supposed to get eye drops; I am not supposed to go for a test; I do not take two of these tablets; why are you prepping my back, they're going to operate on my thyroid; they just gave me that tablet an hour ago, and so on. While experienced health professionals can cite incidents where such concerns were unfounded and the treatment of the patients was correct and proper, professionals also know of cases where patients have prevented errors or otherwise aided in their therapy with timely questions.

Patients should be encouraged to question what is happening to them and to display their knowledge of previous therapy. And it is imperative that patients' protests, questions or suggestions be taken seriously. Is this the right patient? (see error #43, 54, 55, 56, 141); was the order written on the right chart? (see error #18, 21, 30); is this the proper medicine? (see error #29, 106); and is this the right route of administration? (see error #8, 15, 31, 87). Patients should know their diseases or problems, allergies, hypersensitivities, and the name, strength and dosage of their current medications. It has been suggested that patients carry a card with such information and that this information be kept current. Such a method would be useful in taking a complete and accurate drug history and to insure continuity of therapy (see error #7, 122).

A patient should ascertain that the medicine he or she is receiving that appears to be different is the same drug that was previously taken. Patients must be informed about generic and trade names and be aware that different brands of the same drug may not look the same.

Some unit dose hospitals permit the patient, when capable, to be given the unopened unit dosage capsules or tablets to take while the nurse observes. This allows the patient to be the final check in the medication system, and to become more knowledgeable about their medication through reading labels and by means of increased dialogue with the nurse. However, nurses must observe the patient take the medication to prevent hoarding, or forgetting to take the dose.

It is extremely important that hospitals formalize discharge planning. Insuring the proper taking of medication at home is an important component of this procedure. Medications the patient brings with him on admission must be coordinated with discharge prescriptions. Discharge prescriptions must be written in advance of discharge so that time is available for counseling and education[2] (see error #108). Self-medication programs for hospitalized patients have been advocated as a bridge between patient education and self-sufficiency. Ambulatory patients also require counseling by physicians and pharmacists on how medication is to be taken.

Investigating a patient's objections, questions and worries to determine their validity takes time. Patient counseling and education also requires time. If medication errors are to be prevented and if patients are to comply with the prescribed regimens, proper systems must be developed in the physician's office, in hospitals, in pharmacies, and at home with visiting nurses, and time set aside for these activities.

References

1. Mauksch HO. The patient and ancillary hospital personnel. Hosp Pharm Vol 4 No 9 (Sep) p 5 1969.
2. Grissinger SE, Wolfe LW, Cohen MR. A protocol for consultation with discharged patients about their medications. Hosp Pharm 8:175, 1973.

14

Errors Related to Cancer Chemotherapy

Because most of the agents used in cancer chemotherapy exhibit some type of toxicity even in therapeutic doses, inadvertent overdoses can be especially harmful. Conversely, subtherapeutic doses do not give the patient the full benefit of a course of chemotherapy. Cancer chemotherapy is an area in which the majority of pharmacists, nurses and physicians lack specialized knowledge and expertise. For this reason, complete trust in oncologic specialists who do the drug prescribing is commonplace. However, it should be noted that these people make mistakes too, as error #71 demonstrates. In this case, a physician ordered 8 mg of vincristine instead of vinblastine. The pharmacist who received the order failed to question what he suspected to be a high dose because an oncologist wrote the order, and he had not been known to err in the past.

Lack of familiarity with drug dose may lead to error, as indicated in error #24. In this case, a physician incorrectly wrote for a three-day dose of the cancer chemotherapeutic mithramycin to be administered over a single day. A nurse, unfamiliar with the dose, requested the overdose from the pharmacy. An alert pharmacist prevented serious error. Unfamiliarity with drug dose also was a contributing factor in error #71 above.

In error #47, unfamiliarity with a protocol that required follow-up dosing with folinic acid to counteract the toxic effects of methotrexate led to an error. The nurse believed folinic acid to be *only* a vitamin. Since the patient was sleeping when the dose was due, she did not wish to wake him. Physicians, nurses and pharmacists must be especially careful when prescribing, administering or dispensing drugs with which they may be unfamiliar. This is especially true of cancer chemotherapy agents. Appropriate literature review, and/or consultation with a knowledgeable colleague is necessary before use of an uncommon or unfamiliar drug.

Also a problem related to lack of familiarity with dose is that package inserts of marketed drugs may not provide complete current prescribing information. In error #71, a dose of vincristine 8 mg did not seem unusual to the pharmacist, even though the highest adult dose listed on the package insert was approximately 2 mg. The pharmacist had been used to unusually high doses of other drugs routinely used in cancer chemotherapy protocols, which are above the range listed in official product information inserts. He specifically recalled routine doses of fluorouracil far above those recommended in package inserts. New literature on drug dosing of cancer chemotherapeutic agents appears so often that it is nearly impossible to keep abreast of changes. This is yet another reason that those involved tend to put complete faith in the prescribing specialist. A system for keeping health professionals in institutions aware of the most current dosing techniques with these agents is reviewed in error #71.

Error #86 describes five published overdose errors which occurred with vincristine in the San Diego area in a five year period; the death of a 13-year-old who received 32 mg; a seven-year-old who was given a monthly dose on two consecutive days; the death of an eight-year-old who received 6.5 mg; a five-year-old who received 3.5 mg and a seven-year-old who died after receiving a 13.5 mg dose. Another case report cites a three-year-old who received a 6.5 mg dose of vincristine, a tenfold error.[1] A four-year-old patient received 8.75 mg of vincristine, rather than the 1.75 mg ordered when the 5 mg vials were mistakenly used instead of the 1 mg vials (rather than using 1 and ¾ 1 mg vials, 1 and ¾ 5 mg vials were used).[2]

Vincristine is available from the manufacturer in both 1 mg and 5 mg vials. The 5 mg vials were intended for use in institutions which treat large numbers of cancer patients where more than one dose at a time is to be prepared (for several patients at the same time). The maximum adult dose of this drug does not normally exceed 2 mg. The presence of the 5 mg vial helps substantiate a professional's belief that a prescribed or incorrectly calculated overdose may be appropriate. "Why would a 5 mg vial be available if not for these higher doses?" If this package size is necessary and continues to be manufactured, a warning label placed on the 5 mg vial stating that it is for use in preparing multiple doses *only* might help to prevent future errors. It is our opinion that professionals' lack of knowledge renders the 5 mg vincristine package unsafe and this size package should not be marketed.

Labeling used for a container of Cee NU (lomustine) also led to error (H.W. #7).

A good deal of confusion and resultant error is generated by the poor system of nomenclature for many of the cancer chemotherapeutic agents. Much of this confusion is due to the use of several different names for a single agent. The name used first is generally the chemical designation. Occasionally this is abbreviated as a lettered, or numbered and lettered abbreviation, then to a generic or United States Adopted Name (USAN). Finally, there is a trade name. Some examples are: 6-mercaptopurine (chemical name), 6-MP (abbreviation for chemical name), Mercaptopurine (generic or USAN), Purinethol (trade name), and Mechlorethamine (generic or USAN), HN_2 (abbreviated chemical designation), Nitrogen Mustard (synonym and common name), Mustargen (trade name).

Enough confusion, danger and breaks in protocols exist without the introduction of all these names. Davis (Hosp Pharm 1976, 11:36) editorialized on this subject, suggesting that no trade names be assigned to cancer chemotherapeutics. Error #150 describes a mix-up between cytarabine and vidarabine. This occurred following a physician's use of the abbreviation, ARA-A, for the pre-marketing nomenclature for vidarabine (short for adeniol arabinoside). The name ARA-A was confused with cytosine arabinoside, sometimes abbreviated as ARA-C. Two pharmacists mistakenly believed these to be the same drugs and a patient received the wrong drug!

Another problem related to naming has to do with the use of abbreviations. In error #110, a pharmacist confused a common abbreviation for Mustargen (HN_2) with that for methotrexate, MTX. The Mustargen was dispensed for methotrexate and injected intramuscularly. This could have led to serious abscess formation, but fortunately did not, due to infiltration of an antidote (Sodium Thiosulfate) into the injected area when the error was discovered. Abbreviations for drug names should not be permitted. When ordering, the full official or trade name should always be used.

The use of a number prefix before a chemotherapy drug name has led to error. Error #104 describes a death that occurred when an order for thioguanine was written using its former chemical name, 6-thioguanine. Since the manufacturer's bottle is properly labeled only as "Thioguanine," a nurse preparing the dose thought that the number 6 prefix in the physician's written order meant that 6 doses were to be given. A similar error occurred with mercaptopurine (6-mercaptopurine) in error #13. A numbered prefix for any drug name is dangerous and must be discouraged.

Storage conditions for a drug, diluent used for reconstitution, dilution, dose, rate of administration, frequency of administration, route of administration and effects of extravasation, are important considerations for all drugs, but they are particularly important for cancer chemotherapy agents. Since this therapy is in such a state of development and flux, the drugs used are often investigational, or product literature does not reflect current published therapy. This makes it imperative that physicians, pharmacists and nurses have access to the protocols being used, or the published literature utilized by the prescribers. Most hospital pharmacy and therapeutics committees require drug investigators to file copies of their investigational protocols with the pharmacy. The pharmacy should make abstracts of these protocols for nursing personnel who must administer the drug and monitor its effects. These protocols must be checked when investigational drugs are being utilized. Although a drug may already be marketed, prescribing for an unapproved use or dose as part of a study will cause it to be classified as an investigational drug which requires a protocol (see Chapter 4).

References

1. Suskind RM, Brusilow SW, Zehr J. Syndrome of inappropriate secretion of antidiuretic hormone produced by vincristine toxicity (With bioassay of ADH level). J Pediatr 1972; 81:90-2.

2. Casteels-Vann Deele M, Beirinckx J, Baines P. Overdosage with vincristine letter. J Pediatr 1977; 90:1042-3.

15

The Manufacturer's Contribution to Medication Errors

There have been instances where pharmaceutical manufacturers have, through poor naming of drugs, poor label design, and because of the packaging, contributed to errors made by health professionals. These shortcomings have allowed careless or poorly educated health professionals to make some of the many errors reported in this book. The errors were not made because a label, drug name or package size was incorrect, rather, one or the other was poorly conceived. Better planning and execution would have prevented errors. Many of the problems cited have already been remedied by manufacturers. Their presentation here is intended to help prevent repetition.

The Container's Label

Some manufacturers have lost sight of the primary purpose of a label, which is to permit the user (pharmacist, nurse or physician) to identify the name(s), dosage form and strength of their product. This can be seen from various angles.

When designing a package, the company name, and in some cases logo, may be so prominent in location or size that the product name is obscured. The most prominent items on such prescription product labels are thus not in the best interest of safety. One company printed a drug name vertically, making it difficult to read, (see illustration accompanying error #61). We recommend that the manufacturer's name be placed at the bottom of the label so that the most prominent legend on the label is the name(s) and strength of the product. Placing the company name in bold print at the top of the label often creates similarities between labels which encourages careless health professionals to select the wrong container.

Errors have been made because prominence has been given to the fact that a product is to be used together with another product such as "normal saline solution for use with EVANS BLUE" (see error #36), "VIVONEX flavor packet" (see error #68) and "diluent for COL-YMYCIN S OPHTHALMIC" (see error #40). In these cases Normal Saline was used instead of Evans Blue, a flavor was used rather than Vivonex, and a diluent was used rather than Colymycin Solution. Other items less important than name and strength include percent concentration for systemic drugs, needle length, needle gauge, and dosage form (tablet, capsule, suspension, etc.). If labels were reviewed by practitioners who are sensitive to such problems, designs might be greatly improved. However, it should be noted that manufacturers will make label changes when problems are brought to their attention.

The type on the front panel of a label should be kept to a minimum so as to emphasize product name(s) and strength. Legends such as "brand of," "Handy 100's," "Rx Pak," "Tabloid," "preparation of," and periods after the abbreviation ml and mg should be eliminated. The use of the abbreviation HCl for hydrochloride as part of a drug name is very helpful in keeping a label uncluttered. Placing a chemical name in addition to trade and generic names is unnecessary. (See table 15-1 for labeling recommendations for manufacturers.)

When strengths and sizes are specified, care must be taken with quantities less than 1. A zero must be placed before the naked decimal in such cases, (e.g., 0.5 ml). A zero and decimal point must *not* be placed after a whole number, such as 100.0 mg (see illustration accompanying hazard warning #3). In this case 100 mg is the correct designation. In both situations, if the decimal point is not seen, a tenfold error occurs. The danger is that professionals seeing labeling and professional literature with these designations believe them to be proper and adopt them when writing orders, causing serious error (see errors #3, 50 and 98).

Labeling printed directly on glass ampuls is particularly difficult to read. Lighting conditions are not optimal in many nursing areas, and the transparency of ampul labels makes a correct reading difficult (see errors #20, 29 and 32). The pharmacist, who should be in a position to select brands to be purchased, must examine ampuls for label clarity. Printing should be on an opaque surface for maximum readability.

Care must be taken to make sure that the contents per unit of measure are not confused with the contents of the entire container. The designation, "100 mg per ml when reconstituted — 10 ml vial," caused an error when the vial was thought to contain 100 mg, and it contained 1 g (see error #38). Related problems occur when concentrations per liter are expressed on partial fill IV bottles (see error #28).

Ferrous Fumerate labeled only as to elemental iron content of 66 mg caused a threefold error when 200 mg of ferrous fumerate was ordered and three tablets were dispensed (see error #60). A 200 mg ferrous fumerate tablet contains 66 mg of elemental iron.

Table 15-1. Labeling Recommendations for Manufacturers.

Prominent	Subordinate in Size and Placement
— Generic name*	— Manufacturer's name
— Trade name*	— Manufacturer's list number
— Strength or concentration**	— Manufacturer's logo
	— NDC number
	— U.S.P. designation†
	— Legend statement (Rx only)
	— Control number and expiration date
	— Words such as "brand of," "tabloid," etc.†
	— Package size for non-unit dose oral solids and oral liquids
	— Needle length, gauge for unit dose parenterals
	— Designations such as "Handy 100's," "Prescription Package," etc.†

* When the name includes salts such as hydrochloride, sulfate, etc., this part of the name should be made less prominent. The abbreviation HCl should be used when it is part of a drug name.

** Special care must be taken with injections to insure that the amount per unit volume and the contents of the entire container are clearly distinguishable. No periods should be used with the abbreviations ml, mg, mEq, g or mcg.

† Such expressions should be eliminated to reduce label clutter.

Naming Drugs

There are many drug names that sound or look alike (see Chapter 4). Errors have been reported because of these similarities (see errors #12, 39, 50, 97, 106, 121, 146, 150 and Hazard Warnings 6, 10, 11 and 15.) The utmost care must be exercised in selecting and assigning drug names.

Certain trade names create errors. "Ascriptin Tablets #2" was taken to mean 2 Ascriptin tablets, rather than Ascriptin with codeine 15 mg (see error #27). "Elixophyllin Pediatric Elixir" was more concentrated than "Elixophyllin" (see Hazard Warning #8); Slo—Phyllin tablets are not a sustained release dosage form as are Slo-Phyllin Gyrocaps (see error #145). An order for "Estratest HS Daily" is not an order for one Estratest tablet at bedtime, but is an order for *half s*trength Estratest

Tablets which are named "Estratest HS" (see error #118). Care must be taken when assigning drug names.

The use of number or letter suffixes to alter a basic or original drug name leads to error. Anderson[1] has pointed out that errors may result if the proper suffix is not included in the order. This can be seen with V-Cillin and V-Cillin K, Thiosulfil, Thiosulfil-A and Thiosulfil-A Forte, Oxaine and Oxaine M, Pen-Vee, Pen VeeK and Pen-Vee L-A, Bicillin L-A, and Bicillin C-R, etc.

Anderson also points out that in the case of Milpath-200 and Milpath-400, Butiserpazide-25 and Butiserpazide-50, and Pathibamate-200 and Pathibamate-400, one product is not twice or half the strength of the other, since only one of the components of these mixtures varies in strength, while the other or others are constant. This is also true of Tylenol with codeine, Empirin with codeine and Ascriptin with codeine. (See also error #27.)

Errors have occurred when personnel have attempted to give half a dose or 2 doses to accommodate an order, not having the product prescribed.

Color Coding

Users must read labels. A company that attempts to color code its products or groups of products is doing the user a disservice, for there is a limit to the number of colors with distinguishable differences. Colors fade when exposed to light, and some companies cannot reproduce color in successive batches. When a user switches suppliers, those users who have relied on color for product identification may select the wrong item. Errors #9, 10, 29, 32, 77, 114 and Hazard Warnings #12, 13 and 16, relate to users relying on color or appearance rather than reading labels.

However, it is our opinion that color differentiation of related products can be helpful to the user in special situations. For instance, a different color for gentamicin adult and pediatric strength injection, Cordran Cream and Ointment, Cortisporin Otic and Ophthalmic, 5% and 50% Dextrose, Sodium Chloride Concentrate and 0.9% Sodium Chloride Injections, etc. is helpful. Such color differentiation is not a substitute for bold, clear labeling: it is an adjunct which, in certain potentially dangerous or error-prone situations, can prove helpful.

Special bold warning statements are needed for items such as 50% Dextrose, or Electrolyte Concentrate Injections, which are meant for dilution in hyperalimentation or other I.V. solutions.

Package Size

Eli Lilly Company markets two Oncovin products, a 1 and 5 mg vial, both of which are marked as multidose containers. The usual adult dose is less than 2 mg. The 5 mg vial is available for those institutions which prepare many daily doses. Errors #71, 86 and 131 describe how overdoses—some of them fatal—of 6.5 mg, 8 mg, 13.5 and 32 mg of Oncovin were administered. We believe the availability of a 5 mg vial was a minor contributing factor which permitted these erroneous doses to be administered. The fact that a specialist, an oncologist or his agent ordered the dose, that cancer chemotherapy doses are not well established, and that there is a 5 mg vial, contributed to health professionals' failure to heed the recommended doses cited in product literature. Many leading U.S. cancer centers do not stock the 5 mg vial of Oncovin, keeping only the 1 mg vial in supply.

Miscellaneous Problems

The drug enforcement agency (DEA) symbol for class 4 substances, Ⓘⓥ, has been confused for intravenous (I.V.), resulting in unintended intravenous administration (see errors #42 and 109).

A poorly conceived code number imprinted on a tablet has been erroneously interpreted as a strength designation (see Hazard Warning #1).

It has been recommended that when something works, it doesn't need fixing. We have observed that occasionally clear and uncluttered labels with product names and strengths nicely prominent have been replaced with new label designs which are much less readable. The problem seems to be that some designers and marketing personnel fail to realize that there are different requirements when designing a label for an over-the-counter package intended to foster impulse buying and instant customer recognition, than those for label on a prescription drug. The physician, nurse or pharmacist are reaching for a specific drug product, not a design, logo or company name.

The Industry Helps

It should be noted that the pharmaceutical industry has an important role in the effort to reduce medication errors. The industry has made available at reasonable cost, oral solid and liquid unit dose packages, prefilled injectable syringes and a variety of prefilled I.V. admixture drugs. Generally, pharmaceutical labeling is good. Manufacturers are normally responsive to legitimate suggestions for improving labeling to increase safety. They are also very active in supplying educational literature, audio-visual material and seminars.

Drug Product Problem Reporting Program

There is an established mechanism for reporting perceived packaging, labeling and drug product quality problems. First, such problems should be brought to the attention of the pharmacy department so they can be investigated and reported if appropriate. When it is felt necessary to take such a step, the Drug Product Problem Reporting program can be helpful. The program was initiated in 1971 and currently receives approximately 6,000 reports per year from concerned profes-

	Form approved: OMB No. 57-R0059
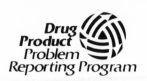	**DO NOT USE THIS SPACE**
Drug **Product** **Problem** **Reporting Program**	DATE RECEIVED
	REFERENCE NO.

1. PRODUCT NAME, DOSAGE FORM, STRENGTH, NDC NUMBER

2. LOT NUMBER*(s)* AND EXPIRATION DATE*(s)*

3. DATE PURCHASED *(If known)*

4. SOURCE OF PRODUCT *(Where purchased, if known)*

5. NAME AND ADDRESS OF THE MANUFACTURER, PACKAGER AND/OR DISTRIBUTOR ON THE LABEL

6. REPORTER'S NAME *(Please print or type)*

7. NAME AND ADDRESS OF PRACTICE LOCATION *(Include Zip Code)*

8. PHONE NUMBER AT PRACTICE LOCATION *(Include area code)*

9. PROBLEMS NOTED OR SUSPECTED

RETURN TO	OR	CALL TOLL FREE ANYTIME
United States Pharmacopeia		**800-638-6725***
12601 Twinbrook Parkway		IN THE CONTINENTAL UNITED STATES
Rockville, Maryland 20852		*In Maryland, call collect (301) 881-0256
Attention: Dr. Joseph G. Valentino		between 9:00 AM and 4:30 PM

FORM FDA 2519 (7/79)

FIGURE 15-1.

sionals. The system is coordinated by the United States Pharmacopeia (USP), funded by the Food and Drug Administration (FDA), and co-sponsored by over 50 pharmacy organizations. The Joint Commission of Accreditation of Hospitals has incorporated the program into its standards and interpretations for pharmaceutical services.

By reporting problems encountered with products utilized in your practice, you are offered the opportunity to exercise your professional judgment.

Reporting can be done by filling out a reporting form (see Figure 15-1), or by calling the toll free number in the continental U.S.A.,

800-638-6725, (or in Maryland call 881-0256). When phoning, one should try to have at hand the information delineated in Figure 1. The USP acts as a neutral intermediary, forwarding copies of these reports to individuals in the Food and Drug Administration and the pharmaceutical firm involved. The proper authorities can be made aware of the problems encountered and are in a position to take constructive action when appropriate. Also, USP will take reported problems into account when revising or devising standards for drug substances and their drug products.

Drug problems include the entire spectrum of problems which might be noted when drugs are received, prepared, dispensed or administered. Examples of packaging and labeling complaints are when carton does not protect the inner container, container does not protect the product, wrong or deficient label, inadequate package insert information, etc. Examples of evidence of poor pharmaceutical quality in the products themselves are broken, crumbling or imperfectly manufactured dosage forms; foreign or particulate matter present; drug solid does not reconstitute properly; off color or off taste, etc. Products with questionable bioavailability and stability may also be reported. The program is not limited to prescription drugs, thus problems with prescription and over-the-counter drug products can be reported. Reports are also solicited on equipment related to drug use, such as IV solution administration sets, infusion pumps and filters.

It is very important that the pharmacy be made aware of labeling or drug quality problems as soon as they are observed or suspected so that, if indicated, the current supply can be removed and a different product substituted.

Reference

1. Anderson DR. The physician's contribution to hospital medication errors. Am J Hosp Pharm 1971: 28:18.

16

Mathematical Mistakes in Calculating Doses

Mathematical calculations are sometimes required to determine the quantity of a drug to be administered. This is true for adult dosing, but it is more common and more critical for pediatric patients.

Error #86 illustrates mathematical mistakes made by physicians in calculating vincristine doses resulting in the death of young patients.

In order to give 1/200 grain of nitroglycerin, 2 x 1/100 grain tablets were administered, a fourfold overdose (Error #74). This occurred because of mathematical weakness in the use of fractions. The drug should have been ordered in milligrams or micrograms, rather than grains (see Chapter 5).

A study[1] was conducted to ascertain the accuracy of nurses, physicians and pharmacists in performing calculations for new born infants. The testing instrument consisted of ten physicians' drug orders for infants of specified ages and weights. The strengths (concentrations) of the available drug preparations were given.

Examples of orders used were: sodium bicarbonate 6.75 mEq added to I.V. for a 1-day-old, 1,500 g patient—sodium bicarbonate being available in 40 mEq/50 ml dosage form, gentamicin sulfate 7 mg, IM for a 4-day-old, 1,200 g patient—gentamicin sulfate being available in 40 mg/ml dosage form, and atropine sulfate 0.015 mg, IM for a 3-day-old, 1,450 g patient—atropine sulfate being available in 0.8 mg/ml dosage form.

Personnel were asked to calculate how much of a drug preparation was needed to administer the ordered dose and whether the dose was appropriate. In contrast to an actual work situation, personnel were not allowed to use reference material. The results are shown in Table 16-1.

Ninety-five registered nurses in a pediatric center were tested, 31 having had more than one year of professional experience; 64 had less than one year's experience. An error was counted only when a computation would have resulted in administering a dose at least 10 times

Table 16-1. Test Results from a Pediatric Center Study of the Ability of Nurses, Pediatricians and Pharmacists to make Mathematical Calculations and Judgments for Neonatal Drug Orders.[1]

	Number tested	Total number of problems attempted	Percent of problems where calculated answers were at least 10 times greater or lesser than correct.	Percent of wrong judgments concerning correctness of ordered doses.	Percent with admitted uncertainty concerning appropriateness of ordered doses.
Registered Nurses					
Experienced†	31	303	12.2%	17%	26%
Inexperienced	64	624	14.9%	14%	51%
Total	95	927	14.0%	15%	43%
Pediatricians	11	110	4.2%	19%	7%
Pharmacists	5	50	0 %	*	*

*Not Stated
†More than 1 year's professional experience

greater or less than what was ordered. Eighty-six percent of the nurses' answers were not in error, as defined. There was no statistically significant difference between the error rate of the experienced vs. inexperienced nurses. Thus in 14% of the calculations performed, errors resulting in at least tenfold overdoses or underdoses would have occurred if the calculated dose had been administered.

The nurses were also asked if the doses were appropriate. Seventeen percent of the experienced nurses and 14% of the inexperienced nurses judged incorrectly (no statistical difference). The subjects were queried about the uncertainty of their answers. Twenty-six percent of the experienced nurses admitted uncertainty, while 51% of the inexperienced nurses did so, (a statistically significant difference, $P = < 0.01$). If these figures are combined, the authors estimate the experienced nurses would have made at least a tenfold error 8% of the time, while an inexperienced nurse would have done so 3% of the time.

Perlstein et al.[1] commented that their study indicated a serious problem in insuring that correct drug doses will be administered to high risk infants. It was difficult to find evidence that drugs are actually maladministered in the hospital study. The authors cited anecdotal incidents unrelated to the study, of infants receiving 0.5 mg of Atropine Sulfate when 0.05 mg was ordered, and 0.09 mg of digoxin when 0.009 mg was ordered, to illustrate that they have experienced problems in this area. The authors found that a misplaced decimal point in the calculation was the most frequent case of error. Also, nurses' careless working of problems causes them to misread their own answers. The third major cause for error was nurses who apparently calculated the problems mentally.

The study noted that calculators may be useful but do not provide a self-evident solution to the problem of decimal point errors made by personnel who are unable to judge consistently the reasonableness of their mathematical results. It was suggested that computer assistance could be helpful in solving the problem; also, that the colleagues should check each others' calculations. It was also recommended that curriculums be altered to place additional emphasis on mathematical calculations.

The study reported that none of the five pharmacists tested made mistakes which would have yielded errors more than 1% greater or less than the dose ordered. Of 11 pediatricians (six board certified neonatologists and five post-graduate fellows in neonatology) who took the ten-problem examination, calculations resulting in at least tenfold errors occurred in 4% of their answers. In 19% of drug orders, the pediatricians made wrong judgments about the appropriateness of doses. In 7.2% of situations they were unsure of the appropriateness of the doses.

Other dose calculation errors can be found in Chapter 14.

We believe the problem of calculating doses can be attacked in many ways. A safe system is to have the pharmacist and nurse make calculations independently to serve as a double check. In critical calculations it is not uncommon for one pharmacist to check the calculations of another. The doses should be prepared and labeled by the pharmacy within the framework of a unit dose dispensing system.

In order to avoid working with decimals, drugs should be ordered and expressed in micrograms, rather than milligrams. If manufacturers' containers are not labeled in micrograms, supplemental labels should be affixed by pharmacy, or such information should be in a form readily available to the nurse on the nursing unit.

Physicians, nurses and pharmacists should work together to formulate charts for commonly prescribed or problem drugs showing, for example, the appropriate doses for a range of body weights, and how much of a given strength of stock solution of the drug this represents. (See Figure 31 in error #71 for an example of how a chart can be prepared to serve as a check to ascertain if a calculated dose is reasonable.)

Pharmacists must be more attentive to dosage calculation problems when teaching nurses and medical students, as well as continuing to stress this area in the pharmacy school curriculum. Professional licensing boards must test to insure competency in this area. As mentioned in Chapter 3, it is appropriate that tests be administered to prospective employes by hospital departments to highlight potential problem areas, and to plan for remedial work and retesting. If the tests have been properly validated in cooperation with the personnel department, they will serve as criteria for employment when administered to applicants.

The study also illustrates that it is essential to have reference material available in the work area.

Miscellaneous Errors and Problems: Accuracy in Publishing

A word of caution is in order about the need for accuracy for those involved in preparing articles for publication. There is a natural tendency to accept as fact what appears in print. Error #120 describes a case where two patients received a tenfold overdose of the narcotic antagonist Narcan. The incorrect dose was obtained from a chart published by a pharmacy school which omitted a decimal point in error. When publishing, make sure everything is checked carefully for accuracy. It is a good policy to have others review the work both before and after printer's proofs are received. Be especially careful with charts and tables.

Confusion Over Midnight

Error #82 reviews a problem involving confusion about the meaning of "midnight" and the abbreviations used for 12 noon (12 PM) and 12 midnight (12 AM). Midnight is considered the beginning of a new day (or new year if it's midnight January 1st). Drug orders that are to start or stop at "midnight" may be stopped or started 24 hours too soon or too late, unless the prescriber and the person interpreting the order understand this term. A similar problem occurs with the abbreviations mentioned. Review error #82 for proper interpretation.

Medical Service Representatives in Hospital Inpatient Areas

It is recommended that hospitals have formal procedures designed to control access by pharmaceutical company Medical Service Representatives (MSR) to inpatient areas and other patient care areas. Their visits may be disruptive to the flow of patient care as busy health professionals are interrupted for product detailing. Representatives who refrain from practicing in an inpatient area because they recognize the potential for being disruptive, are unfairly placed at a disadvantage if others are allowed to do so. Also, prescription drug product security may be compromised. This was the case in error #127, where MSR paid a visit to an inpatient psychiatry unit. A patient removed a number of sample tablets from the MSR's bag and self-administered an overdose. MSRs should not be permitted on patient floors, emergency departments, or other areas where their presence is likely to interfere with patient care.

Reference

1. Perlstein PH, White Cornelia C, Barnes B, Edwards N. Errors in drug computations during newborn intensive care. Am J Dis Child 1979; 133:376-379.

17

Risk Management Aspects of the Medication Error Problem

This chapter covers medication error reporting in institutions.

a. The incident report.

b. A protocol for medication error reporting in hospitals.

c. Charting and medical liability control.

d. Medical liability and post-incident claim control.

e. How to monitor your hospital's medication error rate.

The information in sections a, c and d in this chapter appears with the cooperation of Mr. Charles J. Milazzo, Loss Control Manager, and his staff at Alexis Risk Management Services, Inc., a subsidiary of Alexander and Alexander, 130 East Randolph Drive, Chicago, Ill., 60601. The material was originally published in HELP News, a newsletter published by Alexis Risk Management Services for its clients.

A. The Incident Report*

The American Hospital Association defines an incident as "any happening which is not consistent with the routine operation of the hospital or the routine care of a particular patient. It may be an accident or a situation which might result in an accident." Many institutions define an incident as "All unusual occurrences within the hospital or its physical plant which might result in a liability or any condition, situation, or event which might create a liability for the hospital."

When it is known that a medication has been given or omitted in error, this is considered an incident. An incident reporting policy should be basic to most healthcare institution policy manuals. Incident reporting policy and procedure and in-service education programs regarding incident reporting should be reviewed on a periodic basis to help assure that all important issues, questions and other points have been covered. During medical liability litigation, the inci-

---

*Modified from *Help News*, 1977, Alexis—a subsidiary of Alexander and Alexander, Inc., Chicago, Ill. 60601.

dent report may have a significant bearing on a case. Thus, it is important that all employes be fully cognizant of proper completion technique. The points listed below relate to incident reports and should be familiar to all who are involved with medication prescribing, distribution or administration in hospitals or other health care institutions.

1. *Why do we complete an incident report? What is it for?*
   a. To provide a record of the incident and to document the facts.
   b. To provide a base from which hospital staff can further investigate to determine and evaluate:
      — Deviations from the standard of care, policies, procedures, etc.
      — Corrective measures needed to prevent recurrence.
   c. To provide means of refreshing the memory of those having a direct knowledge of the incident.
   d. To alert hospital risk management staff to a possible claim situation and to respond immediately for complete investigation and documentation.
   e. It is a Joint Commission on Accreditation of Hospitals requirement (see STANDARD V under Pharmaceutical Services in appendix).
   f. The document is often used for statistical analysis and computer input.

2. *Who reports an incident?*
   The incident report should be completed by the individual who has the best knowledge of the incident. In a case where a student nurse or student pharmacist has the most knowledge regarding the facts, he or she should *initiate* the incident report, but the supervising staff nurse would be responsible for its accurate completion.

3. *When should an incident report be completed?*
   Immediately after the incident is discovered. The necessity for immediate reports cannot be overestimated. Obviously, the longer the wait before report completion, the less clear will be the facts. During litigation, an incident report completed two weeks after the occurrence will have little value as defense evidence. Records made "in due course" have much greater weight as evidence during litigation.

4. *Get the facts.*
   The concept of factual documentation should be made clear. To get all the facts, the person completing the incident report must answer the "who, what, where, why, and how" of the incident. But what about hearsay and opinion? These can be valuable for further investigation but must be identified as hearsay, opinion or assumption. This information should be placed on a separate sheet

of paper. Such items may be helpful in disclosing contributing factors or important facts about the incident. In completing the report, only known facts can be documented.

5. *Charting*

The medical record should only document the occurrence, with no reference that an incident report was completed. For example, the nurse's notes should state "65 mg of Darvon administered in error instead of ordered 32 mg. Dr. Jones notified; vital signs monitored as per doctor." Other information may be included as necessary. If the nurse's notes indicate that an incident report was completed, that incident report must be a part of the medical record. We suggest that incident reports not be part of the medical record, but kept in a separate, secure file.

6. *Use of Witnesses*

Most incident report forms have space for the names and addresses of witnesses. For hospital personnel, name and identification that they are hospital employes normally is sufficient. Statements of witnesses should be handwritten, dated, time noted and signed by the witnesses and attached to the incident report form.

7. *Patient's Statements*

If the incident involves a patient or visitor, his or her comments or statements should be carefully recorded, with quotation marks where applicable.

8. *Equipment-Related Incidents*

If a piece of equipment such as an IV infusion pump or IV administration set is involved in an incident, the name of the equipment, the manufacturer, the manufacturer's control number (if applicable), the hospital's control number and other related identification should be documented on the incident report. If there was a *suspected* malfunction, the incident report should relate the facts that indicated malfunction. It is of primary importance in cases of suspected malfunctions that equipment be removed from service and secured for later testing. The hospital may want to have the unit tested to document the function or malfunction of the piece of equipment and may have recourse to the manufacturer or service contractor for subrogation (referring the loss to the manufacturer, service contractor or another third party).

9. *Confidentiality*

All incident reporting must stress confidentiality. The patient has a right to privacy, and incident reports involving the patient should not be freely discussed within the institution; hospital employes have a duty to keep hospital-related subjects confidential. In short, any discussion of incidents apart from professional considerations should not be permitted.

10. Do you write an incident report for a serious case?
A common misconception among hospital staff is that an incident report should not be completed in situations where there would be liability exposure for the hospital. During medical liability litigation, what we do not know may damage our position. The incident report is the basis from which a complete investigation is made. All *facts* of the incident must be documented to objectively evaluate the hospital's position.

Hospital staff should not be reluctant to complete incident reports because of personal liability. The person completing the report is *not* held specifically liable because of having prepared the incident report.

If the incident is serious, it should be reported by phone to the immediate supervisor: Do not wait for notification by the normal paper work flow. Any necessary investigation must be made immediately.

Review of Reports

Healthcare institutions have been found negligent when no action is taken on recurring incidents. Insurance companies and hospital consultants suggest that incident reports be reviewed by:

1. The supervisor of the area involved, 2. Department head of the areas involved, 3. The administrator or assistant administrator, and 4. A hospital safety committee.

Obviously, corrective actions should be taken before the safety committee review. The safety committee responsibility is to determine whether corrective action was taken, whether the action was effective, or if other actions should be taken, and whether corrective measure(s) should be applied elsewhere. It is suggested that only two or three members of the safety committee or incident review sub-committee be responsible for the review because of the confidentiality of the material.

B. A protocol for medication error reporting in hospitals*

In order to define medication errors and delineate lines of responsibility for handling and reporting medication error incidents, one hospital established a protocol for use by various departments. The protocol outlines all procedures that must be followed when an error is noticed and includes forms used for reporting as well as counseling.

Suggested procedure for medication error reporting

Definition: A medication error is considered to have occurred when
1. The *wrong patient* receives a medication.
2. The patient receives a *wrong dose* of medication (less than or greater than the amount prescribed).

---

*From *Hosp. Pharm.* 14:280, 1979.

3. The patient receives a medication at the *wrong time* (this is relative and is deemed an error by the ordering physician when notified). Any scheduled medication administered one hour before, or one hour after it is due, should be reported to the physician.
4. A patient's medication was *omitted*.
5. A patient receives a *wrong drug* (a drug meant for another patient, an unordered drug, etc.).
6. A patient receives an *extra dose* (unordered dose). The extra dose may be in addition to a regularly scheduled dose or a dose administered after the drug was discontinued.
7. A patient receives medication by the *wrong route* of administration, or wrong dosage form is administered.
8. A patient receives a deteriorated (outdated) dose of medication.

A medication error is not considered to have occurred until after the patient has received a drug (or any of above).

Handling of medication errors — who should be notified

When a medication error is noticed, it is important (whether or not injury has been sustained) for the incident to be reported verbally to the physician, charge nurse, and pharmacist, and in writing for use of others (supervisor, legal counsel, etc.).

The standard hospital incident report form should be used to report medication errors (Fig. 17-1.)

Who should report errors

The person discovering the error should report this verbally to the physician as soon as possible. The person having the most knowledge concerning the error should complete the written report. Usually, the person who has committed the error has most of the facts. If the person who committed the error is not present at the time of discovery, or cannot be identified, the person discovering the error should complete the form. Alternatively, a supervisor should complete the form. The person completing the form may be a nurse, physician or pharmacist.

Completing the medication error report form

All parts of the incident report form must be filled out. Special emphasis on legibility is to be made. The report must be factual as to time, place, patient diagnosis, etc. A clear addressograph imprint must be made. Names of witnesses, and those involved in the error, are to be listed. All facts related to the error are to be listed in the report. The reverse side of the report or an attached piece of paper should be used where necessary. *Avoid opinions and hearsay — list the facts only.*

102

INCIDENT REPORT

DIAGNOSIS: _____   Type of Incident _____

_____   Date of Incident _____

O.O.B. Privileges: _____ Amb. _____ Bed Rest _____   Time of Incident _____

Mental Status: Alert _____ Coma _____ Confused _____

Position of Hi-Low Bed: Up _____ Down _____   Signature of Nurse in Charge _____

Position of Bed Rails: Up _____ Down _____   Received in NSO by _____

Resident in Charge of Case: _____   Date and Time Received _____

Outline briefly significant details of the incident. If the patient had any possible injury, include in the report the TPR and BP.

_____

_____

_____

_____

_____

(Continue on Other Side)

Name of all Witnesses

Signature _____   Position _____

A report by the Physician on condition of patient is required in all incidents in which the patient may have sustained injury.

PATIENT'S CONDITION FOLLOWING THE INCIDENT: TIME OF ARRIVAL OF PHYSICIAN

_____

_____

_____

(Continued on Other Side)

Signature _____ M.D.

DIRECTIONS: The purpose of the incident report is to acquaint the administration of all important happenings that might result in lawsuits. Reports are made on lost personal belongings, incorrect administration of medications, abnormal behavior of patients, injury to patients, visitors, or personnel. A supplemental incident report will be required in cases of serious injury or where additional reports are needed to complete the factual picture.
PLEASE USE OTHER SIDE FOR ADDITIONAL INFORMATION

Figure 17-1. Multipurpose incident report.

It is necessary for the responsible physician to make a note on the report describing the patient's condition after the error.

The report bears the signature of the person completing the form and the signature of the physician and charge nurse.

Reports must not be used to berate or criticize another person or department. Only facts surrounding the incident are to be reported. *All reports remain confidential.* For extremely serious errors (patient injury or death), verbal notification should be given immediately to the hospital legal assistant. A supplemental form will be sent by this office to obtain further information. This form is returned directly to the legal office.

After verbal notification has been given to the physician, pharmacist, and charge nurse, and after the incident report form has been

```
                        DEPARTMENT OF PHARMACY
                MEDICATION ERROR AND OMISSION REVIEW FORM

            WHO WAS NOTIFIED:  | | Physician
                               | | Supervisor       | | Charge  Nurse

HOW ERROR OCCURRED:




WHAT COULD HAVE BEEN DONE TO PREVENT ERROR:



            SIGNATURE: _____     R.Ph.

            POSITION: _____
REVIEW BY PHARMACY SUPERVISOR



            SIGNATURE: _____     R.Ph.

            POSITION: _____
```

Figure 17-2. Pharmacy medication error review form. It is forwarded to the appropriate Assistant Director, Department of Pharmacy.

properly filled out and signed, the form is sent to the appropriate nursing patient care coordinator. In cases where medication errors were committed by other than nursing personnel (physician, pharmacist, etc.) the error report should be made available for that person's supervisor. Upon receipt of the report in the Nursing Office, distribution is as follows:

1. Administration (Risk Management Office)
2. Chairperson, Medication Error Committee

Supervision

When deemed applicable, the supervisor of the person who committed the error offers counseling. To assist in this function, the *Medication Error and Omission Review Form* (Fig. 17-2) may be used for pharmacy errors. The offender lists how the error occurred and what could (should) have been done to prevent the error. Nursing personnel are to use their own form (Fig. 17-3). These forms are to be used by head nurses, patient care coordinators and pharmacy supervisors as a counseling tool only.

Education

Many medication errors could be prevented if hospital personnel were aware of problem areas and had more pharmacologic knowledge. The Department of Pharmacy should publicize accounts of cer-

104

```
┌─────────────────────────────────────────────────────────────────────────┐
│                         NURSE COUNSELING SHEET                            │
│                         FOR MEDICATION ERRORS                             │
│                                                                           │
│ DATE _____   TIME _____                                   │
│ Describe the error _____ │
│                                                                           │
│ 1. What medication and dosage (if any) should have been given?   2. What medication and dosage was given? │
│ _____  Time _____    _____ │
│ 3. List any drug allergies _____ │
│                                                                           │
│   WRONG MEDICATION                                                        │
│ 4. Did you:                                                               │
│    a. Check the medication sheet to be sure that you understood the order? _____ │
│    b. Check the doctor's order sheet? _____                            │
│    c. Check chart to be sure medication was not cut? _____             │
│    d. Check chart to be sure this is still a standing order? _____     │
│    e. Have a properly filled out medication sheet? _____               │
│    f. Check the medication three times? _____                         │
│    g. Check the name of the medication Kardex with the pharmacist's label? _____ │
│    h. Check the arm band on the patient? _____                        │
│    i. Give the medication by the proper route? _____                  │
│                                                                           │
│ 5. a. Did the patient question the medication he was given? _____      │
│    b. If so, did you review the doctor's order sheet? _____            │
│                                                                           │
│   MEDICATION OMISSION                                                     │
│ 6. Did you:                                                               │
│    a. Check to see if someone else gave the medication? _____          │
│    b. Check to see if there was an additional medication record sheet? ____ │
│    c. Assume the medication was given and not charted? _____           │
│    d. Check the order sheet for medications not transcribed? _____     │
│    e. Overlook the medication on the medication record? _____          │
│    f. Think the medication should be omitted because the patient was pre-procedure? ____ │
│    g. Bypass the medication because you did not know the action and/or side effects and forget to go back to that drug? ____ │
│    h. Notice any extra medications in the cart draw that were not on the record? ____ │
│    i. Notice any extra medications in the patient's draw that were not on the record? ____ │
│                                                                           │
│ 7. If you wish to elaborate on any point, use the reverse side of this sheet. │
│                                                                           │
│ Signature of Person Filing Report _____ │
│ Signature of Head Nurse _____ │
│ Signature of Patient Care Coordinator _____ │
└─────────────────────────────────────────────────────────────────────────┘
```

Figure 17-3. Form used by nursing personnel to report medication errors.

tain errors in Nursing, Physician and Pharmacist Newsletters so that personnel may learn from the mistakes of others. These reports should not be identified as occurring at this hospital. In fact, they may be accounts of errors that occurred in other institutions.

Disciplinary action

Since so much importance is given to receiving reports of errors, an air of encouragement must persist within the institution. Therefore, it should be understood that error reports are not to be used for punitive purposes. However, when recognized procedures are habitually broken, resulting in errors, disciplinary action may be taken by the supervisor.

Reports of errors in patient's medical record

When a medication error occurs that results or has the potential to result in patient injury, an entry of the medication administered or omitted shall be properly recorded in the progress notes of the patient's chart by the physician responsible for the care of the patient. The note shall include any therapeutic measures taken to correct possible effects of the error. No mention is made that an incident report has been filed.

The medication error committee

A permanent subcommittee of the Pharmacy and Therapeutics Committee has been established for the purpose of reviewing current reports of hospital medication errors. The committee should meet on at least a monthly basis.

From reviews of medication error reports, the committee should recommend new procedures, reinforce existing procedures and oversee the educational effort to reduce the incidence of errors.

The committee members should represent members of departments involved in the drug distribution cycle. It is recommended that the chairperson be a representative from the house staff of the Department of Medicine. Committee members should represent at least:

House staff, Department of Medicine; Pharmacy (1 staff and 1 supervisor); Nursing (1 staff and 1 supervisor); Administration (1)

C. Charting and Medical Liability Control*

Adequate, legible, timely, and accurate records are the first lines of defense once a medical liability claim has been made. In liability litigation, records made *"in due course"* (those made in the regular course of patient care) have great weight as defense evidence. Records, statements, incident reports, charting revisions, etc., made two days, weeks, months, or years after the fact are thought of as *"convenient memory"* and are of very little merit.

According to the statistics of the National Association of Insurance Commissioners, medical liability suits come to litigation, on the average, six years after occurrence. Since the medical records are almost always introduced into evidence in a medical liability trial, the records, when made, must again be adequate, legible, timely, and accurate. In review of the evidence by the court, problems related to the validity of charting are:

1. Whether the particular implications may be drawn from accidental or deliberate inaccuracies in the chart.

---

*From *HELP News*, Vol. 1, No. 10, 1977, Alexis — a subsidiary of Alexander and Alexander, Inc., Chicago, Ill. 60601.

2. Whether there was an alteration of the chart or some other document relating to patient care in order to mislead persons who might review the chart as to what occurred or the distruction of reports or notes.

3. The extent to which the chart fails to indicate therapy orders or specific instructions of the patient's physician were followed by nursing personnel.

When the chart is unreliable as an indicator of care rendered to the patient, it is more likely that the plaintiff will be successful.

The attorney for the plaintiff can seize upon defects in the records and the patient's chart to develop *inferences* unfavorable to the defendants. A trial is, in part, a reconstruction of the past events. The defendants are often relying on the chart and other records as evidence to refresh their memories of what may have occurred three, four, or more years in the past. Inadequate, misleading, or otherwise deficient documents may seriously inhibit the successful defense of a legal action. Let us examine several situations involved in actual litigation and the language of some courts regarding chart-related practices.

Inaccurate Entry: The Case of Hiatt vs. Croce

This case concerned a woman who sustained an injury during and immediately after delivery. The baby was delivered by a nurse in the presence of a physician who had been summoned by the nurse in the hallway just as the baby was being born (he was not the patient's physician). The nurse had been casual in her approach to the indications that delivery was near and failed to call the patient's physician in time for him to perform the delivery.

Hospital records stated the physician who had been passing in the hall delivered the baby for the patient's obstetrician. During cross-examination the nurse testified that she had been advised by her supervisor never to state in the records that she had delivered a baby. When the hospital records were introduced and admitted as evidence the court said, "However, the records are still subject to the jury's scrutiny in light of all of the evidence. The evidence shows that nurse Croce performed the delivery of the baby, and that she had been instructed by her supervisors never to state in hospital records that she had delivered a baby. The jury might have been persuaded that if the records were erroneous in one respect they were erroneous in other respects as well."

There is no way to estimate how often untrue entries are made but their adverse effect upon the defense of the suit when known cannot be overemphasized.

Altering Records: Foley vs. Flushing Hospital and Medical Center

The alteration of patient records also has a significant influence on jurors in malpractice litigation. You can never really cover up. Differences in writing, in type, in the pen or pencil used, etc., will give the alteration away. Remember, if an alteration is suspected, the plaintiff will call in the experts such as a graphoanalyst.

In the Foley case, the court said, "The word 'orally' is in darker type and extends into the right-hand margin, suggesting that it was typed into the letter at some time after the letter's completion." This case involved an infant who suffered a sciatic nerve injury due to an improperly performed injection of Achromycin in the buttock. Several months after the incident, with the subsequent manifestation of motor power impairment, the treating pediatrician, who was aware of a possible claim, made an entry into the records which read, "Achromycin given orally." The word "orally" was in the margin and the fact of the alteration had significant bearing on the eventual loss of the case.

Destruction of Records: Carr vs. St. Paul Fire and Marine Insurance

This case involved a fatal acute myocardial infarction and arteriosclerosis secondary to diabetes which occurred in the emergency room. The patient had come into the emergency room several hours earlier suffering from abdominal pains and vomiting, and he had a history of diabetes. They were unable to contact the patient's own physician at home and the patient was then sent home. Several hours later the patient returned to the emergency room in an ambulance and subsequently died. Some of the emergency room records, including the one concerning this patient, apparently had been destroyed by the staff later that night after the coroner's report had been prepared. The Federal District Court *allowed the jury to "infer from the destruction of the records that, had they been available, the records would have shown an emergency situation existed at the time of the patient's first visit to the emergency room and that he had been sent home without the opportunity to be seen by a physician."*

Absence of Data: Horowitz vs. Michael Reese Hospital/Collins Vs. Westlake Memorial Hospital

The most frequent issue regarding charting in matters before a court is related to the absence of data which, under some circumstances, leads to an *inference* that proper care was not given. Even if the informational gap has been filled by other sources, adverse comments by courts appear in their opinions. For example, in the case of *Horowitz vs. Michael Reese Hospital*, the court stated,

"It must be noted that this evidence comes from a specially prepared report made by the Director of Nursing on May 15 and not from the hospital record. The hospital record should contain all matters concerning the care of the patient and reveals none of the above occurrences for the night of May 12-13. In this case, the infant's temperature was of great importance in her care, as well as in subsequent litigation, because the suit was brought for a central nervous system disorder, allegedly caused from the infant being kept in an overheated incubator for a substantial period of time soon after her premature birth."

In another case, *Collins vs. Westlake Community Hospital*, one theory of the suit was that the hospital was liable because of the failure of personnel to adequately observe the patient's condition and to alert the physician promptly about its deterioration. Critical to this was the question of whether the absence of the entries from 11 PM to 6 AM concerning the condition of the patient's toes indicated that the observation of the toes was not done.

Importance of the patient's chart in malpractice and negligence cases when harm to the patient is asserted to result from neglect by nurses and physicians cannot be overstressed. In some situations, the chart may show it was not the failure of the nurses to observe and report changes that occasioned the harm but the ineffectiveness of the subsequent medical care. The chart can also serve to indicate who, among those responsible for the attention of the patient, failed to meet the standard of competent professional performance.

Common Medical Liability Control Charting Errors

These charting errors can discredit the chart as being an accurate record of the total patient care. One thing to remember is that the plaintiff's attorney will do everything he can to discredit the nurse and the quality of care received. Proper charting and documentation will confirm the quality of professional care given.

1. *Blank Spaces:* When charting, two nurses, on occasion, may be working with the same chart. One may say, "Save me a couple of lines." What results is a squeezed-in writing or blank lines. A lawyer would have no trouble convincing the jury that *if* the notes were legitimate, they would have been charted in a chronological order and not filled in at a later time.

2. *Late Entry:* If you do have a late entry, chart it by stating, "Late Entry," record the time, but put it on the next chronological line down on the chart. Again, do not try and squeeze it in the margin. By putting it on the next line it will indicate how late an entry actually was.

3. *Signs of Erasures:* Erasures infer cover-up in a trial. Simply put one line through any charting error and initial it. Some hospitals require you to write the word "error" over the lined-out area. After "error," the date and signature of the individual should appear.

4. *Accuracy:* One medical liability case involved a six-year-old who suffered a cardiac arrest while on the operating table during a tonsillectomy. The "preop" medication was ordered as 1/450th grain atropine. The nurse charted the medication as 1/150th grain, which would be the adult dose. The next day, when the incident was being investigated and the chart reviewed, the nurse was absolutely sure that

she gave the proper dose but improperly charted that dose. This charting inaccuracy did have a significant role in proving the plaintiff's case.

5. *Incidents: How Do You Chart an Incident?* Document the facts of the occurrence in the chart. Do not chart that an incident report has been completed. If you do not document the occurrence, one could infer a cover-up. Remember, courts allow inferences of guilt from efforts to cover up.

6. *Continuity:* Obviously the charting of patient care must have continuity from day to day. If you chart that "patient was found on the floor again," there had better be matching entries from prior periods.

7. *No Unsolved Mysteries:* If you chart a patient's statement or make an observation that a child pushed a toy into his cast, be sure that you chart your report to the orthopedist, and when the object was recovered. If you do chart that a child was observed pushing an object into his cast, and later a severe infection results, there can be a liability for not taking proper action.

8. *Wording/Terminology:* Be sure to use the proper descriptive terminology when describing a situation:

Bleeding (is it oozing, gushing, or what?)

Discolored (flush, was it a rash, pallor?)

Elevated Temperature (how high?)

Motor Reflexes (what exactly do you mean?)

Do not use such terms as "had a good night," "poor day," "usual day," etc. What is a good, usual, or poor day? It is all relative. State what actually occurred. Document the facts instead of conclusions. For another example, don't chart that the "patient had a marked distension of his abdomen." Measure it and let the people reviewing the chart draw their own conclusions. Do not use the words "apparently" or "appears." One exception perhaps could be "apparently sleeping." The only way you would know for sure is to wake him up. Just chart what you know and observe. Statements such as "his face was apparently flushed," "apparently he has pain all over," "apparently the patient choked," will indicate to a lawyer that the nurse does not in fact know the patient's condition. This is a change in prior theory taught in schools of nursing several years ago. However, we are in a different legal climate today. The lawyer will stringently cross-examine the nurse and the words "apparently" or "appears" will indicate that one did not know for sure.

9. *Avoid Biased Findings:* Do not let the experts' opinion color your observations. In one case, the nurse observed a patient with symptoms of a seizure and the neurological consultant examined the patient and said it was "nothing." No further charting of this patient's symptoms was made until the patient suffered a grand mal seizure and then the problem was identified. Since the neurological consultant said that the patient was not having seizures, the symptoms were no longer

charted and as far as the patient's physician was concerned, the symptoms must have disappeared.

10. *Emotions:* Do not let emotion show up in the charting. In one case where a man was verbally abusive to anyone who entered the room, the charting was spent more in the description of his abuse than in the care given.

11. *Patient Honesty:* One case was reviewed and involved a woman who was in constant severe pain but whenever her family visited her stated that she was "fine." The husband had been taking care of four children at home and the mother wanted to make him feel as good as possible. As soon as the family left, the woman would cry out in pain. If this situation ever went to litigation for one reason or another, the family might infer that unnecessary drugs were given so that the mother might not bother the staff or the family might feel that there was a malpractice for a poor recovery. The family saw "mom" doing fine in the hospital and all of a sudden she took a turn for the worse, "so there must be a malpractice somewhere."

12. *Common Sense:* Common sense and professional expertise are basic in charting. Make sure the nurse reads the patient's history, doctor's admission notes, etc., and make sure she "knows" the patient.

13. *Medications:* Statements in the chart such as "medication given as ordered" means little during liability litigation. If one gave 50 mg of Demerol at 4 PM orally, state exactly what and how much medication you gave, what time, and what route. Chart the medications immediately after they are given, not at the end of the shift.

14. *Punctuation:* Do not forget to punctuate for clarity.

Careless charting reflects careless nursing care and will impress the judge and jury in that manner. Remember, the best defense against a claim is accurate, legible, factual, timely reports. One line of faded ink is worth more than a thousand faded memories. During the trial, if you try to cover up, give double talk, try to avoid the issue, you will actually discredit the defense and can only harm the hospital and you.

References: "Nurses Notes" by Ms. Kerr, RN
Nursing '75 February issue.
"Building a Hospital Defense for Malpractice Litigation" by Bruce Lynn.
"The Influence of Charting Upon Liability Determinations" by N. Hershey, LLB, *Journal of Nursing Administration*, March 1976.

D. Medical Liability and Post-Incident Claim Control*

Timely, organized, aggressive action on potential medical liability claims can determine the course of action and eventual outcome of the

---

*From *HELP News*, Vol. 1, No. 11, 1977. Alexis—a subsidiary of Alexander and Alexander, Inc., Chicago, Ill. 60601

incident. After an incident has occurred, the relative action or inaction that is taken by the hospital administration, Risk Manager, medical staff and employes can determine the success or failure of the case. According to the Illinois Institute for Continuing Legal Education Manual on Medical Malpractice, "all malpractice cases, despite how they may appear initially, have some defensible aspect to them . . . an early, aggressive preparation of the defense in a malpractice case is the best method for a successful conclusion of the case." The strategy of defense (assumption of risk — consent, Res Judica, emergency, statute of limitations, unwarranted action, etc.) is best handled by the hospital legal liability counsel. However, there are specific actions and policies which the hospital staff can implement to protect the liability exposure. This requires action by the hospital administrator(s) and Risk Manager, medical staff, hospital employes and the Medical Record Department.

Administration/Risk Manager

For the purpose of this discussion, the Risk Manager is the person who functions in the capacity of controlling the medical liability program at the hospital at an administrator or assistant administrator level. Risk Management could also be a committee function.

The Risk Manager should have all incident reports, inquiries regarding incidents, significant patient complaints, notification of attorneys, attorney inquiries, claims investigator interviews, subpoena records, etc., directed to his or her attention and should function as the central "clearinghouse" of all such activity.

For each case, the Risk Manager should make a preliminary study of the facts and relay this information to the medical liability claims consultants, the medical liability committee, if any, and then to the hospital's legal counsel if necessary. Under the direction of the hospital attorney, the Risk Manager should direct the preservation of evidence, obtain the facts and coordinate the claim investigation.

In a malpractice case, it is what you do not know about the incident that is dangerous when the case goes to trial. There should be no surprises at a medical liability trial. Thus if a serious incident has occurred, the facts must be documented. These facts can be documented by interview with those having knowledge of the circumstances of the incident, by photographs and diagrams, by interviews with recorded statements, and by properly examining and preserving the records, copies of policies in effect at the time of incident, etc. Again, this should be accomplished at the direction of the hospital's legal counsel, which may insulate the findings of the investigation from falling within the category of "discovery" by the plaintiff's attorney.

The defense effort may rely heavily upon the equipment, records, and other physical evidence involved. There may be possibilities for subrogation or transferring the loss, (if any), to a manufacturer, supplier, service contractor, etc. If functional or chemical tests of the "evidence" are necessary, these should be done in consort with, and at the direction of, the hospital's legal counsel and claim consultants. In short, *all* physical evidence, including equipment-related service contracts, maintenance records, purchasing records, etc., must be preserved in its exact state at the time of the incident in order to properly document and function in a defense posture. It is suggested that a security cabinet or room be designated and utilized for such purposes.

No photographs, inspections, testing, examination, etc., should be permitted without knowledge and consent of the hospital's Risk Manager and legal counsel. If such actions are permitted under the rules of "discovery," then duplication or reproduction of those photographs, inspections, testing, examinations, etc., should be made in order to assist with identification and evaluation of the findings.

As a general hospital policy, employes or staff physicians should avoid discussions of any incident in any context other than the professional care of the patients. It should be made clear that no discussion by telephone or in person of any incident should take place with an attorney, claims investigator, news media, etc., without the hospital Risk Manager being present and without the consent of the hospital's legal counsel. If such an interview is authorized, all those involved should be fully identified, and a complete report of the interview should be filed by the Risk Manager.

Role of Medical Staff

For most all serious incidents involving medical liability or malpractice, the hospital's medical staff would be involved to some degree. Cooperation from the medical staff is needed to:

1. Notify immediately the hospital Risk Management Department of an incident.
2. Preserve the evidence.
3. Give a frank description of the incident.
4. Provide documentation of the exact occurrence.
5. Evaluate the degree of damage done, if any, probability of permanent or partial disability, chances of recovery, etc.
6. Impartially evaluate the merits of allegations in light of documented evidence and work with the hospital's legal counsel to help make informed decisions as to the merits of the alleged case and the defense posture to be taken.
7. Evaluate what possible medical expert testimony may be used for defense, as well as by the plaintiff. This would also include what texts, periodicals, treatises, special consultants, etc., may be introduced to provide information as to the "standard of care."

8. Make all written progress notes, operative summaries, etc., in accordance with proper medical standards.
9. Have no conversations with claims investigators, attorneys, etc., without the approval of Risk Manager and hospital legal counsel.

Role of Hospital Employe

Each employe of the hospital has certain responsibilities to control medical liability potential after an incident has occurred. A hospital employe can play an important part in liability control by functioning in the following areas:

1. Make immediate notification of a serious incident.
2. Implement proper documentation procedures.
3. Preserve the evidence, as previously discussed.
4. Observe the confidentiality regulations of the hospital.
5. Cooperate fully with in-house investigations by the hospital Risk Management staff and the hospital legal counsel.

Medical Record Security Procedure

A special medical record control procedure should be implemented for all cases designated by the hospital Risk Manager as serious incidents, incidents involving suspected medical liability or negligence, cases for which attorneys have requested medical records, or when litigation is filed against the hospital. For such cases, the medical record librarian should follow the procedures listed below:

1. The patient's complete chart should be pulled immediately.
2. At least three photocopies of the complete medical record of the patient should be prepared. The photocopies should be dated and initialed by the person making the copies. The original medical record should be retained in a security file with limited access, or as directed by the hospital's legal counsel.
3. One photocopy will be used by the hospital's legal counsel as defense material, if necessary. The second copy will be used by the hospital's Risk Management consultants in their investigation of the particular incident. The third copy will remain under the *exclusive* control of the hospital medical record librarian in a security file.
4. Thereafter, any request to review the original chart by a doctor, lawyer, investigator, member of the administration, hospital employe, patient, etc., should be authorized only by the Risk Manager and subject to the usual procedures for review of the patient's chart, including proper authorization. A log should be maintained by the medical record librarian of persons requesting the chart and date released to such persons.

The records should not be allowed to leave the Medical Record Department.

5. If the chart was incomplete at the time of the filing of the lawsuit or at the time when the file was designated to be pulled by the hospital medical record librarian, a memo on the original chart indicating the chart deficiencies should also be photocopied.

6. Attempts by the medical staff members to complete the chart which was incomplete at the time of the filing of the lawsuit should be authorized by the Risk Manager, who should seek advice of the hospital's legal counsel as to the appropriateness of completing the chart.

Conclusions

Loss control is concerned with pre-loss prevention measures and loss reduction methods after the occurrence. This discussion is concerned with claim control procedures after an incident occurs. The procedures and topics in this review are meant to be guidelines toward liability control and meant to summarize loss reduction techniques. Your individual organization chart and legal counsel should be consulted to define and accomplish the items listed here. Obviously, many more techniques can be implemented as individual circumstances require.

References: *Medical Malpractice* — Illinois Institute for Continuing Legal Education
Action Kit for Hospital Law — June, 1977.
Medical Malpractice — Houisell and Williams

E. How to monitor a hospital's medication error rate

If a unit dose system is in operation in your hospital, there is a fairly easy method to constantly monitor errors of omission — probably the largest single category of medication errors.[1-4]

The unit dose system allows for greater accountability and monitoring of error rate. Doses returned unadministered at cart exchange, without a reasonable explanation (as judged by the pharmacist) are considered errors of omission unless and until proven otherwise (a nursing-pharmacy communication form can be used to provide explanations). These omitted doses are followed up by the pharmacist. Those considered to be omitted due to error are documented and held. At the end of one week or one month, all dose omissions for each patient care unit are tallied. Some of the reasons for errors of omission have been published.[5] If one knows what to look for, a good deal of time can be saved.

Using data available from the hospital business office, determine how many patient days there were in each patient care unit studied during that time period. This figure, divided into the number of omission errors yields omission errors per patient day. The figure should then be adjusted (obviously where more medications are given per patient day there is a greater chance for error) by determining doses administered per patient day. This may be determined by charges submitted for each patient care unit, an average done once every so often, by sampling or any other suitable means.

To ascertain the error rate for the entire hospital, one would need to determine doses per patient day throughout the hospital. These statistics can then be compared to published studies and to previous studies at your hospital to see how well your system is working. The data may be used to point out troubled patient care units so that corrective action can be taken.

Here is a sample for a 400 bed unit dose hospital.

Nursing Unit	Omission Errors	Patient Days	Omission Errors per pt. day	Doses/pt. day	Percent Omission errors
1	39	1008	0.039	10.2	0.38%
2	55	745	0.074	11.3	0.65%
3	36	1005	0.036	9.5	0.38%
4	172	1179	0.146	12.3	1.17%
5	58	1087	0.053	9.6	0.55%
6	23	1248	0.018	6.3	0.29%
7	17	1341	0.013	6.1	0.21%
8	14	1071	0.013	7.8	0.17%
TOTAL	414	8684	0.048	9.1	0.53%

From these data it can be seen that Unit 4 has a problem when compared with the rest of the hospital. While the doses per patient day are roughly double that of Unit 7, the omission error rate is almost sixfold greater. Compared to omission error rates published in references 1, 2, 3 and 4 (average omission error rate in non-unit dose hospitals was 5.5% and in unit dose hospitals it was 1.1%), Unit 4 is not out of step with the national averages. Apparently the hospital's unit dose system is helping to prevent errors. But one strives for perfection and the figures point out the need for improvement with special attention given to Unit 4. The error rate studies cited in the references were better controlled and would tend to uncover more errors than the system described above. Therefore, one would expect to find a lower rate of omissions in this hospital than in the hospitals cited in the studies.

116

References

1. Barker, KM, McConnell, WE. Detecting errors in hospitals. Am J Hosp Pharm, 1962, 19:361
2. Barker KM. The effects of an experimental medication system on medication errors and cost. Am J Hosp, 1969, 26:324
3. Hynnemann et al. A comparison of medication errors under the University of Kentucky unit dose system and traditional drug distribution systems in four hospitals. Am J Hosp Pharm, 1970, 27:803
4. Shultz et al. Medication errors reduced by unit dose. Hospitals, 1973, 47:106
5. Cohen MR. Discrepancies in unit dose cart fills. Hosp Pharm, 1980, 15:16

18

Recommendations

We can summarize our recommendations for preventing medication errors based on certain patterns which we have observed in the errors which have been sent to us by our readers.

Some simple rules can be formulated and implemented to prevent the following recurring type errors. Following the rules will help you to achieve maximum safety in drug therapy. When you observe fellow employes or colleagues in other health professions using incorrect notation, for example, take time to educate. If you observe incorrect notation in print, as in manufacturer's labeling or advertising or in professional journals, take the time to educate the companies and publishers. You will indirectly be helping to reduce the risk of medication error.

1. Never abbreviate U for unit as it is read as an "O" or "4". Write out "Unit."
2. Never use chemical names—especially names preceded by a number prefix.

Do not use	Use
6 Mercaptopurine	Mercaptopurine
6 Thioguanine	Thioguanine

    The 6 is mistaken for 6 dosage units.
3. Never abbreviate drug names. Use either generic or trade names.
4. Never abbreviate once daily as OD, as it is interpreted as "right eye." Write out "Daily" or "Once Daily."
5. Never abbreviate once daily as q.d., as it is read as four times daily.
6. Never administer more than 2 dosage units to a patient unless you are 100% sure the dose is correct. Check with a knowledgeable colleague or pharmacist.
7. Never leave a decimal point naked, such as .5 ml. When the decimal point is not seen, a tenfold overdose may occur. This should be written as 0.5 ml.

8. Never put a decimal point and zero after a whole number such as 2.0 mg. This should be written as 2 mg. If the decimal point is not seen, a tenfold overdose may result.

9. Always use the metric system; never use the apothecary system.

Other factors which cause, contribute to, or prevent medication errors cannot be corrected simply by formulating rules. Positive steps must come from departmental policy, self-discipline when writing and transcribing orders and when preparing or administering medication, institution of modern drug distribution systems, regulation or legislation by governmental agencies or JCAH, having adequate staff, having qualified staff and having proper working conditions.

Listed below are important considerations in preventing medication errors.

1. Considerable thought and care must be taken in hiring and assigning personnel who will be ordering medications, noting medication orders, preparing medication, dispensing medication and administering medication. This includes: Interviewing job applicants, Testing job applicants, Orienting new employes, Placement of employes, Supervision of employes, and, Quality control checks.

2. Drug floor stock should be minimal. Except for emergencies, at least two people, a pharmacist and a nurse, should review every physician order prior to dispensing and administration. The original order or an exact copy (NCR or carbon) should be reviewed, never a transcription by another person.

3. A properly conceived and monitored Unit Dose Drug Distribution System should be used.

4. A pharmacy controlled I.V. Admixture program should be used.

5. Pharmacy hours of service should be sufficient to meet the needs of the patients, nurses and physicians.

6. Nursing supervisors or physicians should not be permitted in the pharmacy when it is closed. A night cabinet or cart with a limited variety of packaged medications should be available for after hours service. A pharmacist should be on call, the ultimate goal being 24-hour pharmacy coverage.

7. Physicians should not routinely make rounds and write orders at night if the nursing and pharmacy staffs are not adequate at those times.

8. Students and supportive personnel must be supervised and operate within prescribed limits.

9. Handwritten material must be legible.

10. Drug orders must be complete and clear with no ambiguities.

11. Dangerous or uncommon abbreviations should not be used.
12. Verbal orders must only be utilized in emergency situations and when used, extreme care must be used to insure understanding. Such orders should be countersigned by the prescriber as soon as possible, but within 24 hours.
13. Care must be used by manufacturers and the United States Adopted Names (USAN) Council when assigning or choosing drug names to prevent misunderstanding and error from occurring. The USAN must be assigned as early as possible and used in the research literature.
14. Manufacturers should design container labels so that the name(s) and strength of the product are the most prominent items on the label. The company name and logo are best placed at the bottom of the label.
15. Health professionals must be knowledgeable about drugs when they start their careers and must keep current.
16. Adequate reference books must be in the patient care area and pharmacy.
17. Health professionals must understand the medication ordering, dispensing and administration systems in effect. The systems must be in writing in the form of policies and procedures.
18. A drug should not be administered to a patient unless it is clearly indicated for the patient's condition.
19. Patient drug allergies and hypersensitivities must be noted and utilized.
20. Labels must be read purposefully, and completely. Never rely on a glance at gross appearance or color.
21. All drug containers must be completely and properly labeled.
22. Sufficient personnel must be available to do the job properly.
23. Working conditions should be designed to maximize a quiet work area with minimal distraction. Adequate light and ventilation must be present.
24. Before a drug is administered to an institutionalized patient, his or her armband must be checked.
25. Patients must be educated about the drugs they are taking. This includes both institutionalized patients and outpatients.
26. A patient who questions whether he or she is receiving the proper medication, the proper amount, at the proper time of administration, should be taken seriously.
27. Nursing personnel should stay with the patient and observe the patient take the medication.

28. Medication tickets (cards) should not be used as the mechanism for alerting nursing to administer a medication and for charting. A medication administration record form is better suited for this purpose. The nurse's medication administration record form should be taken, along with the labeled unit dose medication, to the patient's bedside area.

29. Medication administration charting should be accomplished immediately after the drug(s) is given.

30. Once dispensed, unless individually sealed and labeled (unit dose package), unadministered medications should not be returned to their original container, rather they should be discarded. Once a closure is removed, large volume parenterals should not be returned to stock.

31. Medication such as pHisohex, hydrogen peroxide or alcohol should not be taken out of their original containers and placed at the patient's bedside.

32. The pharmacy department must be the only department that packages, labels and dispenses medication. No other department should be permitted to use pharmacy labels or containers.

33. Pharmacy personnel must inspect drug stocks throughout the institution monthly. Improperly labeled drugs, outdated or otherwise deteriorated drugs, overstocked drugs or drugs that should not be at the location, must be removed.

34. The pharmacy must exercise care in selecting drug products to be purchased, a prime consideration being clarity of labeling.

35. An effective mechanism must be used to report medication errors. Errors must be analyzed by nursing, pharmacy, medical staff, risk management personnel and administration, with a goal of formulating policies, procedures and systems to prevent them.

36. The pharmacy should maintain copies of cancer chemotherapy protocols and use them to check ordered doses.

37. The pharmacy should double check dosage calculations of physicians and nurses for pediatric patients, cancer chemotherapy and other situations where calculations are involved.

38. When a physician writes an unusual order it should be discussed with nursing and pharmacy personnel. The information should then be made available to all personnel responsible for carrying out the order.

39. Care must be taken by physicians that orders are written on the right patient's chart.

40. Pharmacy should maintain and utilize pharmacy patient profiles for outpatients. This is a chronicle of prescriptions

received by the patient which also lists allergies, hypersensitivities and chronic diseases. This profile should be used to check for appropriateness of therapy and in patient counselling.

Medication errors are costly in human suffering, increased length of hospital stay, professional time taken to investigate the errors, damaged reputations, reduced patient confidence, out of court settlements, court awarded verdicts and increased malpractice insurance rates. The government, third party agents and the public must realize it is costly to provide properly trained health professionals in adequate numbers, working in the proper environment and utilizing appropriate systems. Health professionals must be mindful of the importance of their work, giving it the time and meticulous attention it requires. Patients must become more knowledgeable about their medical conditions and the drugs they are taking.

Appendix 1

Medication Errors

Reprinted with permission from Lippincott's *Hospital Pharmacy*, copyrighted 1975-80. Each error is followed by the number of the volume, page and year in which it appeared in *Hospital Pharmacy*.

Medication error reports

Medication error reports are solicited from readers of HOSPITAL PHARMACY and *Nursing 81* (where the column also appears). All reports are handled in a confidential manner so as not to reveal the source of the error. Written error reports sent to the editor of this column are analyzed by him and the editor of the journal for pertinence, originality and potential as a learning experience for journal readers and others. On many occasions, the sender is phoned to obtain further information to be included in the published version. Sometimes error reports originate as a verbal communication directly to one of us. They are handled in the same manner as written reports.

Because of the impossibility of checking that each error report is factual, we must rely on the good faith of health professionals who report errors. In no case are any of the error reports contrived by us.

In our feature, we will try not to be specific as to who was involved—for instance, staff physician, resident or intern—but rather will simply use the designation physician. This is being done because we want to focus on the error itself, not on exactly who was responsible for it. The same would be true if an error was caused by someone administering a drug. It does not matter which exact category of personnel was involved, the error could have happened to anyone doing the task.

Error 1

An order was written, "4 U Lente Insulin." Because of poor handwriting, the U was mistaken for an O. The patient received 40 units of Lente Insulin.

The abbreviation "U" should not be used; the word units should be spelled out.

Reader Comments

On error 1 (using the abbreviation "U" for units)

In your first medication error report, you warn against the abbrevia-

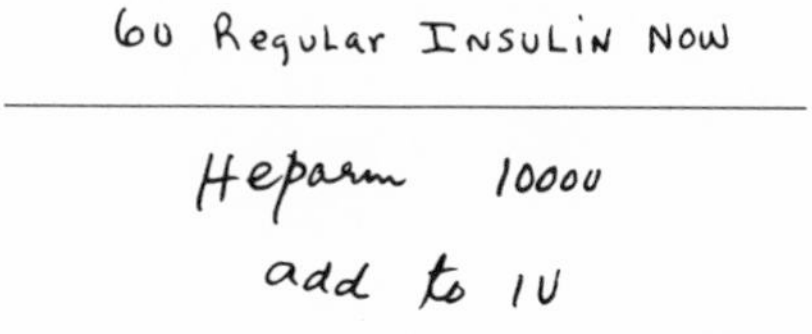

60 Regular Insulin Now

Heparin   10000

add to 1U

Figure 1

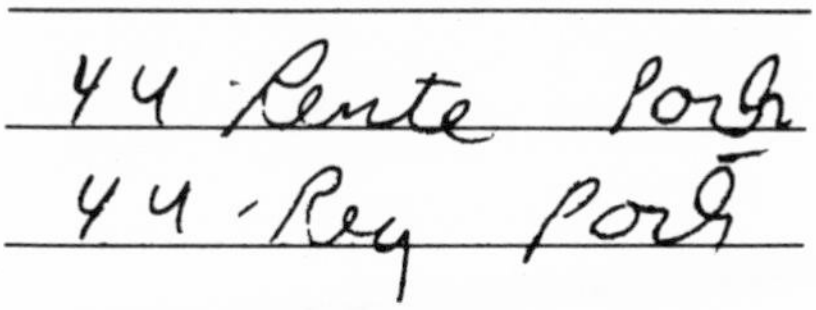

44 Lente Pork

44 · Reg Pork

Figure 2

tion "U" being used instead of writing out the word "units." The problem is that the "U" can easily be mistaken for a zero. The following example of this hazardous abbreviation was responsible for an administered dose of insulin that was tenfold above the dose that was intended. (Figure 1). Your readers should appreciate this illustration. Pharmacists should perform corrective action whenever this type of abbreviation is discovered to be in use in their institutions. This is not a petty matter. The same can happen with heparin.

Variation of U for units

Mention has been made in the past about the hazard of using the abbreviation U for units. The danger is that this may be mistaken for a zero and increase the dose tenfold. For example, 4 U of NPH insulin in script may look like 40 NPH insulin. Even a loop placed on the U's can cause trouble, as Figure 2 shows. One of our readers reported an incident in which doses of 44 units of insulin were listed on medication administration records by drug administration personnel. The astute pharmacist stopped the error before it occurred.

10:120, 1975

Error 2

An outpatient prescription was written
          Florinef #25
          Sig: As Directed

The pharmacist mistook it for Fiorinal. If the handwriting had been studied carefully, the prescription would have been obvious. However, two out of five other pharmacists when asked hurriedly to read the prescription made the same mistake.

Pharmacists must take care in reading prescriptions. The prescribing physician was asked to write legibly, and indicate the desired strength and specific directions in the future. If he had done so originally, the pharmacist would not have made the error. Patient instructions are also necessary for proper compliance.

10:120, 1975

Error 3

An order was received in the pharmacy for "1 mg Synthroid." (Figure 3). When the pharmacist checked the original order in the chart, he found that the physician had ordered .1 mg Synthroid. The decimal point was placed directly on a line on the order sheet and was not obvious.

The error was prevented. The confusion could have been avoided if the physician had written 0.1 mg. Never leave a decimal point naked. All labeling, formularies, and newsletters should also carry out this format. A

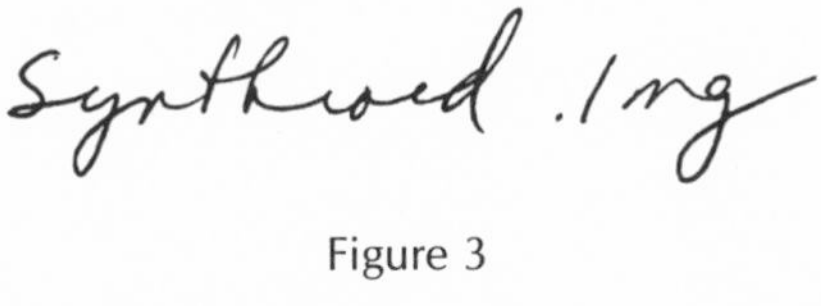

Synthroid .1 mg

Figure 3

124

long-range solution to this recurring problem is the use of the microgram designation for amounts less than 1 mg.

10:120, 1975

Error 4

A physician gave a verbal order for 16 units of regular Insulin. The individual taking the order thought the physician said 60. Sixty units were administered.

This type of error could be eliminated if no verbal orders were accepted for insulin. If verbal orders were required, the individual taking the order should read back carefully to the prescriber, "16, that is, one-six units of regular insulin." Besides hearing the order correctly, the person involved must transcribe it onto the chart of the right patient.

10:120, 1975

Correspondence

About the errors involved in accepting verbal orders

I would like to relate to you an event with which I am familiar that serves to highlight the potential danger inherent when verbal orders are accepted.

A direct order copy was received which read:

"Give Warfarin 40 mg PO HS tonight. v/o Dr. _____/Mr. Nurse

This order was questionable in my mind because the handwriting was not clear; I couldn't be sure whether the nurse meant 4.0 mg (four) or 40 mg (forty). The nurse claimed that 40 mg was intended. Since the patient

was already receiving Coumadin and had not shown signs of Coumadin resistance, I thought that dose was incorrect and promptly called the physician. Of course, he meant four mg. Verbal orders to the pharmacist should always be scrutinized extra carefully. They should be permitted only in cases in which no other alternative exists.

A Reader

Error 5

While in the process of administering medications to a patient, a medication nurse found her patient to be slipping out of bed. She had in her hand the doses of medication to be given to the patient. She hurriedly went to assist the patient back into bed. In doing so, she placed the doses on the night stand of the other patient in the room. After helping her patient, she returned to obtain his medications. The other patient had taken the drugs. The drugs involved were warfarin 20 mg, oxtriphylline 100 mg. and chlordiazepoxide 10 mg.

Prevention

Educational. Those responsible for administering medications must be made aware of situations such as these. Adequate publicity given to such events may help in preventing occurrences. Medications meant for one patient must never be left within reach of another patient.

10:166, 1975

Error 6

In a hospital with a unit dose drug distribution system, the pharmacy received an order for quinidine sulfate 200 mg four times daily. The drug was scheduled to be given at 12 noon, 6 pm, 12 midnight and 6 am. Since the order was received late in the day and because the system involved use of a 4 pm cart fill that contained all drug doses due up until 7 am, the pharmacist was required to dispense three doses of drug (6 pm, 12 mn and 6 am). Commercially available perforated strip packaged unit doses were used.

In the act of dispensing, the pharmacist did not separate the doses. He placed the attached doses in the hand of the individual responsible for administering medications and said, "Give the 6 pm dose now." Believing that the three tablets made up one dose, the individual administered all three doses.

10:166, 1975

Prevention

Educational; procedural. In a unit dose drug distribution system, never permit strip-packed unit dose medications to be dispensed without separating the perforated packages, unless more than one package makes up a single dose. When medications are available commercially, more than one package might be necessary to equal a single dose. Those responsible for administration of medications get used to finding that more than one package makes up a single dose when stapled together or left unperforated, as are large doses of prednisone representing a single dose.

For the sake of clarity when unit doses have to be made up extemporaneously, the entire dose should be placed in one package and labeled with the number of tablets or cap-

sules that make up the dose. An example follows:

Furosemide (Lasix)

60 mg

1½ of 40 mg tablet

Emphasize to all personnel the importance of checking and rechecking and not taking anyone's word for any task related to drug administration.

Correspondence

On error 6 (dispensing unit dose medication strip packs unperforated)

A variation of one of the error reports occurred in our hospital recently that I would like to share with your readers.

In error 6, three doses of quinidine sulfate 200 mg were administered in one dose because the pharmacist dispensed these unperforated unit doses in strip pack form and the nurse thought it was one dose. We had a patient who was scheduled for an operation in the morning. An abnormal EKG was noted in the afternoon before the day of the operation, and quinidine 200 mg every six hours was ordered.

Because it is our custom to dispense a 24-hour supply in unit dose form, the pharmacist delivered four doses to the person giving medications. He handed her the tablets, which were unseparated in strip pack form, and said "Here's the Quinidine 200 mg." The person giving medications thought all four tablets were to be given as the noon dose. The patient received 800 mg. The error could have been prevented if the doses had been separated and if the pharmacist had explained further that each tablet was quinidine 200 mg. Obviously, if the

126

labels had been read, the error would also have been prevented.

A Hospital Pharmacist

Error 7

An order was written for "regular insulin 100 unit." This was to be given daily to a newly admitted diabetic patient. The nurse on duty, surprised to see such a dose, questioned the prescriber who was a graduate of a foreign medical school and had a poor command of the English language. The prescriber confirmed that what was written was the dose to be given.

Prevention

Fortunately, the error was prevented. When the medication nurse requested the dose from pharmacy, the pharmacist became suspicious and went to question the patient further. The encounter with the patient revealed that U 100 insulin was being used. When the physician asked the patient what dose of insulin was being used, the patient said "100 unit insulin." In fact, the patient had been taking NPH insulin 20 units daily. The lesson to be learned is never take anybody's word for anything if you have doubts about a situation. Investigate all situations to your satisfaction. Incidentally, this error would have been carried out had it not been for the fact that this hospital had a unit dose system in which all doses were prepared by pharmacy.

10:167, 1975

Error 8

A patient was to receive Metamucil, ferrous sulfate, and four drops of colistin otic solution in each ear. In transcribing the physician's order to the drug administration record, the following was handwritten for the *ear* drop:

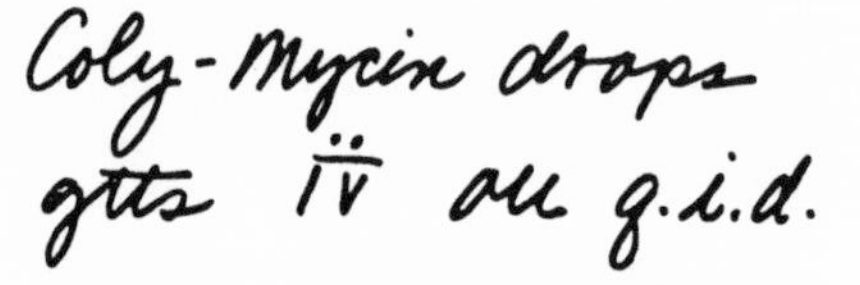

Figure 4

For several days, the drug was administered properly by the medication nurses on all shifts. Then one day a new medication nurse took the drops into the patient's room and administered four drops in each *eye*. The order had been interpreted as O.U., or each eye, instead of A.U., or each ear. After giving the drops, the nurse was leaving the room when the patient called out, "Don't I get any ear drops?" The administration record was consulted and the mistake realized.

Prevention

Educational, procedural. Use of unauthorized abbreviations must not be permitted. In this case the nurse who originally noted the order wrote an abbreviation that was never approved for use within the hospital. Yet almost everyone understood what was meant by A.U. when taken in context with the knowledge that Coly-mycin is an otic solution. They didn't bother to question what was written. Unfortunately, the nurse responsible for the error misunderstood and mistook the A.U. for O.U. It is easy to understand how this error could occur. Personnel must question use of unauthorized abbreviations.

Another important point can be made from this particular error. Although it may sometimes be the case, one cannot expect a patient to prevent such errors from occurring. Even though the patient received the drops in the ear for several doses, the fact that the eye drops were being administered didn't bother him a bit. Patients most frequently put complete

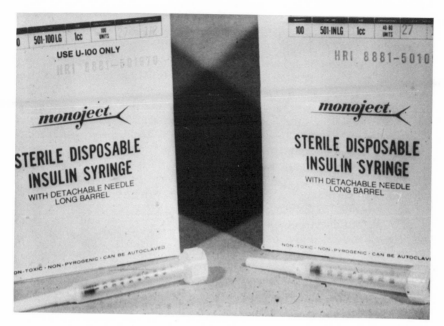

Figure 5

trust in those responsible for their care. Many have been conditioned not to ask questions.

A supplementary label "for the ear" placed on the container by the pharmacy might also have been helpful.

10:202, 1975

Errors 9 and 10

Manufacturers of drugs and hospital supplies may contribute to medication errors. Poor labeling of containers occurs more frequently than one might expect.

In one situation, danger existed because of two similarly labeled large volume parenteral containers, one of 5% dextrose in water and one of 50% dextrose in water. In at least two situations, 50% solution was inadvertently administered for 5% solution.

Inadvertent administration of 50% dextrose could have disastrous con-

sequences, especially in pediatric patients.* If one were to look at the two solutions side by side (especially from a distance as you would if you were choosing the bottle off the shelf), it would be easy to understand the mix-up. Those bottles should never have been stored in proximity. Of course that label should have been read carefully — but it wasn't, and accidents will happen.

This problem has been resolved by at least two manufacturers. One uses red printed warning labels and one uses other means for making the two different concentrations readily distinguishable.

The two concentrations should never be stored in proximity and the 50% concentration should not be available in patient care areas.

*Stanley, C.A. and Baker, L.: Accidental poisoning with 50 percent glucose solution: The danger of large stock bottles. J. Pediatr. 84:270, 1974.

Another situation developed recently with the advent of U-100 syringes. The problem occurred as a result of indistinguishable labeling of syringe cartons by the manufacturer. As may be readily seen in Figure 5, only minute differences of label were visible to differentiate the box of U 40-80 syringes from U-100 syringes. The color of the labeling and the background on the box were identical. In addition, the syringes inside the box were in both instances color-coded yellow to denote needle size. This is an example of the evils of color-coding, since this substantiated the assumption in everyone's mind that no difference existed.

This error occurred in a hospital in which U-100 insulin and syringes were used almost exclusively for over a year. Syringes were distributed to patient care areas by central supply personnel who in turn received the syringes from the hospital purchasing department. The purchasing department had purchased several thousand U 40-80 combination syringes in error.

It is remarkable that these syringes passed through several hands without the error being discovered. No one bothered to read the label carefully, since U-100 syringes had always been sent in the past, and they were always yellow. Unfortunately, several doses of U-100 insulin were drawn up using a U-40 scale. Some of the syringes were even sold to outpatients.

Prevention

Yes, it's true that people involved in these situations did not read the labels carefully and there's no excuse for that, but the poor labeling and color coding certainly contributed to these errors. Pharmacists and nurses must be suspicious of any confusing packaging. Keep an eye open for such material and refuse to use the supplies whenever possible. Resist reliance on color coding.

We all have a responsibility in the name of patient safety to act in these situations. Manufacturers involved must be contacted and must act in a positive manner. If no results are obtained after contacting the manufacturer, the United States Pharmacopeia Drug Defect Reporting System should be used, or it should be used primarily. (See Chapter 15).

10:202, 1975

Error 11

Persons responsible for administration of drugs in a unit dose system get used to single unit packaging and labeling. One package or several packages attached together is always one dose. Labeling must *always* reflect this concept. To explain this, the following example is used.

In a hospital in which a partial unit dose distribution system is used, a medication nurse who had worked in a patient care area with unit dose was temporarily transferred to an area of the hospital in which the traditional system was used. An order was received for "Lasix 40 mg." The nurse checked floor stock and found that there was no Lasix left. She needed it immediately so she called the pharmacy asking for one dose until she could bring the stock container. The pharmacist wanted to help out. He placed 10 Lasix tablets in a small vial and labeled it "Lasix 40 mg." This was received by the medication nurse by way of a messenger. Believing the tablets to equal one dose, she placed all 10 tablets in a medication cup and administered the medication. The nurse later claimed that working with unit dose made her get used to the concept of one package equals one dose.

Prevention

Labeling must be as specific as possible. This is especially true in situations in which a hospital is using a partial unit dose system because of gradual conversion from the traditional system or because of a permanent condition. The label should have read:

Furosemide (Lasix)
40 mg per tablet
10 tablets

The pharmacist should also have communicated the fact that 10 doses were being sent to the unit as a temporary supply and that the 10 tablets were not the single dose that was requested.

10:203, 1975

Error 12

Frequently, misinterpretations of physicians' medication orders cause error. Some physicians are careless about their handwriting; when they carelessly write drug names that look alike, this contributes to the possibility of misinterpretation. The following mixups have been reported as actual occurrences. These misinterpretations may have been made by nurses or pharmacists.

1. Dilantin was taken for Delalutin.
2. Pitocin was taken for Pitressin.
3. Inderal was taken for Isordil.
4. "Cephazolin" was taken for cephalothin.

These drugs may also be mixed up when referred to verbally because they also sound alike. Additionally, in each case dosages may be similar. This increases the likelihood of error. It should be noted that many other examples of look-alike or sound-alike

drugs are published annually in the journal *Pharmacy Times*. (See Chapter 4.)

10:232, 1975

Error 13

Similar to confusion resulting from look-alike or sound-alike drugs, written orders may be misinterpreted because a physician used a name that was not recognized. In this error, an order was written for
6-mercaptopurine 50 mg bid
Six mercaptopurine tablets 50 mg (300 mg total) were administered twice daily. The seriousness of such an error is obvious. Two other drugs that come to mind as having potential for being involved in similar errors are 5-fluorocytosine (250 mg capsules) and 6-thioguanine (40 mg tablets). Other possibilities exist.

Preventing errors from misinterpretations of physician's orders

Clearly, an effort should be made to educate health professionals about drug names that look or sound alike. Care must be taken in writing and referring to these drugs. Whenever practical, interpretation of physician's orders should be checked by another person. For example, orders interpreted by a unit clerk must be checked by a nurse. Orders transcribed by a nurse should be checked by another nurse.

Ideally, the hospital pharmacist should also be able to check these transcriptions. In some clinical pharmacy programs this is done on the nursing unit. This is not practical for most pharmacy operations. However, an excellent way for pharmacists to help prevent these misinterpretations and other errors has been described by Leiman, Rose and Davis in HOSPITAL PHARMACY 8:124, 1973. In this

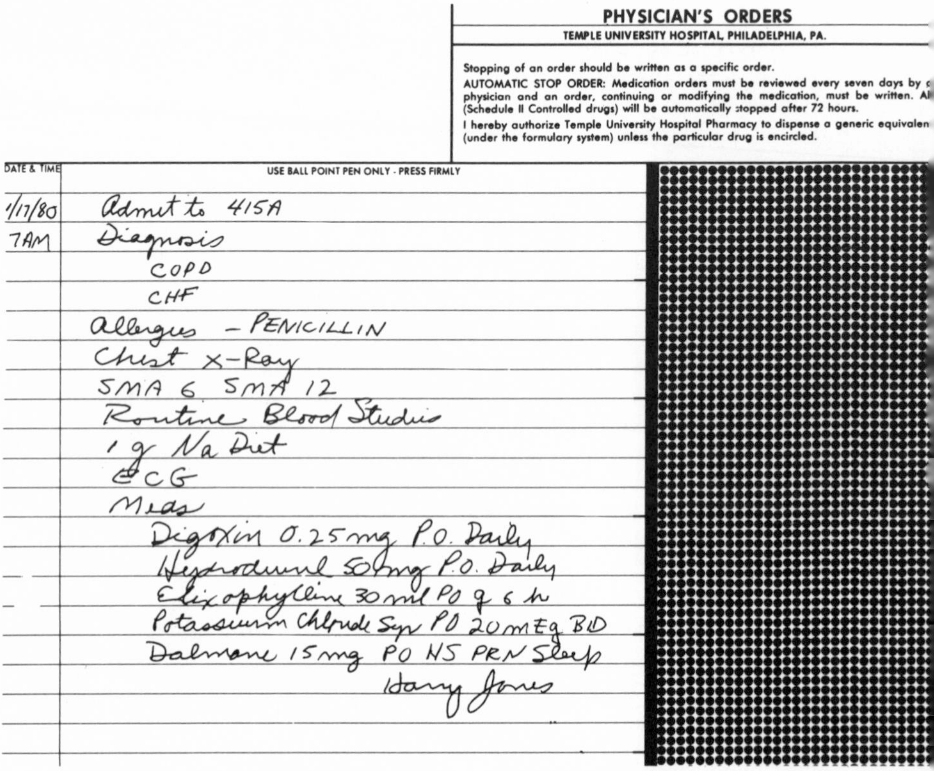

130

PHYSICIAN'S ORDERS
TEMPLE UNIVERSITY HOSPITAL, PHILADELPHIA, PA.

Stopping of an order should be written as a specific order.
AUTOMATIC STOP ORDER: Medication orders must be reviewed every seven days by a physician and an order, continuing or modifying the medication, must be written. All (Schedule II Controlled drugs) will be automatically stopped after 72 hours.
I hereby authorize Temple University Hospital Pharmacy to dispense a generic equivalent (under the formulary system) unless the particular drug is encircled.

DATE & TIME | USE BALL POINT PEN ONLY - PRESS FIRMLY

1/17/80
7AM

Admit to 415A

Diagnosis
  COPD
  CHF

Allergies – PENICILLIN

Chest X-Ray
SMA 6 SMA 12
Routine Blood Studies
1 g Na Diet
ECG
Meds
  Digoxin 0.25 mg P.O. Daily
  Hydrodiuril 50 mg P.O. Daily
  Elixophylline 30 ml PO q 6 h
  Potassium Chloride Syr PO 20 mEq BID
  Dalmane 15 mg PO HS PRN Sleep

Harry Jones

Figure 6. Physician's order form, first page.

system are used two forms, a five-part physician's order form (Figure 6) and a three-part nurse's medication administration form.

When an order is written, the first copy of the full page physician's order form is removed. A "medication instructions" column appears on the right hand side of all copies (Figure 7); this is blocked out on the original physician's order sheet. This column is identical to the "medication instructions" column on the left hand side of the medication administration record (Figure 7).

The nurse locates medication administration record of the particular patient. The right side of the copy of the physician's order is placed *under* the left side of the medication administration record with all blocks

aligned. Medication orders as interpreted by the nurse are entered directly on the medication administration record (top-most sheet, Figure 7). The NCR forms cause the nurse's interpretation to appear on the physician's order form copy (Figure 8). This sheet, which now contains copies of both the physicians original order and the nurse's interpretation of that order, is forwarded to pharmacy. The pharmacist's interpretation of the physician's original order is then compared to the interpretation made by the nurse.

For a complete explanation of this system as well as a discussion of other worthwhile features of the forms used, see the original article.

10:232, 1975

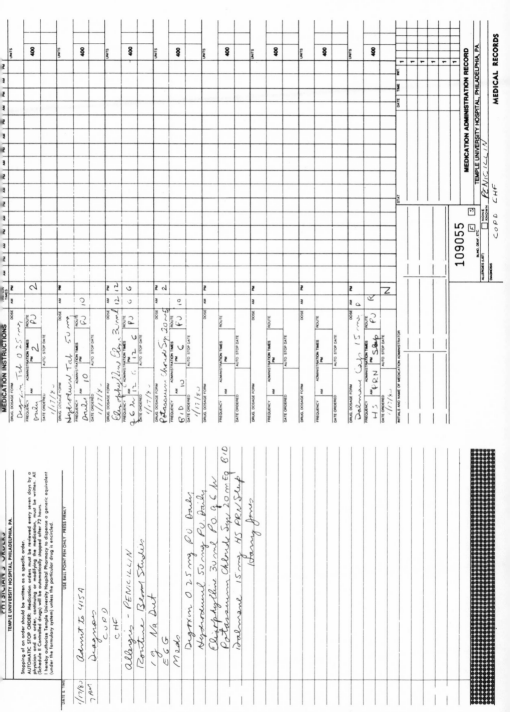

Figure 7. Copy of physician's order form with MAR number entered (left side), aligned with medication administration record, orders transcribed (right side).

PHYSICIAN'S ORDERS

TEMPLE UNIVERSITY HOSPITAL, PHILADELPHIA, PA.

DIRECTIONS FOR REPLACING FORM

A. When last copy is removed:
   1. Strike out remaining unused lines under last order.
   2. Replace with new copy of Physician's Orders form.

B. When form is filled with orders:
   1. Discard remaining unused copies.
   2. Replace with new copy of Physician's Orders form.

DATE & TIME	USE BALL POINT PEN ONLY - PRESS FIRMLY
1/17/80	Admit to 415A
7AM	Diagnosis
	COPD
	CHF
	Allergies - PENICILLIN
	Chest x-Ray
	Routine Blood Studies
	1 g Na Diet
	ECG
	Meds
	Digoxin 0.25 mg P.O. Daily
	Hydrodiuril 50 mg P.O. Daily
	Elixophylline 30 ml PO q 6 h
	Potassium Chloride Syr PO 20mEq BID
	Dalmane 15 mg PO HS PRN Sleep
	Harry Jones

DRUG, DOSAGE FORM		DOSE
Digoxin Tab		0.25 mg
FREQUENCY	ADMINISTRATION TIMES	ROUTE
Daily	2 PM	PO
DATE ORDERED	AUTO. STOP DATE	
1/17/80		

DRUG, DOSAGE FORM		DOSE
Hydrodiuril Tab		50 mg
FREQUENCY	ADMINISTRATION TIMES	ROUTE
Daily	10 AM	PO
DATE ORDERED	AUTO. STOP DATE	
1/17/80		

DRUG, DOSAGE FORM		DOSE
Elixophylline Elixir		30 ml
FREQUENCY	ADMINISTRATION TIMES	ROUTE
q 6 h	12 AM 6 AM 12 PM 6 PM	PO
DATE ORDERED	AUTO. STOP DATE	
1/17/80		

DRUG, DOSAGE FORM		DOSE
Potassium Chloride Syr		20 mEq
FREQUENCY	ADMINISTRATION TIMES	ROUTE
BID	10 AM 6 PM	PO
DATE ORDERED	AUTO. STOP DATE	
1/17/80		

DRUG, DOSAGE FORM		DOSE
FREQUENCY	ADMINISTRATION TIMES	ROUTE
DATE ORDERED	AUTO. STOP DATE	

DRUG, DOSAGE FORM		DOSE
FREQUENCY	ADMINISTRATION TIMES	ROUTE
DATE ORDERED	AUTO. STOP DATE	

DRUG, DOSAGE FORM		DOSE
FREQUENCY	ADMINISTRATION TIMES	ROUTE
DATE ORDERED	AUTO. STOP DATE	

DRUG, DOSAGE FORM		DOSE
Dalmane Cap		15 mg
FREQUENCY	ADMINISTRATION TIMES	ROUTE
HS	PRN Sleep	PO
DATE ORDERED	AUTO. STOP DATE	

BELOW THIS LINE FOR USE BY MEDICATION TECHNICIAN ONLY

TRANSCRIBED BY	DATE	PATIENT'S NAME	ROOM NO.	MED. ADMIN. REC. NO.
Julia Kraft	1/17/80	Frank Stone	415A	055 FS

Figure 8. Transcription that is forwarded to the satellite pharmacy.

Error 14

Error 1 in this series described an order written for "4 U Lente Insulin." Because of poor handwriting, the U was mistaken for an O. The patient received 40 units of insulin. An announcement describing the error requested that all health professionals spell out the word units when referring to insulin doses. One of the hospital's physicians, quick to comply with the request and wanting to leave no stone unturned, wrote the following order:

16 U units reg insulin now

Can you guess how the order was interpreted? Sometimes you just can't win.

10:239, 1975

Error 15

A patient to whom radioactive 131 I was to be administered had the following order written to protect his thyroid gland:

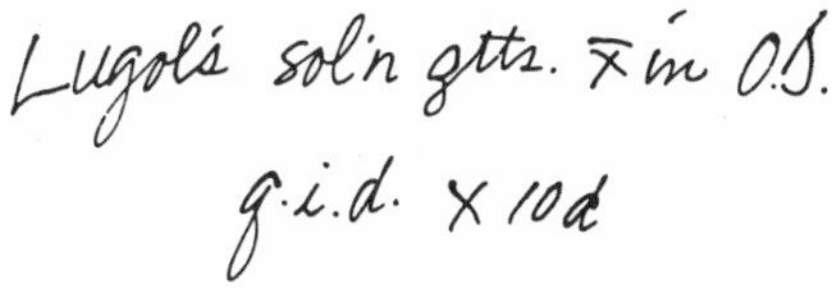

Figure 9

The following morning during rounds the patient was asked how he was feeling. His response: "Pretty good, Doc — except for those eye drops you're giving me. They really hurt." Upon checking, it was discovered that the order was misinterpreted. The physician who wrote the order intended the abbreviation O.J. to be understood as orange juice. Unfortunately, the handwriting was not clear and O.D. or right eye was transcribed onto the medication admin-istration record. The patient received doses on two different shifts.

Once again, the hazards of abbreviation surface.

10:304, 1975

Error 16

After two hours in the recovery room following an operative procedure, a patient was transferred back to his room. Upon reaching the patient care unit, the patient began complaining of pain. An order for meperidine 75 mg IM every four hours PRN pain had been written by the surgeon while the patient was in the recovery room. The dose of narcotic analgesic was administered and shortly thereafter the patient became acutely hypotensive. Upon investigation, it was discovered that Innovar had been administered during anesthesia.

When Innovar injection (fentanyl citrate, droperidol), the combination analgesic-neuroleptic, is administered during anesthesia it is well known that postoperatively, during the recovery phase, doses of narcotic analgesic drugs should be reduced to as low as one-fourth or one-third of those usually recommended. This is to lessen the chance of potentiation of Innovar's respiratory depressant and hypotensive effects. The recovery phase usually lasts for a four to six-hour period. While this information is generally known, in practice, the dosage is not always reduced. This is usually because the physician ordering narcotics postoperatively fails to make the dose reduction because of forgetfulness, because he doesn't feel it's necessary, or because he doesn't know the patient has had Innovar.

The following procedure for assuring recovery period dose reduction of

134

narcotics has been initiated at a hospital where a problem occurred. In the procedure, a label provided by the manufacturer of Innovar is used.

1. Upon administration of Innovar, the anesthesiologist or nurse anesthetist shall immediately affix the notification label provided by the company to the metal front of the patient's chart.

2. After the procedure has been completed, it is incumbent upon the surgeon to note on the label the time period for which Innovar precautions should be in effect. In addition, if a narcotic analgesic is ordered, the physician's order form should reflect an initially reduced dose of the narcotic for the specified time period. An appropriate order would read:

"Meperidine 20 mg IM q 4 h prn pain until 8 PM, then 50 mg IM q 4 h prn."

3. When the patient and patient chart arrive on the nursing floor, the Innovar notification label shall be peeled off the chart at the time of order noting by the nurse or ward clerk and placed directly upon the patient's medication administration record. In addition, the order as written by the surgeon shall be noted.

Two things are being done here. The sticker is being used and the surgeon is writing an order in reduced dosage. If for some reason either procedure is not done, the other will serve as a back-up. As with any procedures, adherence will depend upon several factors, including appropriate supervision. It should be noted that the labels provided have a nonpermanent adhesive and can be used, peeled off and reused several times.

10:304, 1975

Error 17

Floor stock of Vitamin B-12 injection became depleted on one of a hospital's patient care units. Someone called the pharmacy to inform the pharmacist of the shortage. While on the telephone, the person asked if it would be all right to substitute two doses of Vitamin B-6.

On the surface, this situation is certainly laughable. It actually happened. It shows that a real problem exists. Whoever is charged with the responsibility of administering medications needs to be educated. Except for students who are under constant supervision, only sufficiently trained people should be permitted to be responsible for any facet of the medication cycle. We should realize that we can't take anything for granted.

10:305, 1975

Problems with NCR or carbon copies of orders

The advantages of pharmacists receiving direct copies of physician's orders rather than transcriptions made by ward personnel are widely known. These advantages certainly outweigh any disadvantages associated with use of direct copies. However, aside from the obvious situation of orders being less legible when received as copies, there are some other problems. Two of these have surfaced as medication errors.

Error 18

An order was written for the following:

Cytoxan 325 mg
Fluorouracil 325 mg   IV PUSH
Adriamycin 32 mg   TONIGHT

The order was written on an NCR physician's order form with the patient's name addressoplated at the top. The physician writing the order had obtained this patient's form as well as the form for a second patient from an order book in which these were kept.

While the order was being written, the second sheet was inadvertently placed under the first. The order was written with enough pressure to appear not only on the copy of the first patient's sheet, but also on the copy of the second patient's sheet. Both sets of orders were noted, scheduled and requested from Pharmacy. Fortunately, the pharmacist became suspicious when identical orders for cancer chemotherapy were received at the same time for two patients. The drugs were not administered to the second patient.

Prevention

Prevention in this case is difficult. Those using NCR forms must be aware of the possibility of this occurrence. Unless the form is in a chart or a properly separated order book, nothing but the writing surface should be underneath an NCR form when something is being written. Thick cardboard or X-ray film must always separate different patients' NCR forms when the forms are kept in medication books.

I've also experienced a similar occurrence involving a single patient when two blank NCR forms are placed unseparated into a patient's chart. Orders written on the first form will come through on the second. These may be received at a later time when original orders are written on the first page of the second sheet. This is particularly a problem with one-time orders, stats, preoperative seda-

tions and IV orders. These orders may inadvertently be reprocessed. Usually, the writing on the second sheet's copy is just a shade lighter than normal and can often be recognized, but this is not always the case. Be cautious!

10:350, 1975

Error 19

In this case, an order was written on an NCR form for digoxin 0.25 mg p.o. daily. The order was noted, the copy removed and sent to Pharmacy for processing. The drug was dispensed and administered for several days. Signs of digitalis toxicity began to develop in the patient. Digoxin was discontinued.

During investigation of the possible causes of the toxicity, the physician checked the dose that was being administered. He was very surprised to learn that digoxin 0.25 mg was being given. He stated that although this was what he had in mind originally, soon after he wrote that order he returned to the order sheet to reduce the dose to 0.125 mg. He simply inserted the number 1 before the number 2. Unbeknown to him, the order had already been processed, and the copy removed. No one but the physician knew of the dose reduction.

Prevention

It should be noted that this same error could have happened where no NCR copy was being used. The only real prevention is educational. Those who use such forms must know of the problem of changing orders which have already been written. All changes must be completely rewritten. In this incident, a new order

136

should have been written, reducing the dose.

A partial solution would be to use forms with multiple NCR copies that are full pages rather than the commonly used perforated backings. When an order is changed, it will appear on the next page that is received. Unfortunately, this change will not be seen until the next set of orders is written.

10:350, 1975

Error 20

Check Labels on Diluents

How often do nurses, physicians and pharmacists reconstitute unstable powders for parenteral use using diluents from glass ampuls? How often do we pharmacists dispense these diluents, sometimes along with drugs for reconstitution, to the patient care areas? Most of us do it many times during the course of a normal working day.

Now ask yourself how often you really look at the labels on the diluents you use or dispense.

The following actual errors, all involving antibiotic powders, attest to the fact that we're not all doing our job.

A. Clindamycin injection 4 ml ampuls were used to reconstitute a drug. Two doses of powder were inadvertently reconstituted with clindamycin and given.
B. Ampuls of paraldehyde injection 5 ml were found to be attached to vials of antibiotic powders. This was done in the act of dispensing the doses to the patient care area. No doses were mixed, because the error was discovered after the first

ampul was opened and the odor detected.

C. Phenytoin injection (as solution in ampul) was used for reconstitution. One dose of powder was mixed with phenytoin and given.

Prevention

You might ask yourself how these errors could occur. Primarily, they occur because we're more interested in and pay more attention to the drug label than the label of the diluent used to reconstitute the drug. The latter may not even be seen. In all of these examples mentioned the solution in the glass ampul was clear and colorless and appeared to have the same viscosity as water or saline, the most common diluents. All that is really being confirmed is that the solution appears to be water or saline. The labeling of some glass ampuls in which the information is printed directly onto the glass also contributes to the problem. When an opaque background (look at atropine sulfate by Burroughs-Wellcome) or a paper label is used for the printing, readability is greatly improved.

Another factor that contributes to the possibility of this error is poor storage. In one of the cases described (A, clindamycin), the ampuls were stored in close proximity to similarly sized and colored sterile water for injection.

The possibility exists that some IV incompatibilities which you may have learned about (but which are not reproducible) are a result of this. Another possibility is that what was thought to be a drug defect when a precipitate appeared after a powdered drug was reconstituted really was the result of an incorrect diluent being used.

10:352, 1975

Error 21

An error that shows lack of thought

An oncologist intended to have his medical student write an order for chlorambucil (Leukeran) 8 mg daily onto the chart of a patient of his who had Hodgkin's disease. Unfortunately, the student inadvertently wrote the order on the wrong patient's chart, the chart of the patient's roommate. The order was processed by nursing and pharmacy personnel for this wrong patient. The drug was given to the wrong patient for nearly two weeks. A routine blood count done at that time revealed severe bone marrow depression. Treatment had to be started for this person and isolation was necessary.

Prevention

On the surface, it seems clearcut that this was an error caused by a careless student, but let's look closer.

First of all, there was a lack of supervision on the part of the oncologist. Writing orders for prescription drugs is a great responsibility, especially on an oncology service. The hospital had a rule that all orders written by students were to be countersigned by a licensed physician. This was not done. The student cannot be fully blamed.

Secondly, the nurses and pharmacists responsible for the medication orders on these patients did not use their heads. The fact that the patient who received the drug had no neoplastic disease did not enter their minds. In fact, this was not even checked. Here is a perfect example of the importance of nurses and pharmacists obtaining diagnostic information in addition to allergies on their nursing kardex and patient profiles. If this type of information had been sought and used, this terrible error could have been prevented.

We can all think of many other situations in which diagnoses should be confirmed before drugs are ordered, dispensed and administered. It seems so basic — yet if you ask people involved with these errors why they didn't check, their stock answer is: "I didn't have the time. I was just too busy." Let's make it clear that that answer just doesn't hold up in court. If it were one of my relatives who was injured, I know I couldn't accept it.

This serious error injured a patient. At the same time, a patient who might have benefitted from chlorambucil therapy was denied the drug.

10:376, 1975

Errors 22 and 23

Poor handwriting and spelling leads to error

Two more potential errors have been reported that could have been caused by poor handwriting.

Lomotil tablets were nearly given as an overdose because of the following order:

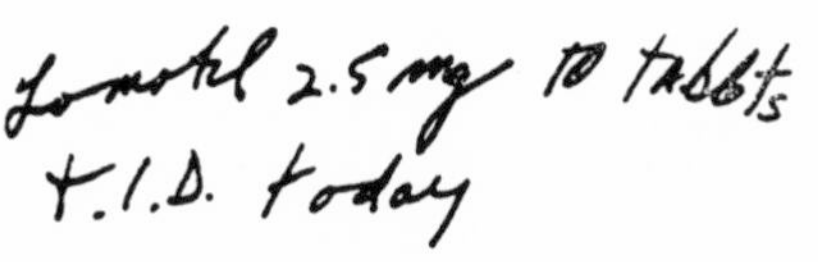

Figure 10

This order was taken to mean 10 tablets three times a day. The physician who wrote the order (an American graduate) used the word "to" instead of "two" to refer to the number of tablets.

Fortunately, in the hospital where this incident occurred, Lomotil was not a floor stock item. When the pharmacist received the request for 10 tablets three times a day, the error was recognized.

138

The following order for Lasix was written:

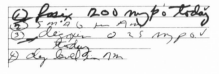

Figure 11

This was interpreted as Lasix 1200 mg to be given orally. This dose did not seem high, since similar doses given intravenously were used in this hospital. Thirty Lasix 40 mg tablets were about to be requested for a single dose when a supervisor arrived. The supervisor became aware of the situation when the person responsible for administering medications complained about having to give so many tablets to the patient for a single dose. The physician was consulted. He acknowledged that poor writing might lead one to believe that 1200 mg of Lasix was written. What he wanted was 200 mg. He had originally written 120 mg but changed his mind. He tried to combine the one with the two to make it look like a two only. If this were an intravenous dose being ordered, it is doubtful that the error would have been caught.

10:376, 1975

Error 24

Error due to unfamiliarity with drug dose

The following order was written for a 64-year-old patient weighing 110 lbs with Stage III squamous cell carcinoma (buccal mucosa) for treatment of hypercalcemia:

Mithramycin 1250 mcg in 1000 ml dextrose 5% in water to run at 150 ml per hour x 3 bottles.

This hospital had a centralized intravenous additive service. The nurse telephoned the service and asked that all three bottles be prepared and delivered to the patient care area. The pharmacist questioned that amount of mithramycin for a single day. Subsequently, the physician remembered the dosage was supposed to be 1250 mcg/day for three or four days — not 1250 mcg in three or four bottles a day. Thus, an overdosage of an extremely toxic drug was averted.

Without an IV additive service this error would almost certainly have taken place. Physicians, nurses and pharmacists must be especially careful when prescribing, administering or dispensing drugs with which they may be unfamiliar. Appropriate literature should be reviewed carefully before the use of an uncommon drug.

10:378, 1975

Errors 25 and 26

Errors of omission: patient refusal

Not administering a medication that has been prescribed for a hospitalized patient is usually considered to be a medication error. There are many reasons for omitting doses of medication. Some of these reasons are: the patient being unavailable at the time the dose was due, a missed transcription of a physician's order and, for oral doses, the patient being given nothing by mouth (NPO).

Another common reason for omitting a dose is patient refusal. Reasons for refusal need to be examined. In some cases, patient knowledge of a previous unfavorable situation which accompanied his taking the drug may be the cause. For example, the patient fears recurrence of a side effect. Wherever possible, those responsible should take the time to reason with the patient to get his cooperation. Perhaps a different drug will be needed. Another reason for refusal is that the patient thinks the drug is not needed. Judgment on the part of the health professional is necessary here. A sleeping patient justifiably may refuse a scheduled h.s. sedation. Yet other drugs that may be refused are essential and again reasoning with the patient will be necessary.

A third reason is that patients may have been made anxious about taking a drug. It may be because they've learned something from a friend or a relative or have overheard or misinterpreted a health professional's remarks about the drug.

The following medication omission reports illustrate another possible way anxiety may be instilled in the mind of a patient — carelessness and thoughtlessness by the person responsible for administering medication.

An alcoholic patient admitted to a hospital began hallucinating and stated that he was driving a bus. Intramuscular paraldehyde was ordered for delirium tremens. Since paraldehyde rapidly attacks plastic, a glass syringe was used. When administration of the drug was attempted, the patient became unruly. It was impossible to inject the drug intramuscularly. The patient was asked whether he would agree to take the drug orally, mixed in juice; he agreed to this. The paraldehyde syringe was taken to the medication preparation area and its contents squirted into a cup of orange juice. The solution was then taken into the patient's room and mixed. As the patient sat up to take the dose, the plastic spoon was removed from the cup. It was completely misshapen. Just then, the cup began to leak from the bottom and sides. A plastic spoon had been used to mix the solution in a styrofoam cup. The patient remarked: "Uh-uh! I ain't taking that stuff. You people are trying to kill me!"

In another case, 10 drops of Lugol's solution (strong iodine solution) was to be administered to a patient before 131 I administration. A cup of orange juice and a dropper bottle of Lugol's solution were taken to the patient's bedside. Ten drops of the Lugol's solution were added and mixed with the juice. The dropper bottle of Lugol's solution was placed on the night stand and the patient was instructed to drink the solution. The patient began to scream; he had seen the label of the Lugol's. A skull and crossbones and the word POISON was prominently written in red. The patient feared the worst. Most laymen, taking the situation at face value, would have, too.

These two actual situations are laughable at first glance but they illustrate how a normal reaction of anxiety is elicited and medications are refused. Are the personnel at your hospital prepared to avoid situations such as these? In both cases, the reaction of the patient to what he had seen was appropriate. The situations could have been avoided with a little forethought by the person administering the medication.

10:442, 1975

Error 27

More errors of order interpretation

Several "mini" errors have been received. The following misinterpretations of drugs ordered deserve publicity in your institution.

Ordered	Error
a. Zactirin 1 tid	Misinterpreted as Bactrim 1 tid.
b. Surbex T bid	Transcribed and administered as such. The suffix "T" was misinterpreted as script Roman numeral one (1). Plain Surbex was administered twice daily.

140

Ordered	Error
c. Mylanta II qid	The suffix II was misinterpreted to mean that two Mylanta tablets were to be administered qid. Mylanta II liquid was actually ordered but no volume prescribed.
d. Tylenol #3 qid prn	Three tablets of Tylenol were administered when needed. What was intended was Tylenol No. 3 (Tylenol with Codeine 30 mg).
e. Ascriptin tablets #2 prn pain	One Ascriptin with Codeine 15 mg was administered. Two Ascriptin tablets were intended.

B, c, d and e above point out primarily the danger associated with the manufacturer's inappropriate choice of names and also the need to educate those involved in ordering, dispensing and administering medication.

10:444, 1975

Error 28

Confusing labeling

Several bottles of extemporaneously mixed total parenteral nutrition (TPN) solutions were prepared with deficient electrolyte concentrations. Only 50% of the calcium listed on the additive label was present. The solutions were also deficient in sodium, potassium, magnesium and anions. Investigation traced the deficiencies to an error in extrapolation of the concentration of electrolytes listed on the manufacturer's label. In the original solution 10% Amigen Injection was used. A volume of 500 ml of this solution is contained in a 1000 ml bottle. (There is presently a 500 ml vacuum to allow for easy addition by suction of 500 ml of 50% dextrose solution as well as addi-

tional electrolytes.) Yet electrolytes are listed on the Amigen label in milliequivalents per liter (Fig. 12). This causes people to think that the concentration of electrolytes as listed is present in the final solution of 1000 ml (500 ml of 10% Amigen and 500 ml of 50% dextrose). In fact, the concentration listed would be in two 500 ml bottles of 10% Amigen.

This error has actually been reported more than once. The potential seriousness of the error is obvious. The error may also happen with amino acid or protein solutions distributed by other manufacturers. In fact, all solutions containing electrolytes list these as milliequivalents per liter—regardless of volume. The error is more likely where partially filled bottles are used, however.

The fault does not lie with the manufacturer. Labeling requirements of the USP force them to label solutions in this manner. New requirements in USP XIX will make it mandatory for manufacturers to list also the osmolarity of electrolyte solutions. Again, this must be listed in milliosmols per liter, which also may invite error.

A better way to label these solutions is in total content per unit of container.

10:444, 1975

Error 29

Always read labels!

An eczematous patient in a dermatology ward complained of severe itching. The patient's physician ordered Phenergan 12.5 mg every four hours PRN itch. A unit dose system which included a drug cart with individual patient bins was used in this hospital. For PRN medications, a 24-hour supply of unit dose packages of drugs were placed in zip-lock bags. The order for Phenergan was received in pharmacy and the PRN bag was prepared and dispensed. A dose was given to the patient when the drug was delivered to the ward. A few hours later the patient complained that no relief of the itching had been obtained after the medicine was administered. He did, however, have an additional complaint, the medicine seemed to cause him to have to urinate three times within a two-hour period. The nurse convinced the patient to give the drug one more try. This time as she opened the bag to take out the dose of Phenergan her eye caught the label of the commercial unit dose package. It read: "Lasix 40 mg." The remainder of unit dose packages were also Lasix.

In another case, a patient in pain as a result of minor surgery was to receive a dose of codeine sulfate 30 mg along with two aspirin tablets. The codeine was obtained from a unit dose, controlled drug supply which was stored in a locked cupboard. After the medication was administered and the preparation area was being cleared, the empty package just used was noted to read "phenobarbital 30 mg." This had been administered instead of codeine.

In both of these cases those persons involved with the medication errors committed would no doubt claim that the reason they dispensed and/or administered the wrong drug was because the drugs are so similarly packaged that they were just assumed to be the correct drug. In the second case, storage in such close proximity also would be stated as a reason for the error. It is true that the medication packages are similar. The Phenergan 12.5 mg unit dose aluminum foil package looks like the Lasix 40 mg unit dose aluminum foil package.

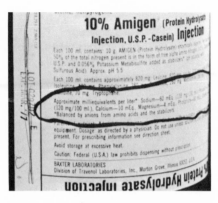

Figure 12. Label for 10% Amigen injection. Note concentration in milliequivalents per liter, although only 500 ml of solution is present in 1000 ml container.

Wyeth's unit dose phenobarbital 30 mg looks similar to unit dose codeine sulfate 30 mg. However, this is not the real reason for the error. The real reason is carelessness. Those responsible for handling medications must learn to read labels. This means that every package should be looked at. Medication administration personnel should get the habit of reading labels at least three times; when obtaining the medication, when administering or dispensing it and when discarding the empty package or returning unused medicine to the storage area.

The pharmacy technician I worked with, Bill Dowd, helped me to develop this habit. One day while he was working with me, a doctor came running into the pharmacy for Benadryl injection, stat. He had a patient who was experiencing an extrapyramidal reaction to a phenothiazine. He gave me a verbal order and left to go to the patient. I quickly obtained an ampul of what I thought was the correct drug, broke it open, drew it up and ran it out to the physician who administered it to the patient. When I re-

142

turned to the pharmacy, I saw that Bill looked bothered.

"What did you give out?" Bill asked. "Benadryl," I answered. He said, "No, it was Pitocin." I looked at the open ampul and sure enough it was Pitocin. I couldn't believe it! I then realized that I really had never looked at the label; I had just assumed it was Benadryl because of the ampul's appearance. The open Pitocin ampul looked just like a Benadryl ampul. "Scared you, didn't I?" Bill laughed. "If you had read the label on the ampul when you took it out of the drawer and when you drew it up, you wouldn't be so scared now. You'd know that you really gave out Benadryl. I just switched it while you were out — just wanted to teach you a lesson."

10:480, 1975

Error 30

Patient identification for drug orders

An order was written for Elixophyllin 30 ml p.o. QID on an NCR order sheet with only the patient's surname handwritten in the space provided for patient identification. The usual address-a-plate stamp was not used. The name appeared to be Brewer. A copy of the order was removed from the original and the drug was scheduled to be given to patient "Brewer." Three doses of Elixophyllin were administered. Later, a physician inquired at the nurses station to find out why the Elixophyllin he ordered for his patient, Mr. Brinson, had not yet been given. The lack of full patient identification on the order form had caused personnel to schedule the medication for the wrong patient. The handwritten name on closer examination did appear to be Brinson and not Brewer.

A similar medication error involving administration of a course of Gantrisin Suspension to the wrong patient occurred because the patient identification on the prescription order was inadequate. Only a first name initial and last name were used (E. Jackson). The order, written for Edna Jackson, was scheduled and dispensed by pharmacy to Ellen Jackson, who happened to be a patient on the same floor.

Those who transcribe and note orders must always use complete identification. If an address-a-plate is not available, at least full first and last names, bed number and patient identification number (chart number) should be used. Pharmacists who receive individual prescription orders should insist on at least this much information before dispensing any medications for a patient.

It should also be mentioned that hospital admitting offices should do all that is possible to separate patients with the same surname into different areas of the hospital. This would also help to decrease errors similar to those described.

10:483, 1975

Error 31

Inadequate labeling by manufacturer

Cromolyn sodium capsules were prescribed for a patient with asthma. The medication, ineffective orally, is administered by inhalation, using a special inhaler provided by the manufacturer. After initial instructions were given to the patient and to floor personnel responsible for medications, the drug was dispensed. The hospital in which this incident took place happened to have a centralized unit dose program with two cart fills daily. Only the capsules were dispensed with each cart fill. The inhaler and instructions remained in the patient bin in the cart along with other oral medications being dispensed. After two days it was discovered that despite the precautions taken to prevent this, several doses of cromolyn had been given orally. Investigation led to the discovery that the error had been committed by a temporary floor-replacement person who was unfamiliar with the use of the medication. This person had not been assigned to the floor at the time instructions were given. The patient was unaware of the error.

Complete information was not given to me with this report. I would assume that the medication record book or the Kardex also listed the route of administration as inhalation. With all the precautions taken at first glance, it's hard to understand how the error could occur. Yet, on closer examination, someone who's used to administering oral medications from unit dose packages could easily make the mistake, unless the Kardex is read completely for route of administration. When it is unwrapped, the capsule certainly appears to be an oral dose. Additionally, there is no notation on the package that the medication is for inhalation use with the special inhaler only (Fig. 13). If the manufacturers of cromolyn sodium had placed this note of caution on the label besides just their company name, errors such as this would have less probability of occurring.

It should be noted that the name of the drug and the strength also is not listed on the package. This is another problem that should be rectified. Pharmaceutical manufacturers should acknowledge that many of their medications are going to be used in unit dose hospitals. Medications that are already unit packaged, such

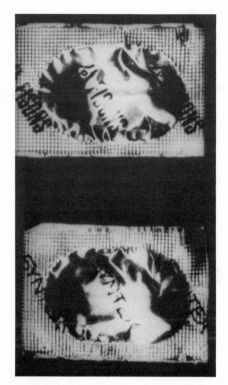

Figure 13. Cromolyn sodium capsules manufactured by Syntex and Fisons. No drug name appears. No notice of caution for inhalation only with special inhaler appears either.

as the above, should be fully labeled. Until the manufacturers comply with these suggestions, whenever cromolyn sodium is dispensed into patient bins for patients in a unit dose hospital, each package should have a label placed on it with the name of the medication, strength and the caution "For inhalation, using special inhaler only." (Note: manufacturers have since made these labeling changes.)

Errors such as this also show that a need exists for internal continuing education programs with in-service training and pharmacy bulletins.

10:483, 1975

Error 32

Mix-up of two different drugs packaged in similar-appearing glass ampuls

A patient for whom pentazocine (Talwin, Winthrop) 30 mg intramuscularly was ordered received a dose of diphenhydramine 50 mg intramuscularly instead. It was discovered that the pentazocine supply section in the patient care area had been inadvertently stocked with ampuls of diphenhydramine manufactured by the Vitarine Corporation.

At first glance the two different ampuls appear identical. Although both are properly labeled, and admittedly the error would not have occurred if those responsible for supplying and later administering the drug had read the label, it is easy to understand how this error happened.

Since Talwin Injection was released in the '60's, the 30 mg dose has been packaged in the same distinctive clear glass ampul with aqua printing and red color break band. The labeling on the ampul is difficult to read. Now, Vitarine's ampul of diphenhydramine is manufactured in a similar-appearing ampul, with the same hard-to-read aqua printing. These ampuls also have a red color break band. The individual responsible for stocking the supply, and later the one responsible for obtaining and administering the drug, were fooled by the similarity in appearance.

Pharmaceutical manufacturers usually attempt to avoid using names for soon-to-be-released drugs that look and sound like those of any that are already marketed. This is done to alleviate confusion. Names of drugs have even been changed to prevent confusion when the written name may resemble that of another drug (Larocin became Larotid because the former was sometimes mistaken for Lanoxin).

An effort must be made by manufacturers to prevent new drug packages from physically resembling those of drugs already marketed. Also, pharmacists who purchase drugs should request a sample of the item before they buy, and look at it for such confusing similarities. Pharmacists should do all they can to help those who administer medications; however, it is the responsibility of these personnel to read labels.

10:526, 1975

Error 33

A nurse and a pharmacist second-guess a physician's order that is incomplete

A physician wrote the following order: "ANTIVERT, one tablet qid." The order was noted as such in nursing records and on the pharmacy patient profile. In the pharmacy, it was assumed that tablets of 12.5 mg were desired. These were dispensed and administered for eight doses. Later, another pharmacist, realizing that the drug was manufactured in both a 12.5 mg and 25 mg tablet size, decided to check with the physician to clarify the order. The physician had intended to have the patient receive 25 mg tablets.

This error would not have occurred had the physician written the prescription properly, indicating strength desired. However, when different tablet strengths are available and the dose desired is not indicated, pharmacists and nurses should not second-guess physicians. No doses should be dispensed in this situation until the proper strength is known.

Many would argue that this was not

really an error; however, the fact remains that the patient did not receive the dose that the physician intended. Primarily a matter of physician education, this type of error is most commonly seen when a drug is marketed in a new strength. Trouble can be expected with such new additions as Hydergine tablets 1 mg and Lasix tablets 20 mg and 80 mg. Physicians must be trained to specify a strength even when only one strength is available, as this can change.

10:526, 1975

Reader comments

About error 33, (a nurse and a pharmacist second-guess a physician's incomplete order)

Regarding error 33 in "Medication Error Reports," the pharmacist dispensed Antivert 12.5 mg instead of 25 mg as the physician intended. This was not in error. Roerig's labeling for this product is Antivert or Antivert/25. Hence, when Antivert is written by a physician, the physician has ordered 12.5 mg. This does not apply to other multiple strength products, but Antivert and Antivert/25 are so labeled.

G.A. Stock, Jr., Pharmacist
Doctors Hospital Inc.
at Stark County
Massillon, Ohio

Editor's reply

I appreciate Mr. Stock's bringing this to my attention. I would agree that this was not a pharmacist-caused error. However, as noted in the report, the patient did not receive the intended dose of 25 mg. Therefore, it was still considered an error, albeit the physician's, for not specifying Antivert/25.

Additional thoughts related to error 33

Until recently, the only strength of acetaminophen tablets available was 325 mg. Since only the 325 mg tablets have been available, even though the dose most often prescribed is 650 mg, many physicians have gotten used to prescribing the drug as "2 tablets" rather than by milligram strength.

Now, however, Philips-Roxane Laboratories has marketed a 650 mg tablet in unit dose packaging. For patient convenience, many hospitals no doubt will purchase and use this product. There is now a strong possibility that if the drug is ordered as "2 tablets," two x 650 mg may be used. To avoid the possibility of medication errors, the following procedure is suggested if your institution uses the new 650 mg tablet:

1. Give adequate publicity to the new tablet strength, stressing that the change is being made for patient convenience.
2. Ask nurses, pharmacists and physicians to use milligram strength *only* when referring to acetaminophen doses. Make sure you or the nurses in your hospital inform physicians of the problem if they write "2 tablets."
3. Enter doses on patient profiles and medication administration records as milligram strength.
4. If an order for "2 tablets" is received, check order transcriptions in the patient care area to see that 650 mg is written — not two tablets. Inform the prescriber.

Error 34
Hazardous abbreviations

The abbreviation CPZ was used to denote Compazine (prochlor-

146

perazine) in the following order: "CPZ 10 mg IM q 4 H PRN." The order was interpreted as chlorpromazine (Thorazine) instead. Several doses were administered in error.

This abbreviation is obviously confusing and should be avoided. If you see it, always check to learn which drug is being requested. Physicians must be discouraged from prescribing or using coined abbreviations. Pharmacists should not use these abbreviations on patient profiles, newsletters or in other communications. Authors should not use these abbreviations in articles or textbooks. Discourage their use at every opportunity.

10:527, 1975

Error 35

Preventing dosage errors with warfarin sodium

A patient with pulmonary embolism was being treated with warfarin sodium. The patient's physician began therapy by prescribing 10 mg doses on the first two consecutive days. Prothrombin times were being monitored. On the third day, although the prothrombin time was reported early, the physician was detained in the Operating Room. He had not ordered a dose of warfarin by the 3 pm nursing shift change time. This was communicated to the 3 pm-11 pm nursing shift during nursing report. One of the nurses was asked to contact the surgeon to remind him to order the dose. The nurse forgot and the patient missed the dose that day.

It has been my observation that of the drugs reported to be involved in medication errors, warfarin sodium is one of those implicated most frequently. This is no doubt attributable to the frequently serious nature of the error. It is too risky for the person who committed the error to try and cover it up. Frequently, overdoses cannot be hidden. Health professionals seem to feel more obliged to report errors of omission or inadvertent administration of warfarin to the wrong patient.

Because of the unique dosing requirements of each patient when therapy is initiated, routine daily doses are impossible. The drug dose may be changed each day and because of this, ordered doses are more easily missed or mixed up with other patients.

A method that has been successful in preventing dosage errors with warfarin has been developed by the pharmacists at Temple University Hospital. A "Warfarin Therapy Record" is kept for each nursing unit in the hospital (Fig. 14). When a patient is first given the drug, his room number and name are listed on the form. Except for the initial dose, before any warfarin is dispensed, prothrombin time must be determined. These values are obtainable from the hospital laboratory. This allows the pharmacist to check against the laboratory value for appropriateness of dose ordered. It also allows for a day-to-day following of prothrombin times; this assists in recognition of possible drug interaction or misreporting of laboratory values.

This form is taped to the metal front of the Acme Visible Line File containing Pharmacy patient profiles for each nursing unit. The listing of names is checked each day and doses and prothrombin times entered on this sheet and the patient's profile. If doses are not ordered by the end of the day, physicians are contacted by telephone and advised of prothrombin time. On discharge or upon discontinuation of the drug, a yellow line is drawn through the patient's name.

ROOM NO.	PATIENT NAME	DATE	$^1/_{13}$	$^1/_{14}$	$^1/_{15}$	$^1/_{16}$							
5398	Ray Close	Dose	10mg	10mg	7½mg	7½mg							
		P.T.	None	18.4	23	20							
5Y1A	Ted Allister	Dose	10mg	10mg	2½mg	7½mg							
		P.T.	none	17	21.8	17.4							
521A	Matthew Reed	Dose		10mg	10mg	7½mg							
		P.T.		None	18.6	21.5							
		Dose											
		P.T.											
		Dose											
		P.T.											
		Dose											
		P.T.											
		Dose											
		P.T.											
		Dose											
		P.T.											
		Dose											
		P.T.											

TUH PHARMACY WARFARIN THERAPY

X-1132 REV. 7/74

Figure 14. Warfarin therapy record.

A form such as this might be useful to nurses if it is not possible for pharmacists to become involved.

Backup systems such as these are developed for patient safety. Let us not forget, however, that laxity on the part of some physicians is why we must do this. Efforts must be made by hospital authorities to correct physician laxity.

10:527, 1975

Error 36

Poor labeling of Evans Blue Injection ampul

A pharmacist asked a pharmacy technician for an ampul of Evans Blue Injection. The technician delivered a 5 ml clear glass ampul containing a clear solution (Fig. 15). Although at first this ampul was thought to be mislabeled, closer inspection revealed some small hard-to-read print-ing. It named the solution correctly as normal saline solution. It was followed by even smaller letters "for use with," then large easy-to-see block letters "Evans Blue Injection, USP." The Evans Blue ampul inventory was then checked.

Although the number of diluent ampuls matched the number of dye ampuls when originally purchased, there were now several more dye ampuls than those of diluent present. It could not be determined for certain whether or not diluent ampuls had been dispensed for dye. The manufacturer of these ampuls should never have labeled them in this manner.

11:22, 1976

Error 37

Incorrect dose of procaine penicillin G administered because its formulation characteristics were not known

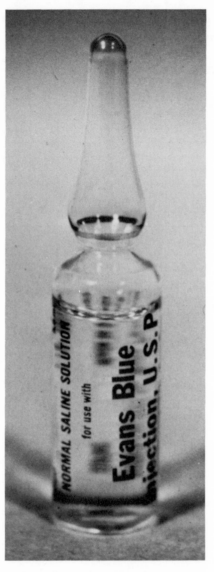

Figure 15

complaint about the "icky stuff" that sits at the bottom of the vial. Unless this person was very careful to not aspirate any of this "icky stuff," it would enter the needle and clog! Apparently, several doses of only the supernatant liquid of the procaine penicillin G suspension had been given by this person.

This incident once again demonstrates that a deplorable lack of basic awareness of the competency of personnel exists on the part of some health professionals who have responsible positions in the drug distribution cycle. Although I have previously pointed out that cases such as these demonstrate a need for more education within institutions, it appears that in this situation, the real fault lies with poor supervision. Someone who does not know what a suspension is, does not read labels. The vial was labeled ("shake well"). The person who does not read this and does not at least immediately question "icky stuff" present in a vial of parenteral medication should not be allowed to be responsible for medication administration. Hospital administrators and department heads have the responsibility to monitor the competency of their employes. When this is not done, errors such as this one and the tragic one reported next are bound to occur.

11:22, 1976

Several days after a 12 ml vial of procaine penicillin G was dispensed to a patient care unit for a specific order, one of the persons responsible for medication administration returned to the hospital pharmacy for additional supply. While waiting for the drug, this person registered a

Error 38

Overdoses of chloramphenicol administered because of poor labeling and uninformed personnel responsible for drug administration.

A letter-to-the-editor in the *Journal of the American Medical Association* reported that at least five patients have accidentally received 10 times the intended dose of chloramphenicol. One patient received a 20 g dose and died 11 hours later. The other patients, including a four-month-old infant, were made severely ill but recovered. In the case in which 20 g of drug was administered, 20 one-gram vials had to be reconstituted. As reported by the authors of the case report, the explanation of the error was misinterpretation of new labeling present on vials of chloromycetin sodium succinate injection by Parke-Davis.

Admittedly, the new label was not designed well (Fig. 16). Whereas the old style label (right) clearly stated that the vial contained 1 g. the newer label stated that, when reconstituted, 100 mg would be present in 1 ml. Unless the label is read very carefully, a quick glance may lead an uninformed person to believe that only 100 mg is present in the bottle. This is apparently what happened in the situation in which 20 vials were reconstituted and administered.

But the poor labeling on the vial cannot be blamed entirely for this incident. How could someone responsible for drug administration give the medication without knowing, or at least questioning someone about, the usual dose? How could someone reconstitute 20 vials of a drug without thinking that something was odd about that? How could someone administer a drug without knowing anything about its side effects and toxicity? It just shouldn't happen.

A person capable of this should have been discovered by a supervisor before being left alone and not permitted to practice until competence could be demonstrated.

A subsequent label change of this product has corrected the problem.

10:22, 1976

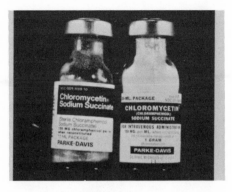

Figure 16

Error 39

Misinterpretation of drug order due to poor handwriting and misspelling by a physician.

The following order was misinterpreted as Doriden (glutethimide):

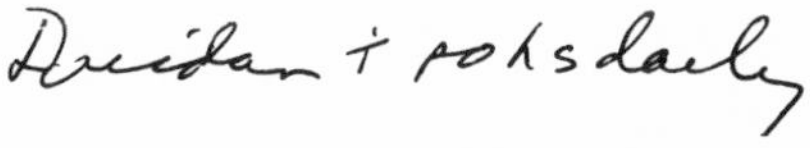

Figure 17

Doriden was given for one dose, after which it was discovered that what the physician actually had intended the patient to receive was Doxidan. The error occurred because of poor handwriting and misspelling by a physician when ordering. In script, the drug names appear similar. The fact that the dose of each drug is usually one dosage unit given at bedtime reinforced the error. If both of these drugs are available at your hospital, publicity should be given to this incident to make everyone aware of the problem.

11:76, 1976

Error 40

Patient inadvertently receives inert ophthalmic solution for treatment of severe eye infection.

150

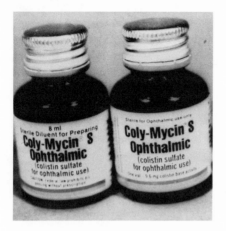

Figure 18

A patient suffering a *Pseudomonas aeruginosa* infection of the eyes was seen by an ophthalmologist, who prescribed colistin sulfate as an ophthalmic solution. This preparation is available on special request from Warner-Lambert Laboratories.

Upon receipt of the medication (packaged as in Figure 18), a vial of solution was removed from the box and the dropper was attached. The medication was then dispensed to the patient care area, where it was used to administer the medication for several days. When a fresh supply was needed and the second vial was removed from the box, it was noted that, unlike the first vial of solution, this vial contained only a small amount of dry powder. Close inspection of the labels on both bottles disclosed that one vial contained active drug for reconstitution while the other vial contained the diluent.

This information on the labels is very difficult to see when compared to the size of the printing of the brand name of the drug. This vial should be clearly marked as DILUENT. Had this been done by the company, a serious error might have been avoided.

Let us not forget to mention once again the importance of practitioners reading labels fully before administering medications. Even though the information is difficult to obtain from the label, it is there, and if read, would also have prevented the error.

11:76, 1976

Error 41
Inert medication dispensed because manufacturer's package was used improperly

An order was received in the pharmacy for Norlestrin 2.5 mg tablets to be given four times daily. The patient for whom the order was written had vaginal bleeding. Tablets were obtained from a partially used blister pack of Norlestrin birth control pills. Seven brown tablets remained out of the original 28 tablets. These were dispensed and administered for the first seven doses. After two days, a fresh package of birth control pills was opened. A different pharmacist dispensed several more doses.

The person administering medications was surprised to see a color difference in the tablets dispensed by pharmacy the second time. The second tablets were pink; this was questioned. It was discovered that the original seven tablets dispensed that were brown in color were actually ferrous fumerate tablets. These remained in the package after the active pills (pink) had been punched out. The birth control pill package was Norlestrin Fe 2.5 mg. Someone had returned the remaining iron tablets portion of the blister to stock. The patient was still bleeding after the seven doses of iron.

This error would have been prevented if stock bottles of Norlestrin had been used instead of the oral con-

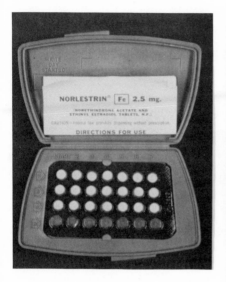

Figure 19

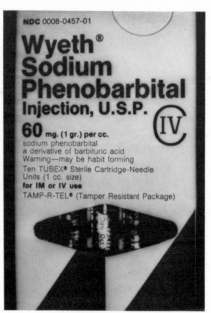

Figure 20

traception package. However, if only the birth control pill packaging was available, the person using the active tablets should have made certain that the remaining iron tablets were discarded. Preferably, the iron tablets should have been punched out as soon as the package was opened for use other than as birth control pills.

11:80, 1976

Error 42

Misinterpretation of controlled-substances symbol

A potential medication error was averted when a pharmacist was questioned by a student nurse about the controlled-substance symbol appearing on a package of ampuls of Winthrop's Luminal Sodium (phenobarbital sodium). The symbol used for phenobarbital injection is ⓋV (see Wyeth tubex product in Figure 20). The interpretation was that the Roman numeral IV was actually the letter abbreviation for intravenous (I.V.).

One might think that this misinterpretation is an extremely rare isolated incident, but my own observation is that this is not so. Apparently, the controlled-substance symbols are not always understood by health professionals who are not pharmacists. Of six such people shown the package in Figure 20 and asked for an interpretation, five made the same mistake as the student nurse.

This could present a problem for people who administer intravenous medications, especially if a physician's order lacks instruction for route of administration: the IV may be interpreted as meaning that the drug may only be given intravenously. I wouldn't be completely surprised if I learned of someone questioning whether or not a long-acting injection or even a noninjectable dosage form could be given intravenously.

Presently, the federal law (Drug Enforcement Agency regulations

152

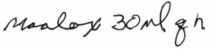

Figure 21

1302.03 through 1302.06) requires that the controlled substances symbol IV or C-IV be placed on commercial labels of containers of any schedule IV drug. The use of the Arabic number C-4 or 4 would be a solution to the problem and should be allowed. Appropriate educational efforts should be undertaken to make the hospital staff aware of the meaning of the symbols. DEA has been contacted. (See Error 109).

11:106, 1976

Error 43

Hazardous unauthorized abbreviation: Q.N.

An order was written for liquid Maalox to be given nightly. The abbreviation q.n. was used by the physician to mean every night (Fig. 21). The abbreviation, in script on the physician's order form of the patient chart, appeared to the nurse to be q.h. Because Maalox is often given hourly to patients with peptic ulcer disease, this further justified to the nurse that an hourly dosage was what was ordered.

Due to the nature of the medication involved, no harm came to the patient because of the error. However, a much more serious error could certainly have occurred because of this abbreviation. The abbreviation q.n. was not approved for use in the hospital. (See also Error No. 8.)

11:106, 1976

Error 44

Wrong route of administration used for kanamycin prophylaxis

A 91-year-old woman was to undergo bowel resection. A surgeon wrote the following order as part of preoperative bowel preparation:

Kanamycin 1 g every hour x 4, then 1 g every 6 hours until surgery.

No route of administration was specified. The first dose was requested verbally from the pharmacy as "Kantrex 500 mg IM." Subsequent doses were scheduled in the nursing medication administration records to be given intramuscularly. When the pharmacist received the written order and saw the dosage ordered, it was obvious to him that the drug was meant to be given orally.

This error could have had serious consequences. The nephrotoxicity and ototoxicity of systemic kanamycin is well know. If the drug were given systemically in the dosage ordered, these side effects would be likely to occur. Because the oral dosage form (capsule) is not appreciably absorbed, this form is used in doses much higher than those used systemically. Its local effect within the bowel lumen reduces bowel flora before operation.

One of the factors which led to this error was that no route of administration was specified by the physician. Because not everyone is familiar with the oral dosage form, and because the use of kanamycin by parenteral route is fairly common, the lack of specification of route of administration led to the belief that the parenteral route was to be used.

Personnel responsible for scheduling and administering medications in this hospital showed a lack of information about the dosage range of kanamycin and about the serious side effects of the drug that are more likely with high doses. If this had been known, the error would not have occurred. (Some hospitals have set policies that require pharmacists to see a written order before any non-emergency drug is dispensed.) The same error could occur with neomycin, which is used similarly.

It should be noted that under a floor stock system, this error would have been continued.

11:107, 1976

Error 45 and 46

Errors caused by not charting doses given at the time of administration

The following two medication error reports illustrate one of the most common causes of medication error in hospitals.

45. A dose of Pyridium was given to a patient by the person responsible for medication administration after the patient had already received the dose from a student nurse. The pharmacist had placed two doses in the drug cart. One dose was supposed to be for 10 am and the other for 2 pm. The medication administration record (MAR) was not in the MAR book because the student had it. For this reason the person giving medications did not check the MAR before giving the dose. After the double dose was given, the MAR was consulted and the student's initials were discovered.

46. Duplicate medication was given to a patient by both a senior floor nurse and an orientee. Both believed that they were responsible for giving medications to the patient. The dosages were not written on the MAR. Two doses of Choledyl 200 mg were involved.

In good drug administration practice, whenever a dose of medication is administered to a patient, the dose should be charted in the medication

administration record immediately thereafter. This standard procedure is in effect at most hospitals.

If a dose of medication is charted before it is given, a potential exists for dose omission should the person who charted it be called off the floor or otherwise distracted before dose administration.

Conversely, if a dose of medication is given to a patient with the intention of charting the dose later, a potential exists for an extra dose of medication to be given to the patient.

Medication errors related to not entering doses at the time of administration are among the most common reported. To prevent these, one must develop a feeling of responsibility to mark down the dose at the time of administering. Never take short cuts.

This type of error occurs when more than one person is involved in giving medications for one particular schedule, or when more than one person is made responsible for stat doses on a single nursing unit. Intravenous medications are commonly involved, since often they are given by a person other than the one assigned to give regular medication. In a teaching hospital, the error is probably more common when teaching is being carried out on the floor and a student is giving some of the medications. Special medication doses such as warfarin or check-daily digoxins are also subject to involvement in these errors, since they are not usually given at the same time as scheduled medications.

11:146, 1976

Error 47

Rescue therapy not given because a professional was unfamiliar with the purpose of folinic acid

A cancer patient was to receive a dose of methotrexate to be followed six hours later by a dose of folinic acid to counteract some of the former drug's adverse systemic effects. Because the order was written late in the day, the methotrexate was not obtained until early evening. The dose was administered soon after it arrived. Although it too arrived, the folinic acid was not administered six hours after the methotrexate as ordered. The dose was held until the next morning. The reason given was that the patient would have had to be awakened and the drug was "only a vitamin."

This error once again shows that a need for in-service education exists. All health professionals involved with medications have a duty to know the purpose of any drug they are handling. Since it is easy to understand how folinic acid could be thought of as "only a vitamin," we should make a special effort to assure that those responsible for drug administration know the purpose of the drug. If verbal contact cannot be made, a label briefly explaining the need for folinic acid might be attached.

Correspondence

Folinic acid rescue therapy

Dear Mr. Cohen:

In Error 47 a patient received a massive methotrexate dose but did not receive scheduled folinic acid rescue on time. This happened because the patient was sleeping when the folinic acid was due and someone, thinking folinic acid was "only a vitamin," didn't want to awaken him. You correctly point out that a need for in-service education exists in institutions that use this type of therapy.

We too have had this error occur in our hospital. Besides effort to educate our staff about folinic acid we have established a policy that has helped to prevent further incidents. The drug is now referred to here only by its official name: leucovorin calcium. Perhaps if this were the case in other institutions, such serious errors would not occur. There is less likelihood of confusing leucovorin calcium with folic acid than there is of confusing folinic acid with folic acid.

(Anonymous)

Editor's Note

I agree that this policy would help to prevent the error. In fact, we use only leucovorin calcium at our hospital. However, you should be aware that I have received a report of a mixup between leucovorin and leukeran. A patient inadvertently received a 5 mg dose of leukeran after methotrexate. The person who administered the drug thought it made sense because it *was* a cancer patient! In this case the ordering physician's poor handwriting led to the error. Perhaps if the full official name, leucovorin calcium, were used, this error might not have occurred.

11:146, 1976

Error 48

Overdose of estrogen given to patient

Premarin 0.625 mg was ordered for a patient. No. 0.625 mg tablets were available in the pharmacy. The pharmacy technician decided that he would give an equal dose by using a number of tablets of a "lesser" strength. Apparently he thought the dose was 6.25 mg. He placed five 1.25 mg Premarin tablets together in a unit dose package and placed these in the patient's bin of a unit dose cart. The pharmacist in charge did not detect the error upon checking the cart. The medication nurse, upon receiving the cart, returned with the dose to question the use of five tablets, and was told by the technician that the dose was correct. The pharmacist was not consulted about the dose by the technician or the nurse, although he was present in the pharmacy at the time. The patient, who had had gynecologic problems in the past, received the dose and exhibited vaginal bleeding three days later. The cause of the bleeding was later discovered and explained to the patient.

Several points need to be made in considering this medication error. First, make every effort not to substitute smaller dose tablets or capsules to equal a larger dose. This must be impressed upon the technicians.

Second, when pharmacists check the carts, they must concentrate and make sure that each dose is correct.

Technicians must be instructed that they are never permitted to judge whether or not a dose is correct. This must be done by a pharmacist. Nursing personnel also must have this impressed upon them.

It has been stated that it is impossible for a pharmacy technician to make an error; only a pharmacist can make an error. This statement is made because it is believed that when the pharmacist checks the work of a technician, he is assuming responsibility for correctness.

11:148, 1976

Error 49

Overdose of digoxin ordered by physician who prescribed using the label on patient's prescription container

An NCR prescription order for digoxin 2.5 mg was received by a hospital pharmacist. At the same time, medications which the patient had brought from home were also received in pharmacy; a digoxin container was among those received.

Although tablets of 0.25 mg were in the vial, it was mislabeled as 2.5 mg. Since, unfortunately, a floor stock system was in use at the hospital, the pharmacist immediately called the patient care area to warn the nurses and halt a possible overdose. The pharmacist was told that the patient had already gone to surgery and that the digoxin dose for the day had been given instead by injection because the patient was being given nothing by mouth.

It was determined that the order for digoxin 2.5 mg resulted because the admitting physician had written the drug order using the mistaken dosage label on a medicine that the patient had brought to the hospital. This was obviously done without much thought as to what actually was being ordered. Obtaining dosage in this manner is a hazardous shortcut that should not be used at any hospital. This mistake, coupled with harried personnel in a hurry to administer drugs without thinking of the consequences of a wrong dose, can lead to serious error.

Once again, the negative aspects of the floor stock system surface. Hospital administrators must support a drug distribution system in which the pharmacist reviews physician orders before any doses are administered to patients.

11:203, 1976

Error 50

Error caused by poor handwriting and a misused decimal point

An order was written for "Hydrocortisone 5.0 mg Daily P.O." Although the handwriting was not good, the order was noted properly by the nurse and the NCR copy was sent to pharmacy. The decimal point in the 5.0 was not visible on the NCR copy. The

156

pharmacist thought the order read "Hydrochlorothiazide 50 mg Daily." The pharmacist asked another pharmacist to verify his interpretation. The second pharmacist did so. A seven-day supply was prepared as an individual prescription and labeled hydrochlorothiazide 50 mg. This was administered to the patient for three days at the hospital.

The pharmacist, the nurse and the physician all played a part in this error. The physician should *not* prescribe 5.0 mg of a drug. In medical practice there is no difference between 5 and 5.0. If 5 mg had been ordered, the error would never have occurred. If the writing had been more legible, the mistake probably would not have occurred.

The pharmacists "guessed" wrong. If they had gone to the patient care area and studied the original order, the medication which the doctor had ordered would have been obvious. In some cases, knowledge of the patient's diagnosis might prevent the error by providing a clue. In any case, there is no room for "guessing." Lastly, when the hydrochlorothiazide tablets 50 mg arrived on the nursing unit, the nurse should have checked the drug against what was ordered and noted that the drug was not ordered for the patient. This should be done routinely before any new drug is administered to a patient.

11:203, 1976

Error 51

Gentamicin dosing interval misinterpreted

An order for a patient with severe renal impairment was interpreted as gentamicin 60 mg IM q 4 hours. The physician intended it to be given every 24 hours.

Originally, the physician wrote "q 14 h." He changed his mind and wanted it administered every 24 hours. To indicate this change, he wrote a two over the one. It appeared as follows:

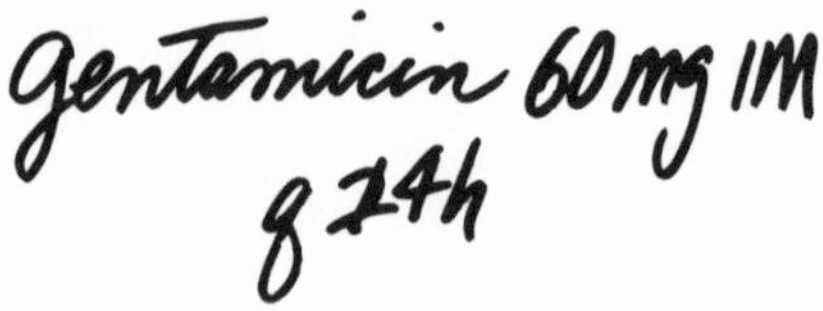

Figure 22

The floor personnel who saw this interpreted the order as q 4 h. Physicians should not change orders in this manner. They should line through, with a single stroke, that which is incorrect and rewrite a correct order. Billingsley (Gentamicin overdosage. *Drug Intel. Clin. Pharm.* 9:618, 1975) reported a q 14 hour dose being misread as q 4 hour as well as a q 30 hour dose read as q 3 h. In both cases, some doses were actually administered at the incorrect interval before the error was corrected. He wisely suggests that physicians consider an increased risk of error whenever normal hospital dosage intervals are disrupted. Where normal dose interval alternatives exist, as they do for gentamicin in patients with renal impairment, this principle should be borne in mind.

Another point to be made is that any individuals responsible for reading the order and administering the drug should realize that a dose of 360 mg daily of gentamicin for a renal patient is incorrect.

These errors probably would not have occurred if pharmacists had reviewed the orders before administration.

11:203, 1976

Error 52

Competency evaluation of medication administration personnel not performed

Postoperatively, an initially reduced dosage of meperidine was ordered for analgesia for a patient who had received Innovar. The dosage was 25 mg IM until 4 pm, then 50 mg IM PRN every three hours. At 3 pm, the patient began to complain of pain.

The person responsible for drug administration obtained the dose of analgesic from the available unit dose narcotic floor stock and administered it to the patient. Moments later, the charge nurse noticed that there was no control form sign-out signature on the appropriate meperidine sheet. The person who had administered the medication was questioned. This person claimed that two sheets had been signed — the sheet for 10 mg syringes and the sheet for 15 mg syringes.

Upon checking, it was discovered that what actually had been given was morphine 25 mg IM. The person administering medications thought that meperidine was just another name for morphine. A check on the patient revealed that respiratory distress had developed and naloxone had to be administered to correct this.

What needs to be mentioned here is that a person with this lack of fundamental knowledge should never have been made responsible for drug administration. Hospital and department administrators have a responsibility to assure competency.

It has been my general impression that pharmacology programs in many schools of nursing are inadequate. The same can be said for hospital medication courses given to licensed practical nurses. Structured pharmacology courses often do not exist. Most often nurses learn about drugs on the job. Pharmacists cannot forget that they have an important job to do in providing continuous in-service education.

A point should be made in hospital in-service programs that whenever more than a single unit-dose syringe is necessary to provide a dose of medication, something may be wrong. If this question had arisen in the mind of the person involved, and a pharmacist or nurse colleague had been consulted, the error probably would not have occurred.

11:242, 1976

Errors 53-56

No check of armbands

One of the most common types of medication error is administration of medication to the wrong patient. Good drug administration practice makes it necessary to identify the proper patient before a drug is given. The most common means of proper patient identification in use in hospitals today is the patient identification armband. However, for various reasons, the identification procedure of looking at the armband is not always carried out. The following error reports illustrate the problem.

53. *"I thought I recognized patient G.W. as being patient M.B."*

Allopurinol 300 mg was given by mistake to a patient in bed A. It was intended for a different patient who had been in bed A previously, but had been transferred without the knowledge of the person giving medications. "I thought I recognized patient G.W. as being M.B. I did not check the patient's armband." The person administering drugs should never rely on apparent recognition of a patient. This presents difficulties for medication administration personnel. It's extremely hard to have to look at the armband of a patient whom you've seen for several weeks in a row. However, momentary lapses in room orientation, which happen to all of us, could result in giving a drug to the wrong patient.

54. *"The patient didn't have an armband."*

A patient in bed A received Lasix and Robitussin that had been scheduled for a patient who was actually in bed B. The patient in bed B was newly admitted; he was supposed to be in bed A. The patient in bed A had no armband; it had been removed during a test procedure earlier in the day.

A rule should be made and adhered to that medication will not be administered to a patient who has no armband. If a patient has no armband, the person responsible for medications should make sure one is obtained before drug administration.

One cannot rely on the patient's response to questions about his surname for the purpose of identification. The following two errors illustrate this problem.

11:242, 1976

55. *"I asked him if his last name was Stankowicz and he said yes . . . later I found out his name was McCoy."*

A patient in bed A was given all of the medications intended for a patient in bed B. When it was noticed that the patient in bed A had no armband, the person giving medications called out the name of the person for whom the medications were intended. It turned out the person in bed A responded positively to the name of the person in bed B (for whom the medications

were actually intended). "I asked him if his last name was Stankowicz and he said, "Yes," so I gave him Stankowicz' medication. Later I found out his name was actually McCoy. Stankowicz was in the other bed."

Patients with organic brain syndrome, poor hearing, who are sedated, etc., may respond positively when addressed incorrectly.

56. *"Sometimes you can't even rely on them telling you their names."*

An IVP prep was to be given to a patient in bed A. The patient had no armband. When asked to give his last name, the patient answered "Williams." This was the correct name as far as the person giving medications was concerned. The prep was administered. Later it was discovered that this patient was not to receive an IVP prep — it was intended for the patient in bed B. This patient's name also was Williams.

Administrators and hospital admission officers should avoid placing patients with the same surnames in the same patient care area, let alone in the same room.

It has been stated that if a patient is not wearing an armband, one should ask the patient to state his name before administering medications. This is supposed to be the method of choice in patient identification if no armband is present. Even this technique is not foolproof. It is my opinion that all patients should have armbands in place at all times and that they always should be used.

Besides medication errors, misidentification has been responsible for laboratory errors, dietary errors, and even autopsy errors.

11:243, 1976

Errors 57-58

Pharmacist should scrutinize drug orders before drugs are given

57. Tenfold dose of cyclophosphamide nearly given

The order for cyclophosphamide in Figure 23 was interpreted by floor personnel as 1000 mg. Administration of this dose was prevented by the hospital pharmacist, who noted that the last zero in the number was actually the loop of the letter "Q" on the line above.

It is easy to see how this error could have happened. The fact that 1000 mg doses of cyclophosphamide are often given intravenously as a part of various chemotherapy protocols could easily preclude questioning of the dose by clinical personnel. A tragedy was averted by the pharmacist.

Additional Comments

Error 57 described an incident in which a pharmacist prevented a tenfold dosing error with cyclophosphamide. The loop of a "q" on the line above the dose made 100 mg look like 1000 mg. Figure 24 shows a similar potential error involving Myleran. Although the physician intended to order 4 mg daily, he claimed that an accidental extra loop on the m of mg made the dose appear as 40 mg. Although 40 mg daily was in fact scheduled and requested by floor personnel, an astute pharmacist became suspicious of the dose and questioned the physician.

Pharmacists involved in preparing doses of cancer chemotherapeutics should always cast a suspicious eye at orders received.

58. Probably lethal doses of lithium given

Although this incident reflects poor medical practice rather than medica-

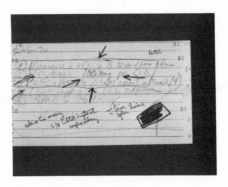

Figure 23

tion error, it illustrates the necessity of having a pharmacist review all drug orders before the drugs are administered to patients.

The patient was a 71-year-old woman admitted to the hospital for severe psychotic depression. The patient had been titrated very evenly with lithium carbonate from a dosage level of 300 mg per day up to a dosage of 1800 mg per day. She had received daily blood tests for serum levels of lithium until the 1800 mg per day dosage had been reached. Then the physician changed the serum level determinations to twice a week. Her blood titers had been averaging 1.2 to 2.1 mEq/liter of lithium during this period.

At this point another physician took over the case and determined that the patient had not exhibited any signs of improvement in her mental status (or at least not enough). He therefore changed the dosage from 1800 mg per day to 2700 mg per day of lithium

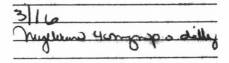

Figure 24

carbonate. No pharmacist reviewed this order; it was dispensed from floor stock for a period of 10 days. Also, after raising the dosage of lithium, the physician made a change in the serum level tests to once a month for some unknown reason.

The patient was admitted to the intensive care unit some 11 days later with lithium overdose symptoms. These included cyanosis, noisy respiration, skin tremors in all areas of the body, elevated temperature, elevated BUN and a serum level of lithium of 3.38 mEq/liter. She died during the next 24 hours before emergency procedures were effective in reversing the condition.

The pharmacist was consulted by personnel only after trouble was noted. To avoid such incidents in the future, the pharmacist should review every order — both those involving the actual medication and those involving the lab tests. In this particular case, if all of the facts had been reviewed by the pharmacist, chances are the change in blood testing or the elevated dose request would have prompted a call to the physician for clarification.

11:281, 1976

Error 59

Outpatient label mix-up

An outpatient presented prescriptions for:
Neosporin Ophth Oint — Apply to each eye at bedtime
Atropine Ophth Soln 1% — 1 drop in left eye 2-times daily
Neosporin Ophth Soln — 1 drop in each eye every 2 hours

The pharmacy labels on the containers of the two eye drops were interchanged. The atropine was labeled "1 drop in each eye every 2 hours,"

and the Neosporin Drops were labeled "1 drop in left eye 2 times daily." The error was discovered the next day when the patient returned complaining of blurred vision.

The pharmacist did not type the contents of the prescription on the label; he relied on the exposed commercial label to identify the product. Had he also typed the name of the product on the label, the chance of a mix-up would have been lessened.

Only one prescription should be worked on at a time. If this were done, the chance for error would be reduced. However, working on one prescription at a time is impractical in a busy pharmacy. If this safety measure is eliminated to facilitate speed, added caution must be instituted in checking the finished prescription.

11:313, 1976

Error 60

Confusing product labeling leads to iron overdose

A physician ordered ferrous fumarate 200 mg. three times daily. The order was filled with Fumasorb tablets (Marion Labs) by a new employe pharmacist. The label was typed "ferrous fumarate 66 mg — three (3) tablets equal 200 mg." As a result, the patient received three tablets three times a day.

Examination of the product labeling revealed the following wording regarding strength: "Each tablet contains: elemental Iron (as ferrous fumarate) 66 mg." The pharmacist interpreted this to mean that three tablets were necessary to obtain the prescribed 200 mg of ferrous fumarate. Previous product labeling listed the tablet strength as ferrous fumarate 200 mg.

The pharmacist who submitted this error to me wrote a letter to Marion

Laboratories protesting the label change from what it had been in years past; the new label was confusing. He received from the company:

"In reference to your letter . . . concerning Fumasorb, we can understand your concern that our product Fumasorb is labeled 'Each tablet contains: elemental iron (as ferrous fumarate) . . . 66 mg' rather than stating (from ferrous fumarate . . . 200 mg).

In previous labeling for Fumasorb, it was listed as ferrous fumarate 3 gr . . . 200 mg. However, the recommended dietary allowance as published by the National Academy of Sciences gives the allowance in terms of elemental iron. Therefore, this being an OTC drug, it is more informative and less confusing for the consumer to have ingredient information consistent with recommended dietary allowance."

It is true that this type of labeling might allow for easier understanding by consumers, but it has led to an error made by a pharmacist. Iron toxicity may have developed. It is difficult to understand why both strength designations cannot be listed on the label. Most other labels of commercial iron salts products list both the amount of salt and the amount of elemental iron that this represents. Fumasorb is listed in American Drug Index as ferrous fumarate (iron equiv.) 66 mg/Tab.

11:313, 1976

Error 61

Overdoses of antibiotic solutions administered because of poor product labeling

An order was received for penicillin V potassium liquid 250 mg q 6 h. Compocillin-VK (Ross Laboratories) was the liquid penicillin V potassium

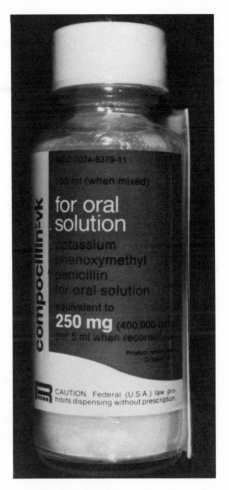

Figure 25

product in use at the hospital. This was sent to the floor after reconstitution by the pharmacist. The person responsible for drug administration was inexperienced and the label was read quickly. Only the name of the product, the strength and the words "for oral solution" were seen on quick glance. Because this person thought that the contents represented one dose, the entire bottle was administered!

Examination of the product labeling (Fig. 25) makes it easy to understand how this serious error occurred.

The label is very attractive for a drug product; imagine the time that went into developing such an artful label. However, it does not vividly present the information that 250 mg is in 5 ml — not in the entire bottle. Notice how poorly visible the "per 5 ml" printing is in comparison to "250 mg." This contributed to the error. This style labeling has been changed.

Of course, the placement of an inexperienced person in such a responsible position was also a contributory factor in this error. This person was not familiar with the product and did not take time to read the label completely.

No information about pharmacy labeling was submitted with this error. No doubt if a pharmacy label had been placed on the container the error would have been prevented.

I received a similar error report involving Ilosone suspension (Dista). A patient was to receive 250 mg every six hours. A 60 ml commercial package of Ilosone 250 mg/5 ml was sent to the patient care area. Again, an inexperienced person read the label as Ilosone suspension 250 mg. The entire 60 ml was administered. Only on the side of the bottle in fine print is the concentration visible.

Pharmaceutical companies have a duty to make sure that product labeling is functional as well as attractive.

A reader comments on Error 61

Mr. Cohen's comment on Error 61 is to my opinion worthless and unfair to the pharmaceutical company and "the inexperienced" person who administered the drug.

He should first look for information of whether the bottle is properly labeled or not before deciding to publish the error.

If I were to look for somebody to blame, the drug distribution system in that particular hospital is first and then the pharmacist who sent that bottle.

A Reader

Reply from Mr. Cohen

I cannot agree that my comments about the serious error that occurred were "worthless and unfair to the pharmaceutical company and 'the inexperienced person' who administered the drug."

The labeling on this product is terrible. The "per 5 ml" print should be as bold as "250 mg." We cannot reproduce the green color used as background over most of the label. This has the effect of de-emphasizing the print in dark ink and makes the "per 5 ml" even less vivid. Even the name of the drug is de-emphasized. The generic name is listed in less prominence than "for oral solution." The brand name is off to the side of the label and printed vertically.

An experienced person would have known that the dose was not the entire bottle. Perhaps the inexperienced nurse in this reader's hospital is less likely to make a similar error because theirs is a children's hospital. Their nursing personnel may be more likely to question such large amounts than inexperienced people in hospitals with an adult population.

I would agree with his comments about placing blame on the pharmacist and the drug distribution system. As mentioned, if the drug were properly labeled by the pharmacy department, I do not believe the error would have occurred. A unit dose system would also have prevented the error. Blame could even be placed on hospital administration, physicians and nurses for not insisting on a safer drug distribution system.

It is a lack of foresight not to see the value of publicizing this error. The shortcomings pointed out can be used by astute pharmacists to prevent similar occurrences. We can hope that pharmaceutical manufacturers will use safer labeling. (M.C.)

Additional Comments

Error 61 described an overdose of Compocillin VK liquid given because someone was confused about the labeling of the bottle and thought that the entire bottle contained only the 250 mg dose that had to be administered. In that error report I mentioned that a similar error was caused by the labeling found on Ilosone Liquid containers (Fig. 26).

I have recently received another report in which an entire bottle of Ilosone Liquid, 60 ml was administered in error. The error occurred in a hospital using a unit dose system. All medications were normally dispensed in unit dose containers. However, the hospital pharmacy's usual supply of unit dose product had run out. As a temporary measure a 60 ml bottle was dispensed. The nursing unit involved was a medical unit in which doses of liquid antibiotic were given infrequently. Employes there were not familiar with the product. Because of the way the product is labeled, it was assumed that 250 mg was present in 60 ml.

The label must indicate 250 mg per 5 ml. Dista Products Co. has been contacted. They stated that they have already started using "250 mg/5 ml" in their promotional material and that their labeling will also reflect the change.

The unit dose pharmacist must place a label indicating patient name, room number, dose and volume required in the event a multidose bottle must be used.

11:313, 1976

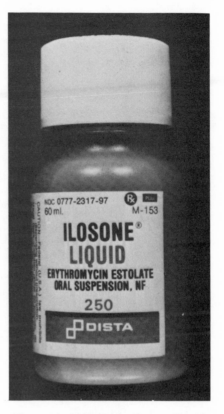

Figure 26. Old label for Ilosone Liquid.

Error 62

Too much knowledge can also be dangerous!

Levothyroxine sodium (Synthroid) 0.5 mg daily was prescribed for a 28-year-old male patient. The hospital pharmacist who received the prescription recognized that this was a high dose and decided to review the patient's chart to make sure the dose was appropriate. He believed that a decimal point might have been incorrectly placed and what the physician really intended the patient to receive was a 0.05 mg (50 mcg) dose.

Upon review of the chart, it was noted that the patient had received surgical treatment in the past for a

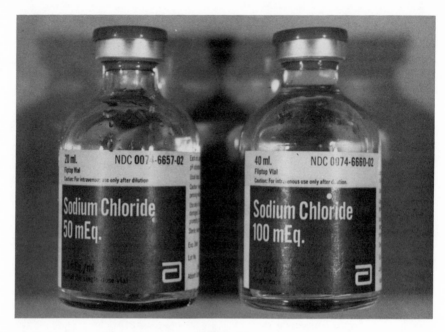

Figure 27

pituitary glioma. The patient also had diabetes insipidus requiring 5 units of pitressin in oil twice daily, and also was on corticosteroids.

The pharmacist theorized that the high dose of levothyroxine was needed because the surgery must have affected pituitary thyroid-stimulating hormone as well. The pharmacist believed the dose of 0.5 mg was appropriate and the patient received it until an order was received to *increase* the dose to 0.1 mg. A check with the physician revealed the error. The physician had indeed incorrectly placed the decimal point. The patient had previously been controlled on 0.05 mg.

Here is a case of a pharmacist having so much knowledge about the patient's clinical situation that the obvious was overlooked. We must all be careful not to fall into a similar trap.

11:435, 1976

Error 63

High concentration of NaCl injection given inadvertently

A cardiac catheterization technician brought a drug requisition to the pharmacy for vials of sodium chloride injection.* The saline was to be used for irrigation of intravascular catheters used during the cardiac catheterization procedure. The pharmacist on duty was a part-timer not completely familiar with hospital pharmacy practice. He looked on the shelf and found vials of sodium chloride (Fig. 27) and dispensed them. They were used by the cardiologists in the lab. The vials dispensed were kept on hand in the pharmacy for the preparation of hyperalimentation solution. They contained either 50 or 100

*(Note: A recent U.S.P. change states the concentration of Sodium Chloride shall be part of official title)

mEq, a concentration 16 times greater than the sodium chloride injection 0.9% that was desired.

This error could have been prevented in several ways. First, the manufacturers should mark the vials more prominently, that they contain a high concentration not suitable for direct injection. A red-colored warning statement on the label would be helpful. The dispensing pharmacist should have recognized the amount of sodium chloride in each vial. If the label had been read completely, the statement (although difficult to see) "Caution: For intravenous use only after dilution" might have been seen. A pharmacist permitted to work in a hospital pharmacy should know the difference between this product and sodium chloride for injection, unless he is under constant supervision.

Error 64

Wrong strength PPD administered because of poor nomenclature

Most hospital pharmacists can recall some confusion when they first learned about tuberculin purified protein derivative test nomenclature.

Since there are three test strengths in existence, it seems inappropriate to refer to the third strength (250 tuberculin units) as "second test strength PPD." Physicians wanting to give the intermediate strength (5 tuberculin units) have been known to order "Second strength PPD," because they think of intermediate as the second most concentrated test. It is potentially hazardous to give a patient 250 tuberculin units when only five are intended. Orders for 250 units for initial testing must be challenged by the pharmacist. Publicity about this problem might be helpful. A recent article in the pharmacy newsletter of Saint Joseph's Hospital in Elmira, New York, addresses itself to this problem. Editor Les Goldschmidt writes:

"We have received many questions concerning the different strengths of tuberculin purified protein derivative (PPD). The nomenclature is unfortunately quite confusing. The available strengths are:

first test strength = (1 test unit)
intermediate strength = (5 test units)
second test strength = (250 test units)

Thus the so-called "Second strength" is actually the strongest of the three tests.

The usual dose is 5 TU (Intermediate). The 1 TU (First) is used in patients who have been shown to be highly sensitive. The 250 TU (Second) is used only in patients who fail to react to the other test strengths. *Under no circumstances should the preparation containing 250 TU/0.1 ml be used for initial testing. (ref: ASHP Formulary Service)."*

11:436, 1976

Error 65

The largest IM dose that should be given is 3 ml

An order was written for vancomycin 500 mg IM q 12 h x 2 days. The physician wrote for the IM route inadvertently — he meant IV. The pharmacist received the order and because of his knowledge of the drug automatically thought the route should be IV.

Rather than correcting the order immediately, the pharmacist drew up the vancomycin in 10 ml of diluent in a syringe for IV use. When typing the label (from the order) he inadvertently typed "IM." He did not reread the label as he placed it on the syringe; he dispensed it labeled "IM," thinking that it would actually be given intravenously.

The person responsible for medication administration read the order and the label on the syringe. She thought it odd to have to give 10 ml of a drug intramuscularly, so she checked with two other professionals. They all agreed that if a doctor ordered it and a pharmacist filled it, it must be ok. The dose was given. The package insert for Vancocin (Lilly) states "Vancocin . . . is very irritating to tissue and causes necrosis when injected intramuscularly; it must be administered intravenously."

The company was contacted and stated that in their experience the major problem with one IM dose was severe pain. The patient had this.

The pharmacist must communicate with the prescribing physician to change orders, even ones that are as obviously wrong as this. I assume the pharmacist intended to tell the nurse to give the drug IV. Would the nurse have done this on merely the pharmacist's word?

People administering medications parenterally should know that most medications cannot be given intramuscularly in a volume of more than 3 ml in one site. If the person even encounters this situation, a mistake should be suspected. Exceptions may be paraldehyde and iron dextran, which may be assigned a 4-5 ml limit.

11:486, 1976

Error 66

Concentrate when checking labels

A pharmacy error involving injectable dexamethasone occurred. It happened in a hospital with a unit dose system in which all injectable doses were prepared centrally by an injection service after orders were received from floor personnel.

An order was written for 1 mg dexamethasone IM bid, and the patient received this dose over a weekend. On Monday, the pharmacist normally in charge of the pharmacy department's injection service was out sick; another pharmacist filled in. An experienced technician working in the injection service drew up the dexamethasone as 2½ ml of a 4 mg per ml solution (10 mg). Evidently, he had in mind a concentration of 0.4 mg/ml. The label placed on the syringe read "Decadron 1 mg." The pharmacist in charge did not notice this error. The pharmacist on the floor also did not notice the error. This amount of medication was dispensed on Monday for both doses. The error occurred again on Tuesday and Wednesday.

On Thursday, the pharmacist in charge of the service returned. He drew up 1 mg of drug correctly in 0.25 ml. When the syringe was sent to the floor, the error was noticed because of the different size of the syringe.

The pharmacist temporarily in charge of the injection service was counseled regarding his absolute responsibility for checking out technician work and concentrating on what is checked. The pharmacists who dispensed the drug should also have concentrated on what they were checking. They should have been especially careful, since a fill-in pharmacist was in charge of the injection service.

11:487, 1976

Error 67

Transient hyperkalemia and cardiac arrest due to incorrect method of potassium administration

A young woman had surgery for repair of a malfunctioning mitral valve. Postoperatively, the patient's serum potassium was noted as 2.7 mEq/liter. A physician ordered 60 mEq of potassium chloride in 100 ml of 5% dextrose in water for her. Fluids needed to be limited.

Instructions were to administer the drug over one hour. The order was given verbally to a nurse, who transcribed the order onto the order sheet on the patient's chart. After the infusion, an additional 40 mEq of KCl in 40 ml was ordered. Shortly after this infusion began, the patient suffered cardiac arrest (ventricular fibrillation was documented on EKG). Resuscitation was successful and a diagnosis of arrest secondary to transient hyperkalemia was made. A contributory factor may have been that the potassium chloride was given piggyback into a central line lying within the superior vena cava.

Standard textbooks recommend that no more than 40 mEq per hour be administered even in the severest of hypokalemias. A maximum concentration of 60 mEq KCl per liter is recommended (*Manual of Medical Therapeutics*, 21st Edition, Washington University School of Medicine, p. 44).* The IV Therapy Committee's guidelines in the hospital where this incident occurred reflected these recommendations. When questioned, personnel working in the patient care area said they were aware of the danger of the practice. However, they claimed that they were assured by the ordering physicians that it was neces-

sary and not dangerous. They had done it before with several patients without problem.

I seriously doubt that this error would have occurred had the hospital's pharmacy department been involved via an IV admixture program. I believe that most hospital pharmacists are aware of the dangers of this type of potassium administration. Other hospital personnel need to be more knowledgeable about the possible hazards of drugs that they use. A plea is made for health professionals to be more critical and not be so accepting of what they believe may be a hazardous physician order.

11:523, 1976

Error 68
Poor labeling of an oral alimentation agent

Some of the medication errors contributed to this column seem unbelievable. However, they have really happened. A report has been received about a patient who was to receive oral alimentation with Vivonex Standard Diet. Vivonex is packaged as a soluble, unflavored powder; a flavor pack is to be added upon use (Fig. 28).

The report submitted describes a case in which the patient was given only the flavoring agent — not the Vivonex. Personnel responsible for mixing the dietary item were not familiar with the product and seeing only the flavor packet thought this was the food and made a solution of the flavor packet.

I believe that poor labeling of the product contributed to the error. The name of the diet product "Vivonex" is in larger lettering than the actual ingredient (flavor packet). A vivid statement such as "must be mixed with

---

*Some hospitals have set up guidelines for using higher concentrations under unusual circumstances. Monitoring of ECG is usually required as is administration by IV control device.

168

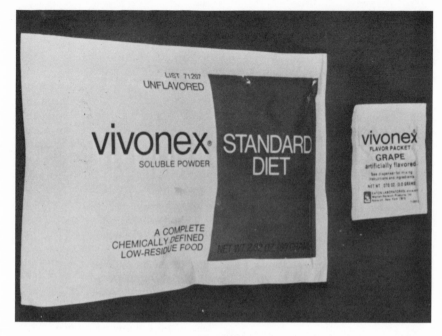

Figure 28

Vivonex soluble powder in solution before use" would also help to prevent such errors. Mixing of dietary products should be left to personnel in the dietary department who must be familiar with the proper directions for preparing nutritional items. In some hospitals the pharmacy prepares and labels this product.

Note: The labeling has since been improved.

11:523, 1976

Error 69

Label clarifications by pharmacy are essential in preventing errors

A myasthenic patient had been receiving 75 mg of pyridostigmine bromide (Mestinon) syrup every three hours. The liquid was dispensed in a pint bottle from pharmacy and labeled "Mestinon Syrup 60 mg/5 ml."

Each dose was given by drug administration personnel as 6.25 ml measured by syringe. After the initial supply of drug had been exhausted, a requisition was sent to pharmacy for another bottle. The second bottle was inadvertently mislabeled by pharmacy as Mestinon Syrup 10 mg/5 ml. The actual concentration was still 60 mg/5 ml. Clinical personnel, using the labeled concentration, drew up 37.5 ml to obtain the 75 mg dose. The patient actually received 450 mg per dose and went into cholinergic crisis.

Perhaps less assumption on the part of drug administration personnel would have helped to stop this error from occurring. They assumed that a different concentration had been dispensed to make it easier to dose the patient through a nasogastric tube that was in place. A change in concentration should have been questioned.

The real responsibility for the error, however, falls on pharmacy. The bottle was labeled only with the concentration. As happened here, a typing mistake or mental slip in listing the concentration can lead to error. Products dispensed from pharmacy must always list the exact dose (mg) and exact quantity (tablets, ml, etc.) to be given if the stated strength of the tablet or liquid concentration differs from the exact dose to be given. A bottle of Mestinon Syrup should state the concentration of 60 mg/5 ml *and also that* 75 mg = 6.25 ml if that is the dose to be given. Other examples are:

Drug dose	Drug strength dispensed	Supplemental label information
Diabinese 500 mg	Diabinese 250 mg	2 tabs = 500 mg
Orinase 250 mg	Orinase 500 mg tab	½ tab = 250 mg
Prednisone 12.5 mg	Prednisone 5 mg tab	2½ tabs = 12.5 mg
Erythromycin 500 mg	Erythromycin syrup 200 mg/5 ml	12.5 ml = 500 mg

Correspondence

Label clarification

Dear Mr. Cohen:

I have rediscovered your journal and find your feature "Medication Errors" very useful for teaching pharmacy students, pharmacists and nurses. However, if I may, I'd like to comment on Error 69, label clarification. The example cited was one in which a dose of 500 mg of erythromycin was prescribed and in which, apparently, a liquid dosage form containing 200 mg/5 ml was dispensed. The supplemental label you suggest, 12.5 ml = 500 mg, is not, in this case, accurate from a therapeutic standpoint. The enclosed copy of a letter from Abbott (reproduced below) explains the discrepancy. It's unfortunate that this information is not made more widely or easily available to pharmacists *and* prescribers.

Henry A. Palmer, PhD
Associate Clinical Professor
University of Connecticut
School of Pharmacy
Storrs. CT 06268

Dear Dr. Palmer:

We are responding to your inquiry concerning the activity of the various oral dosage forms of Erythrocin (erythromycin stearate, ethylsuccinate, Abbott). You also inquired why the Erythrocin Ethyl Succinate dosage (up to 1600 mg per day for children over 100 pounds) seems larger than the Erythrocin Stearate dosages (1000 mg per day for adults).

When the bottle label says "each 5 ml contains activity equivalent to 200 mg of Erythromycin Base," the term "activity" on the label refers to the in vitro assay of antibiotic activity, contained in the 5 ml teaspoon. It does not refer to the absorption of the drug or the resulting levels of erythromycin base ("activity") in the blood stream.

The following comments are pertinent to erythromycin "activity" in the body. Erythromycin base is the only active form of erythromycin; that is, it is the only form which has significant antibacterial activity. Erythromycin stearate, which is a salt of erythromycin, simply dissociates in the gut and is absorbed as the active erythromycin base; however, esters such as erythromycin ethylsuccinate and erythromycin estolate must be hydrolyzed to yield erythromycin base. This in vivo hydrolysis process continues over a period of time; therefore, 100% of the ester is not available as active erythromycin base at any given time. Some of the drug is circulating in the blood in the ester form, which is not active. Our blood level studies were conducted comparing erythromycin ethylsuccinate and erythromycin stearate. The results have shown that a larger dose of erythromycin ethylsuccinate (200 mg and 400 mg) is required to provide active levels of erythromycin base similar to those produced by 125 mg and 250 mg, respectively, of erythromycin stearate. Our dosage recommendations have been based on these blood level data.

In summary, *in the bottle*, 5 ml of Erythrocin-400 Liquid has activity equivalent to 400 mg of erythromycin base. *In the body*, 400 mg of Erythrocin-400 Liquid (5 ml) will provide similar blood levels of erythromycin base (activity) to 250 mg erythromycin stearate.

Fredric B. Bauer
Abbott Laboratories

Helping nurses avoid error

Dear Mr. Cohen:

I am a registered pharmacist with an extensive background in hospital pharmacy and I have a great interest in medication error prevention.

When I receive HOSPITAL PHARMACY, I always review the "Medication Error Reports." Although the existence of such problems is recognized, I am disturbed that not enough seems to be done to prevent or minimize them. I am familiar with the unfortunate habit of many pharmacists of using little effort in labeling a medication. By this habit, they leave a great deal of decision-making to busy and often minimally educated (as far as medications) nurses. Many pharmacists seem to operate on an assembly-line basis, being content with just supplying medications. It appears to me that the pharmacy department should take the initiative to insure that medications are properly utilized, even if such action is time consuming and appears superfluous.

In error 69 you recommended labeling to indicate when fractions or multiples of supplied medications were to be used to provide a required dose. I have often used such labeling. To say that a nurse should be able to calculate a required dose might be sound on an academic level, but the pharmacist should willingly accept the responsibility of guiding the medication administrator.

Here are some ideas I use to try to guide the nurse:

1. If the medication is limited to certain routes of administration, these should be indicated: IV only, IM only, S.C. only. Such labeling could help prevent the giving of medications by dangerous or ineffective routes. Although the same information appears on commercial labels, I place the statement "For sublingual use only" on such medications. Would you believe that once, after supplying medication so labeled, a nurse called the pharmacy claiming she didn't know that nitroglycerin was given sublingually? She thought it was an oral medication.

2. If the medication supplied has specific instructions for consumption, these should be indicated on the pharmacy label even if they appear on a supplied commercial container. (The abundance of directions found, often in fine print, on a commercial container is often easily overlooked). Some examples follow.

   a. "Don't crush or chew"—for enteric-coated or prolonged acting products. This could prevent the altering of therapeutic action of such preparations by a nurse who tries to facilitate patients' swallowing by crushing the medications.

b. "Chew tablets, follow with water" — for tablets that should not be swallowed whole. Examples are Gaviscon, which should effervesce in the mouth before ingestion or Mylicon, which should be reduced in particle size before swallowing, or calcium gluconate wafers that are much too large to be swallowed whole.

c. "Give diluted (with suggested dilution)" — for preparations that should not be consumed in a concentrated form, such as potassium chloride solutions, which could irritate the gut if administered undiluted.

d. "For oral use only, give diluted, measure by drops" — for oral liquids given by drop dosage: belladonna tincture, opium tincture, saturated solution of potassium iodide. Since these medications are normally supplied in dropper bottles, it is necessary to advise the nurse that the contents are for oral use. I know of a nurse who was about to give 10 drops of saturated solution of potassium iodide in the patient's *left eye* because she had misinterpreted the order "SSKI 10 drops in OJ" for "SSKI 10 drops in OS."

Although drop measurement is inaccurate, I usually include the caution "measure by drops" on the label to prevent possible overdosage such as giving 10 ml for an ordered 10 drops. Once a pharmacist that I worked with encountered a nurse who was going to administer 10 tea-spoonfuls of a medication to an infant because she interpreted "gtts" as an abbreviation for teaspoonsfuls.

e. See mixing directions on packets (Label)" — for items such as K-Lor, and Metamucil Instant Mix, which must be reconstituted before administration. Rewriting all necessary directions would be too burdensome; this statement on the label will direct the nurse's attention to the commercial directions and insure that the patient will receive a properly prepared dose, I also used this on Fleet's Phosphosoda, which is recommended to be administered diluted and with a water "chaser."

3. Inclusion of a package insert with each quantity of injectables supplied and a label statement directing the nurse's attention to the insert, such as "See insert for IV use." The supplied insert will provide the nurse with necessary information, such as proper reconstitution, minimum dilution, and rate of administration.

4. Label statement "Use vial once only" to prevent reuse of unpreserved vials (single use) or reuse of unstable products: for example, sodium ampicillin injection which might be reused by a nurse if supplied in a 250 mg vial with the patient getting a 125 mg dose.

5. Try to prevent the same drug from being supplied at the same time from different manufacturers; this creates confusion with different sizes, colors, and shapes of the medication. I label varied colored tablets (Poly*Vi*Fluor, Luride, etc.) with the statement "Comes in different colors." This should allay the fears of the nurse, and prevent possible administration delay because it was thought that pharmacy had made a mistake.

6. All doses should be calculated by the pharmacy and the information placed on the label, not only as you indicated in your January 1977 column for oral medications, but also for injectables and others. For example, in a pharmacy which does not provide syringe medication, a label for a 30 mg dose of Kantrex should be read:

"Kantrex Pediatric Injection
75 mg per 2 ml
2 ml size vial
30 mg per 0.8 ml"

7. All labeling should indicate the strength per dosage unit:

Lanoxin   Lanoxin
0.25 mg per   NOT   0.25 mg
tab.

The first labeling leaves no doubt that the strength is "per tablet," while the second creates doubt as to whether the strength is for one tablet or for the entire contents of the container. A nurse who has been used to giving single doses in a unit dose system might assume that "Lanoxin 0.25 mg" indicated the entire contents of the container. Thinking that five tablets of 50 μg were supplied, the nurse might administer all five tablets.

Also, I would like to comment on the editorial in the same issue on physicians' handwriting. It certainly is an indication of poor medical care when physicians write carelessly, as is too often the case. Many years ago, I prepared an article for a hospital newsletter wherein I suggested that archaic abbreviations be eliminated from use in medication ordering. The symbols for dram and ounce and Roman numerals, especially for five and ten, are too easily confused except when diligently written. The answer, to me, is very simple. Hospital administrators, nursing leaders, and pharmacy heads should join together in insisting that physicians write clearly, or print, or else don't practice

at a particular institution. If physicians were put on notice that their poor writing would not be tolerated, they would have to correct it.

Peter J. Mancuso, RPh
PO Box 42
New City, NY 10956

12:42, 1977

Error 70

KCl given instead of HCl

A pharmacist received an order for three bottles of 1000 ml 5% dextrose and water with 100 mEq of HCl. The rate of infusion ordered was 150 ml/hour. The pharmacist was aware that this was ordered for a renal patient who was alkalotic and who had been hyperkalemic. The patient was anuric and was undergoing dialysis three times a week. The pharmacist had to prepare the sterile HCl solution specially as this is not available commercially.

When the solutions were delivered to the patient care area, the pharmacist was told by personnel there that the solution was no longer needed. They claimed that it had already been prepared from existing floor stock. It was discovered that what had actually been used was 100 mEq of KCl. Approximately 40 mEq had been administered before the pharmacist inquired and the infusion was stopped.

The potential hazard of infusing such a quantity of KCl in an anuric patient is readily understood. The hazards of high-dose potassium infusion were discussed in Error 67. Current recommendations are that no more than 60 mEq of KCl be added per liter of infusion fluid. This happened to be policy in this hospital, but it was not followed. If the person who made the solution had known of the policy, the error would have stopped there. In addition, floor personnel should know better than to administer such a dose to a renal patient. This shows a need for better in-service education.

If all intravenous solution preparations were prepared by pharmacy, the error would not have occurred. Hospital clinical personnel and administrators should support pharmacy-controlled IV admixture services with facilities and enough personnel to do the job.

Lastly, the way the orders were written by the physician (Fig. 29) contributed to the error. If HCl had been spelled out as hydrochloric acid and/or if the physician had explained to floor personnel the reason for using this drug, the error would not have occurred. Since hydrochloric acid is used so rarely, he might have had the foresight to do this. It cannot be overlooked that his "H" looks almost like a "K."

12:42, 1977

Error 71

Errors in cancer chemotherapy

An order was received by a pharmacist for vincristine 8 mg IV push as part of a protocol for cancer chemotherapy. The pharmacist at first thought that the dose seemed high, but he did not check with the prescriber to learn if the dose was incorrect. The drug was prepared and administered to the patient.

Later, the patient experienced peripheral neuropathy and bowel atony that progressed to toxic megacolon (vincristine toxicity). On investigation, the error was discovered. The dose prescribed was a total dose that the prescriber intended to be given over several weeks. The prescriber meant to write for a 2 mg dose.

The pharmacist claimed that he substantiated the dose in his mind,

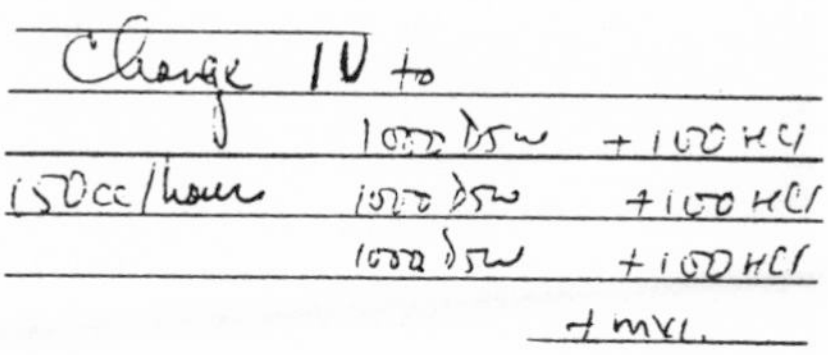

Figure 29. Physician's order. Note "HCl."

because the prescriber was an oncologist and had not been known to err in the past. In fact, another set of chemotherapy orders was written at the same time for another patient and all doses checked out. He further substantiated the dose because vincristine is available in a 1 mg and a 5 mg vial ("Why would 5 mg be available if not for these higher doses?"). Further, the pharmacist was used to seeing unusually high doses of other drugs (above the range listed in official product information inserts) routinely in chemotherapy protocols. He recalled specifically routine doses of fluorouracil far above those recommended in package inserts.

It is important to examine the factors that contributed to this error as well as a few other realities that also lead to errors in chemotherapy. Because most of the agents used exhibit some type of toxicity even in therapeutic doses, inadvertent overdoses can be particularly tragic. Subtherapeutic doses do not give the patient the full benefit of a designed protocol. We have already published several errors dealing with cancer chemotherapy (see Chapter 14).

The greatest problem with chemotherapy is that the entire area is not one in which many of us have a great deal of knowledge. For this reason we may put complete trust in the oncology specialist who orders the regimens. As this error shows, this can lead to tragic circumstances. I believe that the area of cancer chemotherapy is so important that it needs clinical

174

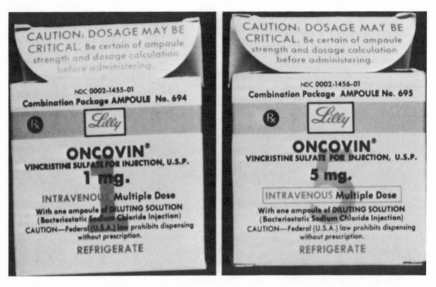

Figure 30. Vials of vincristine sulfate. The 5 mg vial is meant to be used for multiple dose preparation in cancer centers. Its existence may lead one to substantiate an overdose. A warning statement should appear in the labeling that it is for multiple dose *only*.

pharmacy specialists. It is certainly a full-time job trying to keep up with the literature in this constantly changing field. I believe that whenever cancer chemotherapy is used in a general hospital, special ward areas should be set aside so that personnel there become accustomed to the problems of chemotherapy, including techniques, drugs, doses, etc.

Many pharmacists tend to shy away from cancer problems, believing that this is an area that they can never master. The psychological aspects of dealing with cancer patients also leads us to avoid this involvement.

Until clinical pharmacy specialists in the field of oncology become a standard, most of us are still faced with these problems. All doses need to be checked, no matter who prescribed them.

This brings up yet another problem with cancer chemotherapy. Informa-

tion about the drugs — specifically, the doses used in protocols — is often hard to come by. Because doses change so rapidly (often in ranges higher than those used before), the literature may not reflect the changes. We often see unusually high doses of drugs used and this can easily substantiate an inadvertently written high dose of another agent. But we cannot allow ourselves to fall into this trap.

At Temple University Hospital we keep an information book in each satellite pharmacy with all current protocols. Before a new protocol is initiated, an abstract is added to each book; these abstracts serve as a ready reference for checking. The protocol abstract gives us the indications, the drug names, the doses to be used and a dose range for each drug based on body weight or M^2 (Fig. 31). It is listed by protocol number. By mutual agreement with our Oncology Sec-

SEG
Protocol #343

Phase III—Study of intermittent BCNU, cyclophosphamide and prednisone vs intermittent melphalan and prednisone in multiple myeloma and of the addition of fluoxymesterone, sodium fluoride, calcium gluconate and vitamin D vs the addition of placebo for each, and vitamin D

Treatment Regimen: Patients are randomized into Regimen A or B.

Induction Regimen A
BCNU 75 mg/M² IV in 10–30 min.
Cyclophosphamide 400 mg/M² IV push
Prednisone 75 mg/day po × seven days

Repeat every four weeks for six courses

Induction Regimen B
Melphalan 8 mg/M²/day po × 4 days
Prednisone 75 mg/day po × 7 days

Repeat every four weeks for six courses

Maintenance: Responders continue induction regimen at monthly intervals and are randomized to one of the following for 18 months:

A	B
Fluoxymesterone 25 mg/M²/day po	Placebo 1 tab/M² to nearest half tab
Sodium Fluoride 50 mg po TID, AC	Placebo 1 tab po TID, AC
Calcium Gluconate 2 g po TID p.c.	Calcium Gluconate 4 tabs TID, p.c.
Vitamin D 50,000 units po twice weekly	Vitamin D 50,000 units po twice weekly

Dosage checklist

	BCNU 75 mg/M²	Cyclophosphamide 400 mg/M²	Melphalan 8 mg/M²*	Fluoxymesterone 25 mg/M²*
1.2 M²	90 mg	480 mg	9.6 mg	30 mg
1.4 M²	105 mg	560 mg	11.2 mg	35 mg
1.6 M²	120 mg	640 mg	12.8 mg	40 mg
1.8 M²	135 mg	720 mg	14.4 mg	45 mg
2.0 M²	150 mg	800 mg	16.0 mg	50 mg

* To the nearest 1/2 tablet.

Figure 31. Pharmacy-prepared abstract of protocol for cancer chemotherapy regimen.

tion, the protocol number appears on the physician's order or progress notes.

It should be mentioned that much confusion about chemotherapeutic agents is generated by the poor system of nomenclature. The HOSPITAL PHARMACY editorial "No trade names for cancer chemotherapy agents," (11:36, 1976) speaks well to this issue and should be consulted.

Finally, specific for this medication

error, 5 mg vials of vincristine are rarely needed for general use. They are really meant to be used in institutions with large cancer populations where more than one dose at a time is to be drawn up (for several patients at the same time). Stocking these vials in the hospital that sees only occasional use of vincristine should be discouraged. Some consideration should be given by Eli Lilly and Company to labeling the 5 mg vials with a warning statement that this form is for use in preparing multiple doses *only*. Currently, no warning label exists (Fig. 30).

12:70, 1977

Error 72

Inadvertent IV injection of penicillin G procaine

A physician wrote a drug order for 600,000 units of aqueous procaine penicillin G to be given intravenously every six hours. This order was scheduled as originally written, in medication administration records, by floor personnel. The order was then sent to pharmacy for processing and dispensing.

The pharmacist on duty was new on the job; he had not previously practiced in a hospital environment and was unfamiliar with the problems associated with intravenous injections of suspensions. The drug order was entered onto a pharmacy patient profile and readied for dispensing. Just before dispensing, an experienced pharmacist checked the order and the misadventure was stopped.

While trying to contact the prescribing physician, the pharmacists were called by the person who was to administer the drug. This person requested an immediate supply of the

drug since the administration time scheduled had arrived. When the pharmacists questioned this person, they determined that this person in fact expected to give procaine penicillin G intravenously (". . . yes — the white stuff").

That inadvertent intravenous injection of procaine penicillin G may be extremely hazardous to patients is well known. According to Galpin et al. ("Pseudoanaphylactic" reactions from inadvertent infusion of procaine penicillin G, *Annals of Internal Medicine* 81:358, 1974), a potentially lethal reaction might occur due to microembolization of procaine penicillin particles to the lungs and brain, as well as a direct toxic effect of the procaine component. The potential for this reaction may be great, as I have personally reviewed several such physician orders, have received numerous reports of this and have read several articles attesting to the problem.

Anyone involved in the hospital drug distribution cycle (physician, nurse, pharmacist, etc.) must be aware that only clear liquids are given intravenously (an exception would be Intralipid, which is an emulsion). Of course, not all clear liquids are suitable for intravenous use but this should be checked before injection. Colloids and suspensions are also avoided (except amphotericin B and phytonadione injections, which are collodial solutions and appear clear to the unaided eye).

Apparently, confusion over the nomenclature of parenteral penicillin products contributed to this potential error. Confusion exists because penicillin G potassium for injection had a synonym, aqueous penicillin G potassium. Penicillin G procaine is an aqueous suspension and is sometimes referred to as "aqueous procaine peni-

```
NDC 41-128-01              A STERILE SUSPENSION FOR
                           SUBCUTANEOUS INJECTION
                           CAUTION: U.S. Federal Law prohibits
Sus-Phrine®                dispensing without prescription.
                           ADULT DOSE: 0.1 to 0.3ml. subcutaneously.
(EPINEPHRINE               See enclosed circular.
SUSPENSION 1:200)          SHAKE WELL BEFORE USING
                           To obtain a uniform white suspension
5 ml. MULTIPLE DOSE VIAL   LC 12/71              Printed in U.S.A.
```

Figure 32

cillin." This leads some to believe that the product is a solution and can be given intravenously. The confusion would be ended if the terms penicillin G potassium and penicillin G procaine only were used.

12:142, 1977

Error 73

Incorrect route of administration of Sus-Phrine

An error similar to error 72 occurred; this involved the product Sus-phrine. An order was written by a physician as follows, "Sus-phrine 0.3 ml of a 1:200."

A person responsible for drug administration gave 0.3 ml of 1:200 epinephrine suspension (Sus-phrine) intravenously, mixed with 100 ml of 5% dextrose in water. The fact that this is not a clear solution was not noticed. The physician's order in this case was incomplete, since route of administration was not specified. It was assumed that the epinephrine was to be given intravenously.

The patient experienced only tachycardia and headache, and no serious injury. Incidentally, although the package is labeled ". . . for sub-

cutaneous injection" (Fig. 32), no warning appears that it is not intended for intravenous use. Perhaps the manufacturer should consider such a warning, since epinephrine is commonly administered intravenously as epinephrine HCl.

12:142, 1977

Error 74

Since when does ½ + ½ = ¼?

A patient with coronary artery disease had been receiving nitroglycerin sublingual tablets in a strength of 1/200 gr. After therapy was initiated, the nursing unit ran out of this tablet strength. A well-meaning person who was responsible for drug administration did not want the patient to miss any doses. Two tablets of 1/100 gr were later given to the patient when he complained of chest pain. No information was supplied as to how the 1/100 gr tablets were obtained that allowed for a fourfold dosing error.

Remedial education in pharmacy math is obviously indicated here. However, isn't it about time that we drop apothecary dose designations from use in our health care system? If the metric system only were used by health professionals and manufacturers, errors like this one would be unlikely to occur. It is doubtful that two 600 mcg tablets (1.2 mg) would be construed as being equal to a 300 mcg tablet.

12:150, 1977

Error 75

Active ingredient not administered

Officials of a state mental institution pressured the pharmacy department to lower drug costs. Milligram for milligram, the tablet form of Haldol (haloperidol) is less expensive than the liquid concentrate. Since Haldol concentrate was a major item of purchase at the institution, it was suggested that the pharmacist make his own concentrate. After a superficial checking of the stability and solubility, an aqueous preparation was made using the tablets. Tablets were crushed, water added, and the mixture filtered; the filtrate was used.

It was soon noted that the patients did not respond; doses were raised. Eventually, it was discovered that haloperidol is very insoluble in water and that the unused, undissolved material was the active ingredient.

Without the benefit of support from an analytical laboratory and an experienced analytical chemist, pharmacists should not attempt to prepare such extemporaneous dosage forms. A spokesman at McNeil Laboratories notes that haloperidol is very insoluble in water. Only 10 mg of pure drug substance will dissolve in 100 ml of water at pH 5.9. Solubility is further reduced when the drug is combined with excipients used in tablet formulations. He concludes that preparation of a solution from the tablets is not possible.

It cannot be emphasized strongly enough that some pharmacists must not allow themselves to be pressured into dispensing inferior products for the sake of reducing costs. Even if there were no stability or solubility problems, it is doubtful that money would have been saved if the labor and material costs were considered as well as the additional liability being assumed. Alteration of dosage form should only be undertaken when necessary and only after thorough investigation.

The problem cited need never have occurred, since the pharmaceutical industry had long ago come up with a product to meet the need.

12:190, 1977

Error 76

Precipitate injected with careless use of intravenous drug administration equipment

A 70-year-old patient with chronic obstructive pulmonary disease developed acute bronchitis and bacterial lobar pneumonia. Infectious disease personnel recommended an intensive therapy regimen composed of cephalothin and gentamicin to cover the spectrum of the diffused nature of the bacterial infection.

The pharmacy admixture area personnel prepared the drugs in minibags and specifically noted on the labels that the two drugs were incompatible and should not be allowed to mix in any way. The nursing staff was also informed that care was needed in their administration to assure that the drugs were not mixed.

The medications were to be administered via a Y set type of administration device. A blood set was attached to the minibag instead of a regular solution set. After administration of the first antibiotic, there was inadequate "flushing" of the entire set to remove all residue before use of the second antibiotic.

Immediately after the second drug was begun, the patient developed acute respiratory distress and cyanosis. A pharmacist noted a precipitate in the line, immediately stopped the solution and had the tubing changed. Within one hour the patient's symptoms had subsided. The patient mentioned that he noted the precipitate in the tubing; however, he was under the impression that he was being fed intravenously to "help regain strength." It was suspected that the episode was due to accumulation of precipitated drug particles in the lungs in a patient whose condition was already compromised.

This is an example of a drug incompatibility that resulted in a significant manifestation in spite of adequate precautions taken by the pharmacy department's admixture service to prevent such episodes. Prevention of such incidents depends on in-service education of all those responsible for IV drug administration.

12:190, 1977

Error 77

Not reading labels – again

Eleven patients received the wrong ophthalmic ointment due to a packaging error caused by a pharmacist. In preparing the package, the pharmacist depended on color, box appearance and location of product on shelf rather than package label.

An "Eye-kit" had been prepackaged for several months for use by nursing personnel in the care of patients hospitalized for cataract surgery. Of 10 medications contained in the kit, one was Ophthocort ointment (chloramphenicol-polymyxin-hydrocortisone). While packaging a number of the kits, kept in plastic bags, the pharmacist reached for the Ophthocort, which was always kept in the same spot, glanced at the product and placed one package into each bag. Someone had placed chloromycetin ophthalmic ointment where the Ophthocort was normally kept. The packages look similar in color and size. All of the kits contained chloromycetin. In 11 cases, the wrong ointment was subsequently administered by nursing personnel until finally someone noticed the error. When will we ever learn?

12:191, 1977

Error 78

Adding new medications to a patient's regimen requires thoughtful action by a pharmacist

On an admission history, a patient told of an allergy to Mandelamine. It was noted by the physician and a warning label was placed on the chart. It was noted in the nurses' Kardex and in the pharmacist's patient profile. During the course of hospitalization the physician ordered Hiprex. The nurse entered it in her Kardex. The pharmacist entered it on his patient profile and dispensed the medication. The patient had an allergic reaction to Hiprex.

Mandelamine is methenamine mandelate and Hiprex is methenamine hippurate. It is not surprising that a patient who is allergic to one would be allergic to the other. The physician should have known, the nurse should have known and the pharmacist, above all, should have known. This pharmacist must have been entering orders on the profile in a mechanical, non-thinking manner, because he surely knew that both drugs were methenamine salts. The act of adding a new drug to a patient's regimen must always be done with awareness and thoughtfulness by a health professional.

12:250, 1977

Error 79
Experience helps prevent errors

A pharmacist in a hospital with a unit dose system received an order at 8:30 PM for "54 units NPH Insulin." Shortly thereafter one of the floor personnel telephoned about the dose. When questioned, she said the dose was to be administered now. The pharmacist knew that the diabetes of this patient was not controlled; he drew up and labeled the dose.

When a more experienced night pharmacist came on duty, the evening pharmacist told him that the insulin was drawn up and would be picked up shortly. The night pharmacist knew it was highly unlikely that a large dose of this intermediate-acting insulin would be given at night. The physician was contacted and he said he meant to write "54 units of NPH in the AM," although his order did not say "in the AM."

If this drug had been available on the nursing unit, it would have been given and the patient would probably have had an episode of hypoglycemia. If the more experienced pharmacist had not come on duty, the dose might have been given. When asked, the less experienced pharmacist knew the onset, peak and duration of action of NPH insulin but because the patient's disease was not under control and be-

cause he had received a call asking for it, he had been prepared to dispense the dose.

12:250, 1977

Error 80
TesTape – Clinitest Readings

I am writing not to report a specific error, but to bring out a misconception that may lead to potential errors. It is fairly common knowledge to pharmacists and nurses that cephalosporins and a few other agents interfere with copper-reduction tests (Clinitest) for urine glucose and may therefore register a false positive. During the period that these agents are administered, an alternate method of testing urine glucose, such as the glucose oxidase method (TesTape), is usually recommended.

It is important to note that TesTape and Clinitest readings are not interchangeable, in that a ½% sugar concentration is read as a 1+ with Clinitest and 3+ with TesTape.

The potential problem arises when a physician has instructed to change insulin dosages according to 3+ readings based on Clinitest and the nurse or patient is using TesTape. The misunderstanding may lead to overdosing of insulin and possible hypoglycemia.

Physicians, pharmacists, nurses, and patients should be aware of this difference to insure proper insulin use. Perhaps the best resolution to the problem would be to encourage physicians to order insulin coverage based on percentage rather than pluses.

A Pharmacist

Editor's note:

Although most pharmacists are aware of the differences in values between Clinitest and TesTape, the reader's point is an important one and deserves publicity. Pharmacists should take time to explain the differences to other clinical staff when either product may be in use. This problem is one reason why we have elected to use only glucose oxidase strips in our inpatient areas. Note: The manufacturers of these products in cooperation with the American Diabetic Association have recently dropped the "plus" system from their labeling. Only percent will be used.

13:37, 1978

Error 81

Subtherapeutic dose of liquid tranquilizer administered through use of wrong dropper

An inpatient prescription written for fluphenazine HCl (Prolixin Elixir) was filled in the pharmacy in a four-ounce pharmacy glass bottle. It was labeled as 0.5 mg/ml (Fig. 33). Since the dose prescribed was 5 mg, the pharmacist who filled the prescription assumed that a floor employe would use a dose measurer to pour 10 ml of the 0.5 mg per ml liquid. However, someone, apparently thinking it would be more convenient to use a dose-graded dropper to measure the dose, placed a dropper from an empty bottle of Stelazine Concentrate into the Prolixin bottle (Fig. 33). The dropper cap fit perfectly. The measurements on the Stelazine Concentrate (10 mg per ml) dropper are 10 mg, 8 mg and 5 mg. Each of several doses of 5 mg was measured by using the 5 mg increment on the Stelazine dropper. The dose actually administered then was 0.25 mg of Prolixin, a good deal less than the 5 mg intended.

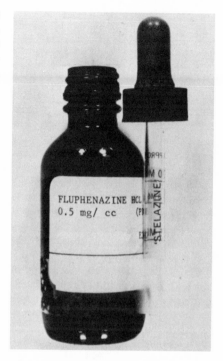

Figure 33. Fluphenazine bottle and Stelazine dropper.

Several factors contributed to this medication error. First and obvious is that droppers meant for one particular medication are not interchangeable for use with another. They should not be used to cap a bottle of another drug, even on a temporary basis, such as if the original non-dropper cap was lost or broken. The dropper itself in this case clearly stated "Stelazine." If this had been read, perhaps the error would not have occurred.

The labeling placed on the bottle in the pharmacy is also open to criticism. The label should have stated the volume of elixir necessary to administer the 5 mg dose. If prepackaged unit doses of liquids were utilized, this type of error would not have been possible.

Correspondence

On exchanging droppers

A reader writes:

In medication error 81, the error in attaching a wrong dropper to a bottle was discussed. This involved a single patient.

In a facility like ours (a mental health facility), an error of that nature may likely involve many patients. On one ward, personnel interchanged a Navane Concentrate dropper with a Loxitane Concentrate bottle by mistake. A Loxitane dropper is calibrated as 25 mg/ml, while the Navane dropper is calibrated as 5 mg/ml. This could lead to patients receiving high doses of Loxitane and low doses of Navane. However, no evidence of administering with wrong droppers was found. Right away as a precautionary measure the pharmacist checked all the caps and a memo was put out to all nursing personnel. This memo deals with all the liquid concentrates used at this hospital and the potential danger of interchangeability of the caps.

TO: All Nursing Personnel

The Nursing Procedure entitled "Oral Medication," on page 64 of Hospital Procedure Manual is supplemented by precautions pertaining to the following major tranquilizer concentrates:

Loxitane C
Serentil
Mellaril
Sinequan
Navane
Thorazine

Each of the calibrated droppers for these medications has a cap that is interchangeable with the various medication bottles indicated. However, each of the graduated glass tubes is plainly marked with the name of the medication it was intended for.

Haldol Concentrate and *Permitil* Concentrate (White's brand of Prolixin) have identical caps. However, Haldol's glass gradu- ated tube is marked "Haldol." Permitil's glass graduated tube has no markings indicating it is for Permitil.

Stelazine Concentrate and *Sparine* Concentrate have the same size caps. Stelazine's glass graduated tube indicates it is for use with Stelazine. Sparine's graduated glass tube has no markings indicating it is for use with Sparine.

It is imperative that every individual working with one of these concentrates inspect the glass tube each and every time medication is prepared to be certain that the indicated dropper is in the proper bottle.

cc: Each Ward
    Each R.N.
    Each Att. Supv.
    Pharmacy
    Asst. Supt. Medical
    Chairman P & T Committee
    Chairman Procedure Committee

A Reader

12:348, 1977

Error 82

Confusion about midnight

Serious consideration should be given to publicizing the actual meaning of the term "midnight" and the abbreviations used for 12 noon (12 PM) and 12 midnight (12 AM).

A real problem exists when medications are ordered so that the first or final dose occurs at midnight. The danger is that the person ordering the drug or persons responsible for scheduling the order may not always agree about whether midnight is the beginning of a day (it is) or the end of a day (it is not). Thus a possibility exists that a patient may receive a drug for an extra 24 hours or have the drug discontinued 24 hours too soon. For example, how would you interpret the following order?

Decadron 4 mg IV q6h until midnight
6/2/77.

Some would assume that the last dose should be given at midnight between 6/1 and 6/2 (correct). Others would assume midnight between 6/2 and 6/3 (wrong—but ask your colleagues). The ordering physician may also be confused about the meaning of midnight, adding to the chance of error.

According to the Time Service Division of the Naval Observatory in Washington, D.C., this is a common problem. They recommend the following solutions (in order of preference).

1. Designate midnight using the dates falling before and after midnight 12 midnight on 6/2 should be listed as 12 midnight (6/1-6/2).

2. Use schedules (have physicians orders) that specify 12:01 or 11:59 (this seems impractical for hospitals). This system is used by railroads.

3. Use military time systems: 0100 (1 AM) to 0000 (12 midnight). This system is in use by airlines and the military. Unfortunately most people (including military personnel) believe that 2400 is the last number in the system but there's no such number—it's 0000 or 0 h. This makes one think it is the end of the day, which it is not.

To me, the most practical system for hospitals would seem to be suggestion number one. However, at our hospital we have gotten excellent results by publicizing that midnight is the beginning of a new day. This is listed in our department's procedure manual and is known and followed by our pharmacists and nurses.

Another issue which is confusing is whether midnight is 12 AM and noon

is 12 PM (right) or vice versa (wrong). Again, different people have different opinions. This can also lead to medication error. The National Bureau of Standards recommends that because of their ambiguity, the abbreviations 12 AM and 12 PM never be used. They suggest the terms noon and midnight be used instead, or more precisely, 12 noon and 12 midnight with no abbreviation.

12:348, 1977

Error 83

Abbreviation OD for "daily" should be banned

Unfortunately, the abbreviation O.D. meaning "once daily" or "daily" is in common use. The hazards of this abbreviation are obvious to pharmacists. A danger exists that a liquid meant for oral use could be given in the right eye. When a "q" is added to the abbreviation (q.o.d.) to mean "every other day," the danger is that this may be mistaken for q.i.d., or every day. I recently received a report from a pharmacist citing yet another misinterpretation of "O.D." This one nearly caused a death.

A prescription was written by a physician for Lasix 40 mg, 1 O.D. Unfortunately, I could not get a copy of the prescription to include in this article as an illustration, but according to the pharmacist, the misinterpretaion occurred because the period after the "O" looked more like a slash. Also, the 1 was so close to the "O" that he thought it was a 10. The prescription was interpreted as Lasix 40 mg, 10/d.

After receiving Lasix 400 mg daily for several doses, the patient became severely dehydrated and was admitted to a hospital with electrolyte im-

184

balance. The fact that 400 mg daily doses of Lasix are not uncommon helped to substantiate the dose in the pharmacist's mind. The error was discovered when the pharmacist investigated further.

A campaign against the use of "O.D." to mean "Once Daily" should be undertaken in pharmacy newsletters. There is no acceptable abbreviation for "daily." The word must be spelled out.

12:363, 1977

Error 84

Coined names

Several years ago, a relatively inexperienced evening pharmacist received an order for "Black and White, 30 ml hs prn." The only black and white the pharmacist knew of was scotch. The whiskey had been stored by the pharmacy for some time and was dispensed occasionally by physician order. This is what was dispensed. No complaint was voiced by the patient. The physician who wrote the order claimed that "everybody knows that Black and White is a laxative mixture containing the equivalent of 5 ml of aromatic cascara fluid extract and 30 ml of milk of magnesia." It is easy to understand how coined names and abbreviations evolve.

Obviously, everyone does not know what these unique "nicknames" mean, thus errors occur. Health professionals waste time clarifying orders and therapy is delayed as a result. Community pharmacists are particularly vulnerable when they receive prescriptions for coined named drugs which are familiar only to those who work within the institution where the physician practices. For example, our dermatologists routinely prescribed "T.M.C.," an abbreviation

for triamcinolone. I personally received several calls from community practitioners asking what this was.

An unbelievable situation was reported to us concerning coined names. When topical solution mixtures of three antibiotics were being used in hip surgery, a lazy physician ordered "chicken soup" rather than spelling out the lengthy formula. Nurses and pharmacists know what the orthopedist wanted. But can you envision this medical record being used in a court case, or even worse, chicken soup being used? I have also received orders for "pink lady" (tincture of belladonna, Maalox, and phenobarbital elixir), "dynamite" (Dulcolax) and I'm sure others which I can't recall.

Most Pharmacy and Therapeutics Committees have rules on the books stating that no chemical symbols be used in writing orders and that there be an approved list of abbreviations (this is a JCAH requirement). When a complex formula is consistently prescribed, a descriptive name for this product should be approved by the Pharmacy and Therapeutics Committee for use only within the institution. The name and exact formula must appear in the Formulary. Every effort must be made to resist creating such unofficial names.

Note on Error 84

Coined names

In Error 84 we discussed the problem that "coined names" for drugs present. One coined name illustrated was "chicken soup," an epithet given in one hospital to irrigating solutions of Neomycin and Bacitracin. We recently received word from a Catholic hospital that they too use a coined name for this antibiotic solution. It is referred to as "Holy Water."

12:427, 1977

Error 85

Illegible handwriting

An order was sloppily written before angiography for Seconal 100 mg IM. This order looked like Demerol 100 mg IM. Demerol was administered. The procedure was cancelled one day and subsequent surgery was postponed until the next week. Hundreds if not thousands of dollars were wasted by this delay, not counting the increased anxiety which must have been suffered by the patient. Sloppy handwriting is no joke.

12:427, 1977

Error 86

Vincristine medication error – 3 deaths

In error 71 a vincristine overdose was cited. Kaufman, in the *Journal Pediatrics* (89:671, 1976), reported the following five vincristine overdose cases.

1. A 13-year-old received a 32 mg dose. The order was written by a new intern on the service. The patient died.
2. A 7-year-old was given a monthly dose on two consecutive days by a physician unfamiliar with the protocol. The patient recovered.
3. A 5-year-old received 3.5 mg (a fourfold error) because of a mistake in calculation. The patient recovered.
4. An 8-year-old received 6.5 mg because of a decimal error. The patient died.
5. A 7-year-old received 13.5 mg due to a decimal error. The patient died.

Kaufman states, "The most important consideration in regard to vincristine overdosage is prevention. All of the cases presented here involved physicians who had little experience with the uses and dangers of vincristine. Be_____ nal dose of vincristine is _____ roximately 0.06 mg/k_____ to make a large er_____ r what seems_____ ug. It is imp_____ ed in treat_____ erapeuti_____ ten- tial d_____ er to mini_____ acci- dent,_____ wing guide

1. _____ han- dl_____ nts sh_____ e of th_____ gh a la_____ edi- at_____ e re- ce_____ , ad- m_____ ould never be co_____ ne task.

2. Charts of normal doses of chemotherapeutic agents should be available in all nursing stations and wherever drugs are prepared or administered.
3. All chemotherapeutic doses should be fully calculated and recorded in the chart by a member of the hematology-oncology service. The dose should be written in mg/kg concentration,* total dose, and volume: 0.06 mg/kg x 33 kg = 2 mg = 10 ml/1 mg x 2 = 20 ml.
4. Chemotherapy should be given only by an experienced physician who can check the dose and concentration before it is administered. As with many other chemotherapy agents, vincristine must be given intravenously. Extravasation into the skin causes severe and painful burns.
5. Stock only small dose vials of vincristine (10 ml = 1 mg). This greatly reduces the opportunity to

---

*Or mg/m^2. (ND)

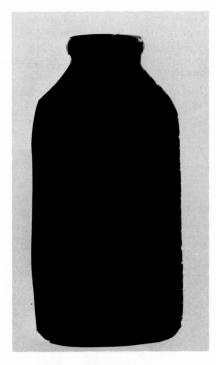

Figure 34. Actual label on cocaine-epinephrine solution for topical use. Important auxiliary labels are missing. Misspelling and overtypes are characteristic of poor labeling.

1. Pharmacists should always receive a copy of the physician's order.
2. Pharmacists should maintain copies of cancer chemotherapy protocols.
3. Pharmacists should maintain patient profiles with patients' vital statistics, diagnoses, and drug regimens.
4. With this information the pharmacist should function as a monitor of dosage calculation and dosage interval and should insure that the order is written for the proper patient before the drug is administered.
5. An experienced pharmacist should prepare and label the dose.

12:499, 1977

give a massive overdose. The maximum single dose of vincristine is usually 2 mg.

Careful observance of these guidelines should minimize the opportunities for accidental overdosage."

Four of these five cases were recognized in three San Diego hospitals since 1970. How many overdoses of vincristine in other San Diego hospitals went unnoted? In the state of California? How many were there in the US during this 5-year period?

We would like to add several additional recommendations to those of Dr. Kaufman:

Error 87
Need for auxiliary labels

A hypertensive patient came to an accident ward with a nosebleed. Physicians there chose to treat this patient with nasal packings of cocaine-epinephrine solution. An intern told a nurse (who had been recently hired) to "get this patient 10 ml of cocaine-epi solution;" he was to apply it topically. However, the nurse was not familiar with the drug and administered 10 ml (1 g) orally to the patient (a 10% cocaine solution).

A call requesting information about cocaine-epinephrine absorption, blood pressure effects, etc. was received in the pharmacy. Fortunately, as it turned out, practically all of a cocaine dose given orally is hydrolyzed and not absorbed. Epinephrine is also broken down and not absorbed. The patient's vital signs taken at 10 minute intervals showed no real changes in blood pressure; heart rate increased by 10 beats per minute. A literature search turned up information that deaths have occurred with as little as 40 mg being injected intravenously.

Although this error demonstrates again that people do not always have all the information they need when prescribing or administering drugs, another point should be made. In this situation when the bottle was obtained from the emergency department (Fig. 34), it was noted that no auxiliary label such as "For external use only" or "Not to be swallowed" was affixed. If these labels had been attached, no doubt this would have offered the nurse enough guidance to prevent the error. Make sure such labels are attached to all external prescriptions you fill.

Believe it or not, I've also received a report about "one cup of pHisohex" being ordered. According to the source, this too was administered orally!

12:518, 1977

Error 88

Reconstituting unit dose suspensions of antibiotics

I received the following comment from a reader:

"The volume for reconstituting *unit dose* antibiotic suspensions is never accurately measured in our pharmacy. The rationale for this is that the patient will take the entire contents of the vial at one time so the volume need not be any specific amount. The labeling on the V Cillin and Keflex unit dose suspension vials indicates the amount of drug in milligrams only. However, the label on Abbott's Erythromycin Ethyl Succinate suspension reads 200 mg per 5 ml. Most of the time these vials are reconstituted by our pharmacists with more than 5 ml.

"A nurse was supposed to be administering 800 mg of erythromycin suspension, that is, four vials. Instead she gave 20 ml (4 x 5 ml), which turned out to be less than four vials and thus less than 800 mg of erythromycin suspension. I believe that Abbott's labeling is misleading. I have written them expressing my belief and concern about this particular product.

"This error report could be interesting to your readers, as this might be occurring at other hospitals, too."

After receiving this pharmacist's letter, I wrote to Abbott Laboratories and they replied:

This is in response to your inquiry regarding the labeling used on E.E.S.™ Granules/Erythrocin Ethyl Succinate Granules in unit dose vials. You asked the reason a specific volume of water is required for reconstitution of the product and why "200 mg erythromycin activity per 5 ml" is claimed instead of "200 mg/vial."

The label claim and reconstitution instructions are related to the assay procedure used by the Food and Drug Administration during the certification process for this antibiotic. The procedure outlined in *Code of Federal Regulations*, Title 21, Part 452.125c(b) requires that a sample be reconstituted as directed in the labeling. An accurately measured volume of the reconstituted suspension is then removed for further dilution and assay. The assay does not measure total erythromycin per vial. Rather, it measures erythromycin per unit of volume. For the assay to be meaningful and reproducible, it is necessary to use a specific volume of water for reconstitution. The addition of 4.7 ml (1 level capful) water provides a suspension containing 200 mg erythromycin activity per 5 ml.

I hope this information adequately answers your questions.

Ronald N. Sheptak
Abbott Laboratories

It appears to me that the only way to alleviate the problem is to reconstitute the vials with 4.7 ml or else dispense the unit dose vials to the patient care area unreconstituted.

12:525, 1977

Error 89

Misinterpretation of poorly written physician's order

A 70-year-old woman, an insulin-controlled diabetic, was receiving 80 mg of prednisone daily. This dosage had been administered for two weeks. The patient's physician wanted to begin withdrawal of the steroid and wrote an order to "decrease prednisone 5 mg daily."

A ward clerk transcribed the order and the new dose listed was 5 mg daily — not 75 mg daily. This was checked by a nurse who evidently interpreted the order in the same way. The following day the patient received only 5 mg (her insulin dosage remained the same).

Later that day, the patient collapsed and the hospital resuscitation team was called. Administration of glucose assisted in reviving her. Blood glucose at the time of collapse was less than 50 mg per ml.

The situation could have been prevented by a more clearly phrased physician's order. What should have been written was "Decrease prednisone by 5 mg daily," or better yet, "Decrease prednisone to 75 mg daily." Nursing personnel must also be aware of the need for gradual withdrawal from corticosteroids when patients receive such high doses for more than a week.

12:525, 1977

Error 90

Error caused by mistranscription of penicillin dose

An order for penicillin G potassium injection, 3,000,000 units was mistranscribed by a ward clerk as 3,00,000 units. This led ward personnel to administer only 300,000 units.

A remedy would be to list such doses as "3 million units."

12:525, 1977

Errors 91 and 92

Floor stock kills with the aid of doctors and nurses

A 45-year-old man was operated on for an inguinal hernia. Ten hours postoperatively he had not yet voided urine. Floor personnel called the patient's physician, who at the time was involved in an emergency. In a rush, the physician gave a verbal order for "Urecholine 25 mg, stat." Five 1 ml vials, each containing 5 mg, were drawn up into a syringe. The person administering the drug assumed that it was to be given intramuscularly. The physician did not specify route of administration and the only form this person was familiar with was the injectable which she had seen in floor stock. The drug was given intramuscularly. Vivid warnings on the vial label and box (subcutaneous use only) were not seen. The physician's intention had actually been oral administration.

Shortly after the dose was given, at the change in shift it was mentioned that the dose had been given. Later, a nurse making routine patient rounds found the patient to be restless and diaphoretic with an elevated blood pressure. The patient told the nurse that he had been given an injection in his buttock to make him urinate.

When the error was discovered, atropine sulfate 0.6 mg IM was given and the symptoms were reversed. This patient was lucky. Most pharmacists are aware that the package insert for bethanecol carries a warning that signs of cholinergic overdose — even cardiac arrest — may occur if the drug is given intramuscularly. Once again we see the problem of not reading labels. This must be publicized.

In addition, it is the pharmacist's continuing responsibility to the hospital professional staff to provide in-service education. A point should be made about bethanecol injection — the only route of administration is subcutaneous. The differences in dose range must also be made clear. While we are at it, we should publicize the drug's pharmacology and major contraindications, such as asthma.

Another point — the fact that five vials of medication were used to prepare the dose — needs to be examined. Health professionals must learn to question single drug doses that require multiple vials, tablets or capsules. This also occurred in the following medication error report. These patients were not as lucky as the one just mentioned.

In error 38, a series of incidents was described, in which five patients received large overdoses of chloramphenicol injection due to misinterpretation of poor labeling by the manufacturer. The person responsible for administering the doses believed that each vial contained only 100 mg when actually 1 g was in the vial. She was led to believe this because the labeling on chloramphenicol vials stated "100 mg chloramphenicol per ml." The "per ml" was easily missed. Even though "10 ml package" was noted elsewhere on the label, it was assumed only 100 mg was in each vial. So for each 1 g dose, 10 vials were used. For a 2 g dose, 20 vials had to be reconstituted. One patient died and four others were injured. The company has since changed the labeling.

What is particularly frightening is that someone reconstituted 10 or 20 vials of drug to prepare the dose. Whether or not this person questioned a colleague about the need for 20 vials to make a single dose is not known. But surely something must have seemed wrong. There are very few instances in which more than one or two dosage units are needed to make a single dose.

I do not think any incident could speak more for the crying need for all hospitals to have a unit dose drug distribution system with little if any floor stock used and with the pharmacy being responsible for preparation of all drug doses. For added safety, 24-hour pharmacy service should be available in hospitals in which drug orders are common at night. All drug orders must be reviewed by a pharmacist before any drugs are dispensed.

Unfortunately, this type of error is not uncommon. In one week I received two similar reports. In both cases the patient died.

In a teaching hospital, an order was written by a physician for "cephalothin 60 mg IV and gentamicin 1 g IV." Obviously he had transposed the respective doses of the two drugs, but someone actually prepared a 1 g dose of gentamicin from 13 vials. The dose was given IV push. This occurred at 2 a.m. Initially, the patient had a respiratory arrest; however, he was resuscitated. Later, renal failure ensued. Furosemide provided no increase in urine output, and neither did a subsequent dose of mannitol. The patient developed congestive heart failure, pulmonary edema and lactic acidosis, then eventually died.

In another case, a physician prescribed 10 mg of haloperidol by mouth for one of his patients, who was a drug addict. The patient had been uncooperative and threatening. When

190

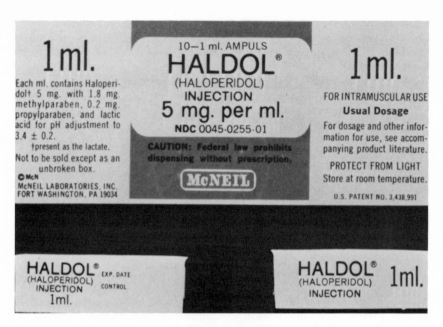

Figure 35. Labeling on front panel of box containing 10 ampuls (above) indicates that each one ml ampul contains 5 mg. However, on box edges (below), there is no strength designation. The 1 ml was misinterpreted as 1 mg.

the oral tablets were given, the patient spit them out. The physician was contacted and gave a verbal order to change the route of administration to intramuscular. The person responsible for drug administration went to floor stock supplies and found 1 ml ampuls of haloperidol injection. Because of the labeling (Fig. 35) on the side of the box, she believed that the ampul contained 1 mg of drug. Since she only had the eight ampuls in stock, she drew up two syringes of 4 ml each (4 ampuls per syringe) and administered these intramuscularly. She then went to the pharmacy for two more ampuls to make up the 10 mg dose. It was then that she learned that actually each ampul contained 5 mg. She had already given a fourfold overdose. She ran back to the floor to find a patient with absent blood pressure. Resuscitative measures were un-

successful. It was later learned that the patient had significant tissue levels of barbiturate and narcotic: this no doubt contributed to death from the haloperidol overdose.

Pharmacists who work in hospitals without unit dose programs must try to convince their administrators and board of trustees of the need for this system of drug distribution. Mentioning cases such as these might be helpful in supporting your point of view. Also, we must work in educating our drug administration personnel to question any doses that require more than one or two dosage units for a single dose. This is especially true in hospitals with floor stock systems. Physicians must exercise proper care in writing orders as they are responsible for their actions.

12:598, 1977

Error 93

Subtherapeutic insulin doses given through improper syringe/needle preparation

A patient was admitted for treatment of diabetic ketoacidosis. As part of the patient's therapy, six units of regular insulin were ordered to be given every six hours intramuscularly. The doses of insulin were prepared and administered by a house staff physician and a medical student.

After several doses, the patient had not responded clinically and blood glucose measurements also showed no improvement. A staff physician ordered the IM insulin to be discontinued in favor of low dose continuous infusion of insulin.

However, in speaking to the medical student, the staff physician learned the reason for the failure with IM insulin. Since only Becton-Dickenson 1 ml insulin syringes (with epoxied needle) were in use in the hospital, intramuscular injections could not be given because the subcutaneous (25 g x ⅝") needle could not be replaced with a needle suitable for intramuscular injection. For this reason, tuberculin syringes were used. Regular insulin (U-100), 0.06 ml was drawn into the syringe using the attached *intradermal* needle. The needle was then removed from the syringe and replaced with a 21 g x 1½" needle. Obviously, as each dose was given intramuscularly, almost all of the drug remained in the newly affixed needle.

This error simply points out that everyone does not know about the potential for the problem illustrated. We should be aware of this and be prepared to provide training to all professionals.

13:37, 1978

Error 94

Gallstones PRN for pain

A patient underwent a cholecystectomy. On the first postoperative day, laboratory personnel brought to the patient's bedside a 7 dram prescription vial containing the gallstones that had been removed. The patient's 23-year-old husband erroneously understood the people from the laboratory to say that this was medication for pain. For the postoperative pain, the husband gave the patient her own gallstones as pain medication. When the error was discovered (no pain relief, I assume), the container was inspected; it had no label.

Many hospital pharmacists will not dispense empty prescription containers or labels to other hospital departments. This is a good rule. Only the pharmacy should dispense or package (JCAH standard).

The pharmacist who sent this report to me swears it's true. Perhaps *this* is what is meant by recurrent gallstones.

13:124, 1978

Error 95

Tetracycline – Maalox combined as a suspension

In a hospital using a unit dose system, a call was received in the pharmacy from a medication nurse. She requested that a single dose of Maalox 15 ml and tetracycline 500 mg capsule be delivered to the floor to replace doses that had been wasted. The pharmacist asked the nurse why they were wasted at the same time, since instructions had been given to the nurses to space doses of the two medications because of the interaction potential. In fact, the scheduled administration times in the nurses' records were appropriate — they had been seen by the pharmacist.

The reason given was that the patient was having trouble swallowing the tetracycline capsule, so it was being mixed to make a suspension with the Maalox. The mixture evidently was spilled. Even though the pharmacist had cautioned floor personnel when the medications were first started about the potential interaction, this information did not reach all nurses or the medication Kardex.

The problem could have been avoided initially if the pharmacists had been told that the patient could not swallow capsules. Tetracycline syrup could have been dispensed (it was subsequently) to be administered at the proper time. Pharmacists should encourage the nurses to provide such patient information.

A short note sent to the floor with the first dose, explaining the reason for separating the doses, could have been clipped on the drug administration record.

13:124, 1978

Error 96

Filtering injectable suspensions

This came from a hospital with a complete pharmacy-coordinated parenteral preparation system.

At this institution, pharmacy technicians extemporaneously prepare all scheduled injectables. A patient was admitted to the hospital with a diagnosis of acute asthma attack. Among other therapies. Sus-phrine 1:200, 0.5 ml subcutaneously every eight hours was ordered. Pharmacy policy dictates the use of a five-micron filter needle whenever procedures involve glass ampuls. The pharmacist cautioned the technician to shake the am-

pul well before aspirating the drug: however, he failed to mention not to use a filter needle.

The patient received three doses before the technician questioned why the drug was cloudy in the ampul and clear in the syringe.

There are two major points in this error:

1. Suspensions obviously should not be aspirated through filter needles.

2. Pharmacists responsible for checking large numbers of injectables should be more alert for less commonly ordered injectables which require procedures unfamiliar to technicians.

A similar incident involving pitressin tannate in oil has happened.

13:124, 1978

Error 97

Verbal order, lack of knowledge and floorstock = amytal for mannitol

In a large hospital, a patient who had had cardiac arrest was being treated for edema after the acute period. A physician gave a verbal order to a nurse to administer 25 g of mannitol. The physician left the floor and returned 10 minutes later to find the nurse drawing up Amytal (amobarbital sodium) from numerous ampuls. Fortunately, the physician realized what was happening and prevented the potentially lethal error.

In Errors 91-92 we discussed in detail the potential for error when someone who prepares a single dose of medication finds that he needs more than one or two dosage units (vials, capsules, ampuls, etc.). Something just might be wrong and unless the person preparing the medication is familiar with using more than one or two dosage units, they should stop and check fully.

The potential error once again points out the hazard of verbal orders and a floor stock system that allows drugs to be dispensed without the order first being reviewed by a pharmacist. A complete lack of knowledge of pharmacology by a person responsible for preparing and administering drugs is also of note.

13:240, 1978

Error 98

Lethal dose of colchicine administered because physician wrote for 1.0 mg

A patient suffering an acute attack of gout was seen by a physician. The physician ordered "colchicine 1.0 mg IV now." (Fig. 36) The decimal point was not seen by the nurse reading the order and she interpreted the dose as 10 mg. A syringe containing 10 mg was prepared from stock and administered to the patient. The patient eventually died from the overdose.

In Error 50 we discussed the problem of using a zero after a decimal point when referring to drug doses. The physician should not prescribe 1.0 mg of a drug. In medical practice there is no difference between 1 mg and 1.0 mg. If 1 mg had been ordered, the patient would not have lost his life. Pharmacists have the responsibility of working to eliminate this writing habit from their institutions.

One company's efforts to reduce medication errors

In Error 98 a problem caused by a physician writing for 1.0 mg of colchicine is addressed. Pharmaceutical

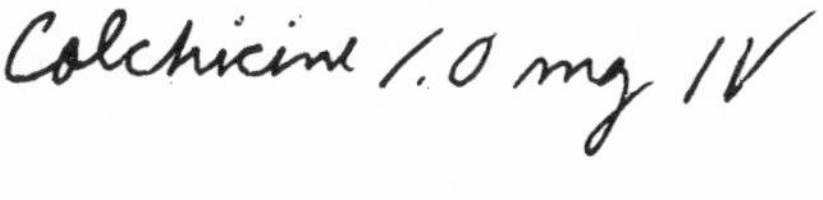

Figure 36

manufacturers have contributed to this problem because they sometimes label their products in this fashion (with a zero after the decimal).

Upon seeing such printed labels and advertisements in journals, label readers may assume that this is a proper method for designating a drug dose in handwriting. One company that has been receptive to change suggested in this feature is Sandoz Pharmaceuticals. An example of their old and new labels is shown in Figure 37. Pharmacists should appreciate their concern.

Pharmacists who observe such labeling should write to the manufacturer and ask them to drop the zero after the decimal.

13:240, 1978

Error 99

You cannot dispense based on half a drug name

An inexperienced recent graduate of pharmacy school received a prescription for Zetar Shampoo to be used two to three times a week as a shampoo. The only Zetar product at the outpatient pharmacy that he was familiar with was Zetar Emulsion. He dispensed the emulsion.

A week later the dermatologist sent the patient back to the pharmacy to have the mistake corrected. Zetar Shampoo has 1% whole coal tar in a lathering shampoo, whereas Zetar emulsion has 30% whole coal tar in a water dispensable and washable base. The emulsion is nonlathering

194

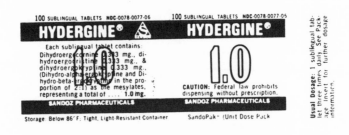

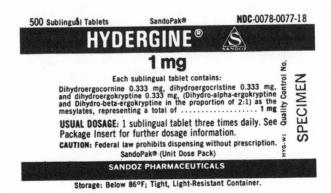

Figure 37

and intended for addition to a bath or direct application to a lesion. You can imagine what the patient thought when she tried to use the nonlathering emulsion as a shampoo.

Even experienced pharmacists are not familiar with all products and are capable of making mistakes if they dispense medication on the basis of half a drug product's name. Inexperienced pharmacists certainly might not be familiar with some products. Inexperienced pharmacists must be supervised by experienced pharmacists or errors will surely occur. Many times physicians are imprecise in writing prescriptions, but the greatest majority of times they are precise. Zetar Emulsion is not Zetar Shampoo!

13:241, 1978

Errors 100 and 101

Tincture of opium should be banned

Serious errors occur because of confusion surrounding the products tincture of opium and paregoric (camphorated tincture of opium). Many people are unaware of the differences between these two products.

An elderly physician wrote a prescription for "camphorated tincture of opium" to be given in a 5 ml dose every four hours for diarrhea. A 1 oz dropper bottle of "opium tincture" was already in the narcotic drawer on the nursing unit. The medication nurse asked another physician if the two were the same thing. He said yes.

The patient was given a 5 ml dose of opium tincture (equivalent to 50 mg morphine). Some time later when a duplicate copy of the original order

Table 1. Morphine contents of opium tincture and paregoric

	Morphine contents of opium products	Single dose
Opium tincture	1 ml = 10 mg	0.6-1.5 ml
Paregoric (camphorated tincture of opium)	1 ml = 0.4 mg 5 ml = 2 mg	5-10 ml

was received in the pharmacy, one of the pharmacists called the nursing unit to find out if they needed the camphorated opium tincture. The error was then discovered. The patient suffered no ill effects from this error in dosage.

It is difficult to substantiate a continued need for tincture of opium. We have several other effective oral narcotic analgesics and antidiarrheals. Because of the similarity in the names of tincture of opium and camphorated tincture of opium there is a real potential for mix-ups by personnel unfamiliar with these products. It seems that tincture of opium is not widely used today: however, many hospitals and community pharmacies do stock it. Since paregoric is still widely prescribed in and out of the hospital, I would favor deletion of tincture of opium as a pharmaceutical product. In fact, perhaps all tincture dosage forms should be questioned; speculation leads me to believe that the solution can evaporate, leaving super concentrations of active drug. Hospital pharmacists should discourage the use of tincture of opium in their institutions and should consider dropping it from their formulary and inventory. It should never be stored anywhere other than the pharmacy.

Manufacturers of tincture of opium (if they are to continue manufacturing this product) should at least place a warning on the product label which cautions that the product is not to be confused with camphorated opium tincture (paregoric), since the morphine concentration in tincture of opium is 25 times greater (see Table 1). Pharmacists who choose to maintain supplies should consider such supplementary labeling now.

A second error reported involving opium tincture is an example of how a physician's error in prescribing almost led to injury. It again demonstrates a lack of knowledge of the product by some hospital personnel.

A physician wrote an order for "Tincture of Opium gr X q 4 h prn." A nurse transcribed this order onto the patient's medication record and called the pharmacy for the dose. Fortunately, no floor stock of this product was kept. When the pharmacist received the order, he called the physician for clarification. The physician apologized and asked the pharmacist to change the order to 10 drops per dose.

13:252, 1978

Error 102

Nitroglycerin ointment: a little dab won't do you

A 50-year-old man with angina pectoris was started on topical nitroglycerin therapy with nitroglycerin ointment 2% (Nitrol, Nitro-bid). Therapy was to be started with a prescribed dose of one inch of ointment ribbon applied at bedtime (sublingual nitroglycerin was used during the day). The nurse responsible for drug administration brought the order to the pharmacy to be filled. While dispensing the drug, the pharmacist briefly described how the drug was to be correctly applied. This information came as a surprise to the nurse; she confessed she had used the drug incorrectly on two previous occasions. She simply had placed a dab of ointment on the measuring paper and spread it with her finger to the prescribed number of inches!

It would be prudent for the pharmacist to check with the nurse when this drug is dispensed to make sure the correct application method is known. Of course, all patients must also be given this information.

Incidentally, the reason the ink on applicator papers is printed backward is to prevent application of the ointment ribbon to the inked side. The ink might smear onto the patient upon application.

13:252, 1978

Error 103

Strict verbal order procedure prevents serious "error"

A nurse received a telephone call one evening from a Dr. Smith, who was known to be a surgeon on the hospital staff. Dr. Smith requested that his patient, Mrs. Jones, a 78-year-old, 90 lb. female, be given one dose of digoxin 0.5 mg IV. He explained that his patient was to be operated on in the morning and that he wanted the digoxin given prior to the surgery. He asked that it be administered soon.

The nurse, who had just begun working on this particular nursing unit, remembered that hospital policy required all verbal orders during evening and night shifts to be given to the nursing supervisor. She explained this to the caller and asked for and was given a telephone number for her supervisor to contact him.

When the phone call was returned by the supervisor, a plumber's office answered. The supervisor then obtained Dr. Smith's telephone number from the directory (a completely different number from the one given during the original conversation). Dr. Smith was contacted and claimed he never ordered any drug by telephone for Mrs. Jones although he was her physician and she was due for surgery in the morning. Another physician caring for Mrs. Jones was contacted and he too denied ordering the digoxin. The original caller turned out to be an imposter.

It was speculated that someone wishing to do harm to the patient made the telephone call. Precautions were taken to protect the patient during the remainder of her hospitalization.

We previously discussed the hazards of verbal orders in Error 4. Many hospitals have rules which do not allow verbal orders to be given by telephone. Some hospitals at least have restrictions. Where verbal orders are permitted, they should be limited to the following circumstances:

1. Verbal orders for emergencies, in response to requests for analgesia, treatment for fever spike or patient injury.

2. Verbal orders resulting from nurse or pharmacist initiation. If verbal order is initiated by physician, the person accepting the order must be assured it is valid. The physician's voice should be well known by the person accepting the order. The order should be consistent with the patient's problems.

3. The order must be clearly un-

derstood and must be repeated back to the physician. The order must be transcribed on the appropriate patient's medical record.

13:358, 1978

Error 104

Nurses should not be permitted to remove items from pharmacy after hours

A physician wrote an order for "6-thioguanine 160 mg every 12 hours" for his patient with leukemia. At the time the order was written, the pharmacy had already closed for the day. However, the physician requested that the drug be started in the evening. The floor nurse contacted her supervisor who had a key to the pharmacy and routinely obtained needed items after hours.

The supervisor obtained the order and went to the pharmacy for the drug. She found thioguanine tablets (40 mg per tablet) in the storage area. Since the prefix "6" was not on the drug label, she rationalized that the physician actually wanted 6 doses of thioguanine 160 mg given to the patient. She removed 24 tablets from the bottle, thinking this was one dose, and recorded this on a dispensation sheet left for this purpose by the pharmacy. Upon returning to the patient care area, she asked another nurse how she would interpret the order. She too interpreted the order as 6 doses of 160 mg. The dose was then administered.

The following morning, when the pharmacist arrived and discovered that 24 tablets had been removed for a single patient, he telephoned the nurses and the ordering physician about the error. Further doses of thio-

guanine were cancelled. The patient developed bone marrow depression shortly thereafter. About two weeks later, the patient expired. It was not clear whether the death was a result of the disease or the drug overdose.

The nursing supervisor became so upset over the incident that she resigned and vowed never to return to nursing.

Confusion resulting from orders using unrecognized names for medications has been discussed previously (Error 13). As a result of this error, the institution where it occurred, no longer accepts orders for 6-thioguanine, 6-mercaptopurine, 5-fluorouracil, etc. Only the recognized generic or trade names are used.

More important, however, is that a non-pharmacist was permitted to enter the pharmacy and obtain the needed drug after hours. If orders are routinely written after pharmacy hours, the pharmacists and nurses should demand that provisions be made to extend those hours.

Certainly, anticancer drugs should not be ordered when the pharmacy is not open if it is intended that they be given that evening. The safe double-check system (pharmacy-nursing, nursing-pharmacy) cannot operate then.

Where extended hours are impossible or not practical, a separate stock cabinet or cart located outside of the pharmacy should be maintained. The cabinet should be stocked with prepackaged items in quantities, enough for starting a patient only. The stock should be mutually agreed upon by nursing and pharmacy. Any item ordered that is not kept in this stock should not be available, or alternatively, a pharmacist should be on call.

13:358, 1978

198

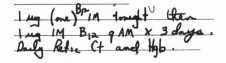

Figure 38. Confusion over microgram designation.

Error 105

Multivitamin ophthalmic suspension

Following a physician's written order for "Multivitamin Suspension 5 ml O.D.," someone poured 5 ml of the drug in a patient's right eye. The error was discovered when the head nurse was questioned about what to do about the excess suspension that didn't get into the eye and mentioned that it was very sticky.

During a counselling session with the person responsible for the error, it was mentioned that the reason she placed it in the right eye was that the order said "O.D." She had been told previously by the hospital pharmacist that the abbreviation O.D. meant right eye and never was to be used to mean once daily. She claimed she was just following hospital policy. The prescriber, the dispenser and the one who administers drugs must all follow a policy in order for it to fulfill its purpose. A policy is not a substitute for thinking.

13:414, 1978

Error 106

Clonidine given instead of clonazepam

A Hazard Warning in this column cautioned about the potential for confusing clonidine with clonazepam. Both drugs were marketed in the United States around the same time. Besides their easily confused names, their dosage ranges overlap. I have recently been made aware of such an error in a pediatric case.[1] A 3½ year old child inadvertently received an overdose of clonidine (five to 20 times the usual adult dose per day) for five days. Clonazepam had been prescribed but clonidine was given instead (0.25 mg in the morning and 0.5 mg in the evening). Fortunately no adverse effects were observed.

To avoid problems, besides legible handwriting, close attention should be paid to the patient's diagnosis to learn of the condition for which the drug is to be used.

Reference

1. Patnode, R. E. et al.: Prolonged clonidine overdosage in a child. *J Pediatrics* 90:848 (May), 1977.

13:414, 1978

Error 107

Writing microgram in script

The abbreviation for microgram is official in the U.S.P. XIX (general notices, page 9) as μg or mcg. While μg presents no problems when the abbreviation is used in type, it often looks like mg when used in script by handwriting. I believe that this has been the cause of many medication errors. A medication error report received by me was due to this easily mistaken abbreviation for microgram. A physician intended his patient to receive 1 microgram of Vitamin B-12 for a Schilling's test. The order appears in Fig. 38. The pharmacist and nurse read the order as 1 milligram and this is what was administered.

To avoid this problem, the only abbreviation used for microgram should be mcg. The U.S.P. and all medical facilities should consider dropping μg as an approved abbreviation.

Medication error error

Correction: 1 mg, not 1 mcg

Even among grand master chess players it is not unheard of for a move to occur that is so obvious not even a rank amateur would miss it. Yet, the grand master would miss it. There's a term for this. It is called "chess-blindness." I am a victim of "pharmacy-blindness." Everyone knows that the dose of B-12 for a Schilling's test is 1 mg (not 1 mcg as listed in Error 107). The original letter I received and edited had mentioned that a Schilling's test "was also scheduled." The dose of 1 microgram was a trial dose — not a Schilling's test dose. "A diagnostic trial of B-12 can be used to detect the presence of B-12 deficiency without concealing folate deficiency in patients with megaloblastic anemia. This is accomplished by administering 1 mcg of cyanocobalamine ... IM daily for ten days while maintaining a diet low in folate and B-12 content." (AHFS 88:08).

Unfortunately, "Schilling's test" stuck in my mind, was reduced to paper and was never really looked at again. The physician did want 1 microgram but not for a Schilling's test.

13:446, 1978

Error 108

K-Lyte in the eye

Along with two prescriptions for eye drops, a patient discharged from the hospital's ophthalmic service received a prescription for K-Lyte: "Dissolve one tablet in ½ glass of cold water and take daily." The patient returned a week later complaining of this "eye wash!"

It is understandable that under the conditions described above the patient thought the K-Lyte was a topical preparation. What was needed was pharmacist counseling of the patient and a prescription label which read "Dissolve one tablet in ½ glass of cold water and drink once daily." Physicians must be as clear as possible when writing prescription directions.

13:446, 1978

Error 109

DEA class IV symbol misinterpreted

In Error 42 I discussed the potential for misinterpreting the DEA class IV symbol (IV as I.V. (intravenous). I expressed concern that an intravenous dose might be given instead of a prescribed IM dose of medication if someone thought the symbol meant that the medication should be given intravenously.

Recently, while expressing this concern during a talk I gave on medication errors, someone volunteered the following error:

A prescription was written for 10 mg of Valium to be given intravenously in a hospital. The nurse who received and transcribed the order had recently returned to nursing after an absence of many years. When she went to obtain Valium from stock, she spotted 10 mg tablets. On the label was the DEA class IV symbol. She crushed the tablet in a mortar, added sterile water, drew the dose up in a syringe and administered the solution intravenously.

When this error was subsequently discovered, the reason given by the nurse was that before she left nursing, she was used to preparing injectables from hypodermic tablets. The DEA class IV symbol substantiated in her mind that the tablet could be given intravenously and must have been a hypodermic tablet.

No information was given as to any adverse effects on the patient.

We should make every effort to familiarize our staffs with this symbol and its real meaning. This should be done during orientation of new hospital employes. The Drug Enforcement Agency must come up with a better symbol.

13:446, 1978

Error 110

Mustargen given instead of methotrexate

A pharmacist working in a pharmacy-run Injection Preparation Service, received an order for "MTX 30 mg IM now." For some reason, even though he knew better, he thought of Mustargen as being the needed drug. The abbreviation MTX signifies methotrexate. He reconstituted three 10 mg vials with one milliliter of sterile water for each vial and prepared a syringe containing 30 mg of Mustargen in 3 ml, thinking that this was actually methotrexate. The drug was to be administered to a psoriasis patient on a dermatology patient care area where methotrexate injection was commonly used. The pharmacist handed the syringe to a nurse and mentioned to her that for some reason he just didn't think everything seemed right. He was leery about administering the drug intramuscularly. The nurse assured him that methotrexate was given I.M. frequently and that everything was all right. But when the nurse looked at the pharmacy-prepared and -labeled syringe, she was surprised to see a different color and volume than she was used to seeing. However, since the syringe was properly labeled and was prepared by a pharmacist, she assumed that everything was correct

and administered the drug in the patient's buttock.

Approximately two hours later, the patient began complaining of buttock pain. The nurse then became suspicious and called the pharmacist, and it was then realized that Mustargen was administered—*not* methotrexate.

Immediate attempts were made to find information about how the effects of this necrotizing agent could be reversed. A one-sixth molar solution of sodium thiosulfate* was infiltrated in 5 ml doses in five spaces around the area of injection. No other therapy was discovered. Even the manufacturer of Mustargen was unable to be of help.

Contrary to what was expected, the patient miraculously suffered no toxicity from the dose or from the local effects as long as one month later.

Several things need to be examined about this incident in order to prevent similar errors in the future.

First of all, the abbreviation MTX should not have been used. This is initially what made the pharmacist think of Mustargen. The pharmacist who sent me this error report wrote that although he knew better, he confused in his mind a common abbreviation for Mustargen (HN_2) and this led to the error. Medications must always be prescribed by their official name.

Secondly, if the pharmacist was thinking that something didn't seem right, he should have had a colleague check the work he was doing. An examination of the vials used (Mustargen) by another pharmacist would have prevented the error.

Finally, the nurse who received the syringed and labeled medication

_____

* Prepared as described in the Mustargen package insert

from the pharmacist put blind faith in the pharmacist's work. I believe that pharmacists have fostered this feeling on the part of nurses and that this can be dangerous. The nurse recognized that a different color and volume of liquid than she was used to seeing with methotrexate injection was present in the syringe. Yet she failed to question the pharmacist because she trusted his work. One of the advantages of unit dose systems with prepared syringed injections is that a double-check exists before the patient receives the medication (pharmacist and nurse).† This would not be true if the nurse prepared the injection. Errors in volume for the particular drug or route of administration are more easily discovered with a double-check, and color differences may be questioned to learn if the wrong drug was prepared. But the nurse must question any recognized discrepancies.

Perhaps pharmaceutical manufacturers could be of help to hospital personnel in preventing errors with syringed parenterals. Since unit dose is rapidly becoming a standard of practice, companies, where possible, should make all of their parenterals available in unit dose form. Where this is impossible, as in the situation described above, perhaps mini-labels could be packaged with vials or ampuls which could be attached to prepared syringes by the pharmacist (some companies already supply printed labels for drugs commonly added to I.V. solutions). If the pharmacist in the case described had had such a label available and used it, the nurse would have read "Mustargen" and recognized the error. I think such

labels would also help to reassure nurses who are concerned about administering an injectable which they didn't prepare themselves.

13:521, 1978

Error 111

Catch 22

A pharmacist received the following note from drug administration personnel, along with a bottle of unadministered medication:

"The patient was sleeping soundly and I was unable to awake him sufficiently to administer his lactulose."

The pharmacist who sent me this error report added "and patient will not wake sufficiently until you give the lactulose!"

Those responsible for drug administration should be taught that lactulose is used in the treatment of hepatic coma.

Remedy

1. Pharmacology courses should be taught in nursing schools.
2. Pharmacists should give pharmacology courses as part of nursing in-service in hospitals.
3. Pharmacists should discuss pharmacologic topics in nursing newsletters.

13:523, 1978

Error 112

Hazardous abbreviation – q.d.

A physician's drug order read: Lasix 80 mg q.d. The period after the "q" looked more like an "i" than a period and the order was transcribed as qid (Fig. 39).

Despite electrolyte changes seen in lab tests over the next few days, the patient continued to receive 320 mg of

---

† For a further discussion of the advantages of pharmacy-prefilled syringes, see Chapter 9.

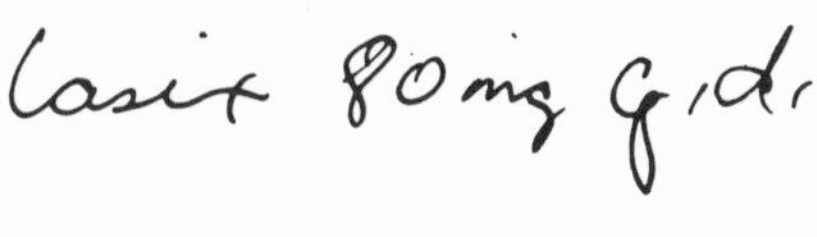

Lasix 80 mg q/d

Figure 39. Physician's drug order: q.d. or q.i.d.?

Lasix for five days before the error was discovered by a medication nurse who questioned the need for such a dose of furosemide on a scheduled basis.

The physician is guilty of sloppy work. Not only did he originate the error by using an abbreviation that is hazardous, he did not pick up the electrolyte changes that occurred.

Health professionals should be encouraged not to use the abbreviation "q.d." There is no safe abbreviation for once daily, since o.d. means right eye.

It is of interest to note that in England q.d. means four times daily.

13:578, 1978

Error 113

Medications should be administered separate from nasogastric feedings

A patient was receiving nasogastric feedings every four hours. The patient's medication regimen included phenytoin, phenobarbital, multivitamins and a stool softener. All medications were in liquid form so that they could be administered through the patient's nasogastric tube. For the nurse's convenience, the tube patient's medications were held until one of the nasogastric feedings was due. In this way, the tube had to be unclamped and irrigated less frequently.

The liquid medications were routinely poured into a cup and mixed with the feedings.

One evening the patient had a grand mal seizure. A check though the patient's records indicated that whenever the patient became distended, the nasogastric tube was aspirated. Also, whenever the patient did not appear to tolerate a total feeding, part was aspirated soon after the feeding. However, this was often done by a nurse other than the one who administered the medication-feeding mixture. In short, no one had any idea how much phenytoin and phenobarbital was actually being absorbed!

Medications should be administered separate from feedings or health professionals should at least be aware of the significance of giving medications with nasogastric feedings. Suctioning of medication not yet absorbed is one possibility. Another is inactivation or absorption prevented by the feeding.

13:578, 1978

Error 114

Pentobarbital-phenobarbital tubex mixup

Several letters have been sent to me regarding mixups in dispensing and/or administration of Wyeth's Tubexes of pentobarbital sodium and phenobarbital sodium. The letters point out that these drugs not only sound similar and have similar spelling, but also have identical packaging. Most of the writers go on to say that they have written the company requesting that some type of color code system be developed for labeling tubexes — especially to make the difference between pentobarbital and phenobarbital easily recognizable.

While I can understand how color coding might be helpful here, it should be pointed out that there is no substitute for reading labels. If people who work in hospitals weren't lazy about reading labels, there would no doubt be quite a decrease in the number of medication errors committed. For this reason, I hope Wyeth Laboratories does not begin color coding its Tubex line because this would foster laziness. Our efforts should go into teaching people to read labels.

13:578, 1978

Error 115

Dr. Daly – please be careful!

A patient received eight units of NPH insulin for two successive days although the physician intended the patient to receive a different dose on the second day. On checking, it was found that personnel had recorded the physician's insulin order as a daily order on the patient's medication administration record. The physician intended this as a one time only dose (8 units SC in AM). Unfortunately, he signed his name on the same line as the insulin order (Fig. 40). Also, unfortunately, his name was Daly. Fortunately, the error in this case was insignificant, but I can certainly think of more serious possibilities.

Dr. Daly was informed of the problem and is now aware of the potential for error caused by his surname. He will be careful to sign his name on a separate line and also to use his first name. Now he just has to be taught not to use the abbreviation "U" for units.

13:579, 1978

Error 116

Use proper abbreviation for gram

A three-year-old child with a provisional diagnosis of meningitis was admitted one evening to a hospital

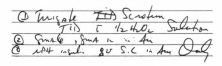

Figure 40. Confusion arising from surname.

with a pediatric service. The pediatrician left an order as follows:

Ampicillin 1 gr IV stat, then 0.5 gr q6h IV.

The nurse working in the pediatric service that evening had little experience with pediatric cases and normally worked in another area of the hospital. She was under the impression that pediatric patients, for the most part, received lower doses of drugs than adults and therefore assumed that the pediatrician wanted the patient to receive one grain of ampicillin for the first dose, then one-half grain per dose. She called her supervisor to have him order the drug, and he verified that this was probably what the pediatrician wanted. The nurse then administered the 60 mg dose.

Later the physician who ordered the drug arrived to see the patient, and was then questioned about the dose. He said that he meant 1 gram. The remainder of the stat dose was made up, and the patient then correctly received 500 mg of ampicillin every six hours.

Several errors were made which prevented the child from receiving the full dose of medication.

First, it would have been better to question the pediatrician directly rather than the supervisor. This could have been done by telephone. As it turned out, the supervisor was merely second-guessing the physician. It would be helpful if physicians would present written orders to the responsible nurse, allow time for the nurse to review them and for answering any questions. In the long run, this step would save time (and medication errors) for all.

Second, it would have been helpful if the nurse had some knowledge about the therapy of bacterial meningitis in pediatric cases. Seemingly large doses of antibiotic are required. This speaks to the hazard of "pulling" nurses from one area of the hospital to another when a specialty is practiced. It is a common practice, and the risk should be considered.

And last, the error was really initiated when the pediatrician used the wrong abbreviation for "gram." USP XIX recognized only small g as the official abbreviation for gram.

13:648, 1978

Error 117

Obsolete abbreviation leads to error

A nurse's medication card read: "Triaminic syrup 3T p.o. qid." A student nurse interpreted this dosage to be 3T or 3 tablespoonsful. Instead of 5 ml, a pediatric patient received 45 ml of the medication. Aside from extreme drowsiness, the child had no other ill effects. He was observed for 24 hours. The student nurse had questioned her instructor and a team leader; yet she was told to go ahead and give the dose.

Obvious advice is to insist upon proper terms and symbols. There is no longer any use for the apothecary system and its abbreviations. The metric system has taken over in medicine.

Although these apothecary abbreviations are not to be used, unfortunately, they are still found sometimes in doctors' orders and are transcribed on to medication records. We should campaign against their use—obviously for good reason.

A nurse with whom I consult on occasion, told me that she was taught that capital "T" meant tablespoonful and small "t" meant teaspoonful. She said these abbreviations are also used in cooking. The physician's apothecary abbreviation for the number one looked like a capital T. The sign for dram looked like a 3.

Correspondence

To the Editor:

I wish to comment on your Medication Error Reports Numbers 116 and 117.

While I agree with your observations on both of these incidents, I feel you should have also pointed out the role of the pharmacist in both situations. Pharmacy-based preparation of doses, as done in a well designed unit dose distribution system, may also have prevented these errors. In addition, comparison of pharmacy and nursing transcriptions of physicians' orders may have prevented these errors.

I enjoy your column very much and hope you continue this very worthwhile, enlightening series.

Thomas N. Brown, RPh, PharmD
Assistant Director of Pharmacy
Programs & Systems Development
Harper-Grace Hospitals
3990 John R.,
Detroit, MI 48201

Editor's reply:

Dr. Brown is correct. Because these comments could be made about most errors we publish, we do not always mention them (MC).

13:648, 1978

Error 118

Brand name of drug causes error

A pharmacist received an order for "Estratest H.S. daily." The pharmacist, who rarely had a call to dispense the drug, sent one Estratest oral tablet for bedtime use. Eight days later, an alert nurse noticed that Estratest H.S. was the brand name for Estratest half-strength oral tablet. The pharmacist had assumed the ordering physician wanted the full-strength tablet at bedtime. Estratest oral tablets contain:

Esterified estrogens 1.25 mg
Methyltestosterone 2.5 mg

Reid-Provident Laboratories, Inc., manufacturers of the product, have been notified. I see nothing short of a name change preventing similar errors with this product. At least, "half-strength" should be spelled out instead of abbreviated "H.S."

Addendum: Reid-Provident Laboratories responded to my letter by saying that the error was due to the pharmacist's unfamiliarity with the product. They saw no present need for a name change. I have reported this to the USP-FDA Drug Defect Reporting Program (M.C.)

13:710, 1978

Error 119

The hazard of "borrowing" medications intended for one patient to administer to another

An order was received by a pharmacist for carbenicillin 5 g IV q 4 h. Prior to dispensing the first dose, the pharmacist checked the patient's drug profile and noted that there was a record of the patient having had a reaction with penicillin administration in the past. Before calling the prescribing physician, the pharmacist went to the patient care area to find out what type of allergic reaction the patient had experienced previously. Upon reviewing the chart, he learned that the patient had developed an urticarial rash and shortness of breath with penicillin in

the past. Before calling the physician with this information and a suggested change in therapy, the pharmacist mentioned the situation to the charge nurse. *But the nurse had already given the patient a dose of carbenicillin.* It was learned that the dose had been obtained by "borrowing" a dose from another patient. Upon checking the patient, the nurse and pharmacist discovered that an allergic reaction had again developed. Treatment was required, and drug therapy was changed to other antibiotics.

This error illustrates a real problem that may occur as a result of "borrowing." Any hospital pharmacist can probably cite similar situations. Publicity must be given within our hospitals about the potential hazard.

Modern drug distribution systems are set up so that the pharmacist is able to review routine drug orders prior to administration of the first dose. Not only overlooked allergies are discovered in this manner (in conjunction with use of well kept patient profiles) but also errors in drug dose, route of administration, choice of drug, etc. Many times it is critical that the patient not receive even the first dose. These modern systems are overridden when a nurse takes it upon herself to "borrow," and this may lead to error and patient injury.

"Borrowing" does not occur with new orders only. In a unit dose system, a nurse may "borrow" from another patient's drug cart bin when she can't find an item in the bin of a patient for whom that item is intended. Nurses may not realize that by reporting a missing item, rather than by borrowing another patient's dose, she may be preventing an error. The pharmacist may have missed the original order, or whoever transcribed the original order may have written it on the wrong patient's medication administration record. Or perhaps the

206

pharmacist didn't put a dose in the bin because the drug was discontinued, yet the medication administration record still lists the drug in error. The practice of borrowing will perpetuate the error in any of these cases. We must place emphasis on the serious hazard this practice presents.

Good communication channels must be maintained between pharmacy and nursing.

13:710, 1978

Error 120

If it's in print, people will take it as fact.

Two patients suffering from narcotic overdoses were admitted to a hospital emergency room. Because of the emergency situation, the attending physician utilized an antidote chart in determining the antidote and dose to be used. The chart, produced by a pharmacy school, called for "Narcan (naloxone) 4 mg IV, IM or subcutaneous." On the basis of this information, both patients received large overdoses of the drug. The chart listed a tenfold overdose due most likely to the omission of a decimal point.

The error was communicated to personnel who work at the school where the chart was published. This should serve as a warning to all of us. People tend to take as fact what they see in print, whether it be on a chart or in a published paper. I have also received word of an error occurring in a chart on doses of cancer chemotherapeutics.

If you are ever involved with publishing, check everything you do for accuracy. It is a good policy to have several people review your work both before and after proofs are received

and then again before the final version is distributed.

14:38, 1979

Error 121

Names given to anti-cancer drugs.

A pharmacist working in the inpatient dispensing area of a hospital pharmacy received a physician's order for

mithomycin C 15 mg

The pharmacist noted mithramycin 15 mg on a patient medication profile. However, he did have enough knowledge of mithramycin dosing to check what seemed to be an unusually high dose. Checking the mithramycin package insert and calculating a dose based on the patient's weight, the pharmacist arrived at a total dose of 1.5 mg. The pharmacist figured that the physician had misplaced a decimal point in his calculations. He then called the physician's office to apprise him of his discovery. To the pharmacist's surprise, the physician claimed that he had ordered mitomycin C 15 mg — not mithramycin. He had misspelled the drug. Mitomycin C was a name used before the current official name, mitomycin.

This is another example of how names assigned to anticancer drugs have caused confusion and, although not in this instance, serious errors. Mithramycin and mitomycin just appear too similar in handwriting. This mixup had the potential for real tragedy.

Davis has discussed the problems associated with brand names being assigned to cancer chemotherapeutic agents (*Hosp. Pharm.* 11:36, 1976), but problems also exist with official names. With the proliferation of new agents the whole problem will get worse.

The USAN Council and the U.S.P. are concerned about this issue, but they have no control over trade names. Serious consideration must be given by manufacturers when establishing trade names so that they are not confused with official names of other drugs. Perhaps changing some of the current names: mithramycin — Mithracin® (Pfizer) and mitomycin — Mutamycin® (Bristol) is in order.

14:38, 1979

Error 122

"I take the pink one"

A woman who appeared to be in her 70's (she was 81) walked into a resort city pharmacy with a prescription for "Synthroid Tab., One Daily," written by her hometown cardiologist. The woman was a seasonal resident in this resort city and had completely run out of the medication. The pharmacist told her he could not dispense the prescription since many strengths of Synthroid were available. She stated that she had been taking the "pink one." The pharmacist showed her the 200 mcg tablet, and she assured him that was what she had been taking for five years. The prescription was dispensed.

She took 200 mcg Synthroid for 27 days when she was hospitalized with symptoms consisting of weight loss, loss of appetite, tachycardia and tremors. She was also taking digoxin, Lasix, Dyrenium and Benemid. She had a 30-year history of heart problems and had had a pacemaker for four years. The strength of Synthroid that she had really been taking right along was 25 mcg, not the 200 mcg she identified. When questioned, she stated that she thought the orange-colored 25 mcg Synthroid was pink.

When shown the orange and pink tablets side by side, she stated, "I'm just not good when it comes to colors." She could see there was a difference in the colors, but she would still say the orange tablet was pink.

What would you have done with this woman in distress, who apparently knew what she was doing?

Try to call the out-of-town cardiologist who may or may not have been available?

Asked to see her old prescription container?

Called her local pharmacy?

Given her two or three tablets until her physician called or until you reached the physician?

Told her you were sorry but the prescription could not be dispensed without her physician calling you?

Dispensed the 200 mcg tablets identified by the patient?

You already know that the last choice is wrong. What would you do for this nice, grey-haired senior citizen? We would like to hear from you. In the meantime, please educate your medical students and physicians to write complete prescriptions.

Correspondence

To the Editor:

In response to your request for comments on Error 122, I would like to offer the following, based on three years of experience in retail pharmacy in a resort area of Vermont. Out of necessity, I had to develop my own policy and procedure with this recurring situation.

I would first obtain the address and/or telephone number of the patient's physician and local pharmacy. If I could get the label of the previously filled container, much time

208

could be saved in confirming the identity of the medication with the physician or pharmacist. In any case I would never take for granted that the patient knows what he or she is taking.

Patients unable to supply me with this information were politely asked to see a physician at our local health center.

Dispensing prescription medications without confirmation can result in therapeutic as well as legal and, in some cases, ethical problems.

Stephen R. Jones, RPh
Director, Pharmacy Service
St. Luke's —
Memorial Hospital Center
Utica, NY 13503

To the Editor:

Here are my thoughts in reply to your Medication Error 122. Having spent nine years in retail practice in addition to currently practicing in the hospital setting, I have encountered similar problems to the one you set forth in the article. In this situation I would have asked to see the patient's old prescription container, as the first move in establishing exactly what the patient was taking. But container or no, the ethical pharmacist is compelled to call the physician, whether it is an out-of-town call or not, in order to obtain a valid prescription. It is lamentable that there are a certain number of practitioners in the profession who are either unable to fulfill the letter of the law (which would have protected them from this liability), or so eager to make a fast buck at the expense of performing in a professional manner, that the welfare of the patient has become secondary.

William Duffy, RPh
St. Francis Hospital
6161 S. Yale Ave.
Tulsa, OK 74136

To the Editor:

I would like to make a comment on the letter by William Duffy (Error 122), which appeared in your correspondence section in the July 1979 issue (Hosp. Pharm. 14:429). In his letter he states, "It is lamentable that there are a certain number of practitioners in the profession who are either unable to fulfill the letter of the law (which would have protected them from this liability), or so eager to make a fast buck at the expense of performing in a professional manner, that the welfare of the patient has become secondary." I feel what is really lamentable is that the dispensing pharmacist did not use better judgment in the filling of this prescription, but what also is lamentable is the conclusion drawn by Mr. Duffy and the publication of his letter in your fine journal. I've found nothing to indicate that the pharmacist in Error 122 was out to make a fast buck, intentionally break the law or was not concerned about the patient's welfare. These conclusions are illogical and cannot be substantiated with the information given. What Mr. Duffy and your journal have succeeded in doing was to take an error presented to you in good faith, to be presented as a tool for learning, and use it as a slap in the face to those pharmacists who happen to practice in the retail setting. I don't believe these error reports should be used for vicious or destructive attacks on any health profession or group. I too work in a hospital setting and find these error reports helpful in my practice. Having worked in the medical field 13 years I know that many errors that occur are not reported because of fear of reprimand. I hope that Mr. Duffy's letter will not discourage others from reporting errors to your journal.

Kenneth L. Thompson, RPh
Hampton, VA

Editor's reply

I can certainly appreciate Mr. Thompson's concerns. He is right; there was nothing in the original error report to indicate anything other than humanitarian motives on the part of the dispensing pharmacist, regardless of the ill-fated results. Information provided for Error 122 was sent to me by a relative (a health professional) of the patient involved, not the pharmacist. There are times when discussion of an error will be critical of the person who sent in the error. On occasion, it seems to me that an error has been reported to me as a confession and a means of relieving guilt feelings. For these and other reasons, they are published anonymously.

14:102, 1979

Error 123

"The attending told me that's what he wants"

The pharmacist received an order for acetic acid 40% irrigation solution. Thinking that a nurse had transcribed the order incorrectly, the pharmacist contacted the nurse who confirmed that a 40% solution was requested. A call to the prescriber, a medical resident, was then made. The resident confessed that he had never used this solution before but he was sure that was the strength his attending physician told him to order. The pharmacist suggested that no solution be made until the resident confirmed the order with the staff physician. The resident himself later checked on the order, and it was changed to a ¼% irrigation.

Fortunately, in this case an experienced pharmacist was on duty to prevent what might have been a serious situation. One must shudder to think what might have happened had there been an inexperienced pharmacist

or worse yet — no pharmacist — involved.

As a pharmacy practitioner, it has been a little disheartening to me over the years to receive nonsensical, often dangerous orders written by house officers who have no explanation or justification other than "the attending told me to order that." They should feel enough responsibility to the patient to at least ask "why?."

14:102, 1979

Error 124

Label oral liquid syringe dispensers properly

A physician prescribed Lasix 40 mg I.V. every eight hours. On the third day of filling the unit dose cassette drawer for that patient, a pharmacy technician filled the order with Lasix oral solution 40 mg. The solution was prepared in a BAXA Oral Liquid Dispenser. The dispenser looks like a syringe for injectable use but the syringe tip will not accommodate a needle. The syringe has clearly imprinted on it "For oral use only." The technician placed a label on the syringe which read "Lasix 10 mg/ml, 4 ml." The pharmacist responsible for checking the cassette did not detect an error nor did the nurse who checked the cart at the time of cassette exchange.

The oral dose was administered intravenously by a nurse. Although the dispenser cannot be fitted with a needle and does not in any way fit properly into a luer receptor of an I.V. cannula, it was inserted into a luer receptor of an I.V. cannula and held so that the liquid contents were pushed through the line without leaking. Apparently, the nurse believed that the syringe tip was malformed and never realized that the syringe was intended for oral use only.

Following the error there did not appear to be any adverse effects. The nurse on the next shift noticed the error in the two other syringes for that day. She used floor stock parenteral Lasix for the next dose but did not communicate the error to her staff or pharmacy. The third shift again detected the error and reported it to pharmacy where it was immediately corrected.

Approximately forty hours after the oral dose was administered, a Code Blue was called on the patient and resuscitative efforts were unsuccessful. Although hospital personnel are of the opinion that there was no cause and effect relationship between the sequence of events and the patient's death, this does leave the hospital in a precarious position. Until the time of death, the patient had been responding well, and new orders had been written changing parenteral medications to oral forms.

Hoechst-Roussel, manufacturers of Lasix oral solution, have never before been informed of such an event occurring. Cultures of oral liquid dispensers from the same batch revealed no bacterial growth.

The occurrence of this error should serve as a warning to all of us who use oral liquid dispensers, such as the BAXA device, to be extremely cautious to prevent mixups. When these syringes are labeled, a precautionary auxiliary label "Warning: for oral use only—Not for injection!" should be placed prominently near the drug name. The warning printed on the syringe barrel apparently is not always enough. Of course, use of regular parenteral syringes for packaging oral solutions should never be allowed.

14:102, 1979

Error 125

Epinephrine HCl 2% not equivalent to epinephrine bitartrate 2%.

A patient with open angle glaucoma was admitted to the hospital. As part of his medication regimen, his physician ordered Epitrate 2% ophthalmic solution. The pharmacist did not have Epitrate (epinephrine bitartrate, Ayerst) in stock. Instead, he dispensed Glaucon 2% ophthalmic solution (Alcon), a preparation of l-epinephrine HCl. The amount of epinephrine base contained in a 2% solution of the bitartrate salt is 1.1%, while Glaucon 2% is approximately 2% epinephrine base. The products are interchangeable only when the percentage of epinephrine base is taken into account.

Glaucon 1% should have been dispensed to approximately equal Epitrate 2%.

14:163, 1979

Error 126

Be cautious with prescriptions written by other than the actual prescriber

The pharmacy received an outpatient prescription with three drugs listed on the same blank. It was for hemorrhoidal suppositories, Compazine suppositories 25 mg, and Doriden tablets (no strength indicated). The technician receiving the prescription gave it to a pharmacist because Doriden is not on the Formulary, and because a controlled substance was written on a "polyprescription."

The pharmacist noticed that it was written by someone other than the prescriber, yet signed by the prescriber. He walked to the clinic and found the clinic nurse and the physician together in the office. The clinic nurse admitted to writing the prescription, and was not aware that Doriden was a controlled substance or that it was not a Formulary item. The doctor acknowledged that it should have been on a separate prescription blank. The pharmacist offered Dalmane 15 mg or 30 mg as a possible stocked substitute. A prescription for Dalmane 15 mg was written and signed by the doctor in the presence of the pharmacist. The pharmacist called the patient back to the pharmacy to explain that the "sleeping pill" would be different. The patient said that she had gotten some there just last week, and added that they were "little brown pills." When the pharmacist questioned this, she said, "yes, little brown pills for your bowels." The pharmacist asked if she had received Doxidan capsules and she said that was correct. This information was then verified by the pharmacist in the patient's chart (medical record). The physician was contacted by telephone, and he authorized Doxidan.

The office nurse had misread the original order for Doxidan.

The story related above is not uncommon. "Busy" physicians sometimes place too much responsibility on and too much faith in the clinic nurse without adequately supervising their work. The patient ultimately bears the burden of this practice.

Had the Doriden prescription been written on a separate prescription and if it were a stocked item, this patient would have been the victim of a drug error. If she were accustomed to taking her laxative during the day, the results might even have been disastrous.

Pharmacists should actively question any prescription that looks "irregular" in any way, especially if it appears to be written by someone other than the person who signed it.

Physicians are responsible for adequate supervision of office personnel and must read and agree with orders they are countersigning.

Error 39 discussed the potential for mixing up Doriden and Doxidan when orders are handwritten poorly.

14:163, 1979

Error 127

Medical service representatives should be banned from inpatient areas

Many hospitals have rulings designed to keep unescorted pharmaceutical company medical service representatives (MSRs) out of inpatient areas. Their presence there must be controlled because their visits may easily be considered disruptive to the flow of patient care as they stop and detail their products to busy health professionals.

Another important reason for this control has recently come to my attention by way of a medication error report sent by a reader.

On an inpatient psychiatry unit a MSR paid a visit to detail one of his products. He stopped a physician working there and began talking. He put his "bag" on the floor and opened it to remove samples of his product. While he was talking to the physician, one of the patients sneaked up to the bag and removed two boxes of drug samples. No one saw the patient do this. She went back to her room, opened the packages and swallowed an overdose of the tablets. Shortly therefter, a nurse on a routine check noticed the emptied sample boxes in the patient's room. Syrup of ipecac was administered immediately, and broken tablets were found in the vomitus that followed. Fortunately, no harm came to the patient.

212

This incident likely would have placed the hospital and the drug company in a very bad light if a lawsuit had been initiated. A patient could have died. The hospital did have a policy that prohibited MSRs from being in inpatient areas but the policy was ignored.

All hospitals should have such policies and they must be strictly enforced. MSRs should know that if they cannot abide by this rule, they will be reported to their companies and banned from other hospital areas where they are permitted.

14:278, 1979

Error 128

Misuse of tincture of opium causes 100 mg morphine dose to be administered.

In Errors 100 and 101, two serious incidents involving tincture of opium were described. This drug has been confused with camphorated tincture of opium (paregoric) because their names are so similar. Many people are unaware of the difference. The danger is that tincture of opium contains 25 times more morphine than paregoric. The following documents yet another reported error with tincture of opium. This one led to three additional days of hospitalization.

An older physician prescribed tincture of opium, 10 m̊ q 4 h prn diarrhea. The pharmacist who received this order was concerned that minims abbreviated as m̊ might be taken as ml. The head nurse was called to warn her of this archaic symbol. The drug administration record was even noted with this warning. The drug was appropriately administered initially. However, in spite of the warnings, a 10 ml dose was administered during the next shift. Subsequently, another 10 ml was administered. The error

was detected. The drowsy patient was transferred to I.C.U. This patient spent an extra three days in the hospital as a result of the error.

This hospital now dispenses tincture of opium in 7.5 ml dropper bottles with a statement on the label, "Usual dose, 0.6 ml Q.I.D." Consideration should be given to removing tincture of opium from hospital formularies because there is no need for it and it can easily be confused with paregoric (see Errors 100 and 101).

It must also be noted that the archaic apothecary system of measurement contributed to the error. "Minims" was confused with milliliter. This system should no longer be used.

14:366, 1979

Error 129

Bactrim – Bactrim DS dosing mixups

Several readers have forwarded error reports involving dosing mixups with Bactrim (trimethoprim-sulfamethoxazole) and Bactrim DS (Double Strength) I assume that Septra and Septra DS tablets would be involved in the same type of error.

Because this drug combination has been so widely prescribed as regular Bactrim (or Septra) in two tablet, twice daily doses, nurses have become accustomed to seeing these orders. However, when the double strength tablet was released, many hospital pharmacists began stocking and dispensing this single tablet. But not all nurses have been made familiar with this newer form. When "Bactrim 2 tablets, b.i.d." is ordered, Bactrim DS may be dispensed, and the pharmacist assumes that the person administering the drug will know that DS means double strength and will substitute one of these for two regular Bactrim tablets. Unfortunately, this is not always the case. When several days' supply of Bactrim DS is dispensed, two of these tablets might be used per dose. A reader who sent such a report to me discovered the error when an empty container was returned to pharmacy twice as soon as it should have been. In unit dose systems that have 24-hour cart fills, both double strength tablets would be placed in the bin each day. Another reader, one who works in a unit dose system, mentioned that he was called on two different occasions for "missing" evening doses of Bactrim (both DS tablets were given in the morning in error and none was left in the bin for the evening dose).

A remedy for this would be to dispense only exactly what is ordered. This is what will be transcribed on the nurses' medication administration record. If this record lists "Bactrim two tablets" the chance for error is great if Bactrim DS is dispensed. Alternatively, if you have excellent communication with your nursing staff, you might be able to assure yourself that they are all aware of the two tablet strengths and that the mixup is unlikely. Both manufacturers should make an effort to educate nurses to the differences in these widely prescribed tablets.

Correspondence

To the Editor:

I would like to comment on your Medication Error Report Number 129 (Bactrim-Bactrim DS dosing mixups).

This problem manifests itself daily in the practice of hospital pharmacy. When we instituted our unit dose program four years ago we found an important need for a mechanism to communicate changes in dosage forms and substitutions to both our physicians and our nursing staff. At that time it was found that the most effective and convenient way was via

---

CHMC - PHARMACY DEPARTMENT
Drug Omission Form

Date _____

Patient Name _____ Rm. _____

Item Ordered

☐ Temporarily out of stock.
  Will be supplied on _____

☐ Not a Formulary Item (See comment)

☐ Verify: Dose _____ Directions _____ Strength _____

☐ Doctor Consulted (See comment)

☐ Substitute provided (See comment)

☐ Medication order discontinued (See comment)

Comment: _____

_____

_____

_____

ATTACH TO PATIENT'S CHART UNTIL PHYSICIAN IS CONTACTED

Figure 41. Drug Omission Form used at Cherry Hill Medical Center to record drug substitutions and changes in forms of dosage.

---

a "Drug Omission Form" This form can either be attached to the patient's chart to make a physician aware of a change or problem, or it can be placed in the patient's medication cart drawer. This will serve as a constant reminder to the medication nurse of any change that has been made. A carbon copy of this form is attached to the patient's profile form in the Pharmacy, and serves as a permanent record of any change.

In this time of increased cost awareness and more liberal substitution laws, it is no longer practical to carry every dosage strength and form so a pharmacist can "dispense only exactly what is ordered."

In the case of Bactrim ii tablets b.i.d., a 24-hour supply of Bactrim DS would be sent to the patient with a Drug Omission Form that indicates the substitution and gives proper dosing instructions. (See Fig. 41.)

This has been found to be a very effective mechanism of communica-

214

tion, and has greatly reduced the number of phone calls requesting more medication due to dosing errors.

I enjoy your column, finding it both worthwhile and necessary to stay one step ahead of potential problems. I have recommended to nursing students that they read your column, hoping that it will help stop errors that are becoming all too common.

Herbert R. Henney III, RPh
Staff Pharmacist
Cherry Hill Medical Center
Cherry Hill, NJ 08002

14:366, 1979

Error 130

Do not write patient name and bed number directly on labels of unit dose products

After a unit dose cart supply was checked and delivered to the patient care area by a pharmacist, he received a new order for ampicillin 500 mg PO q 6 h. The pharmacist took three doses, enough to last until the next cart fill, and placed them in a zip-lock bag. He wrote the name of the patient and bed number on the bag and sent it to the nursing unit for the nurse to place in the patient's drug bin on the cart. The pharmacist did not notice that, earlier in the day, someone else had dispensed those very capsules and had written a name and bed number directly on the label of one of them. When the medication was later discontinued, the capsules were returned to stock but the name and bed number were not crossed off.

Upon receipt, a nurse removed one dose from the bag, then administered it to the wrong patient—the same patient for whom it had already been ordered and discontinued. Later, when the nurse saw the name and bed number written on the zip-lock bag,

she discovered that an error had been made. She wrongly assumed that the name and bed number written on the unit dose package label identified the patient for whom it was intended (she remembered seeing an earlier order for that patient, but was unaware it had been discontinued). Of course, if the nurse had followed procedure by checking the patient's medication administration record, the error would not have occurred, but the name and bed number on the label contributed to the error. There is a danger that similar errors could occur with stat doses, and other miscellaneous, one-time-only items, as well as with drugs dispensed to update unit dose carts before the next fill.

One of the major cost-saving advantages of unit dose packaging is that dispensed but unadministered medications may be returned to stock for reissue without fear of loss of identity or hygienic conditions. But writing the patient name and bed number directly on the label of non-routinely dispensed doses may later lead to error if the dose is returned. This practice should be discouraged. A supplemental label that can be torn off if the drug is returned would be more acceptable. Alternatively, all doses delivered after normal cart fill should go directly into patient bins or should be placed in zip-lock bags, which are then labeled. If returned, the doses may be removed and returned to stock.

14:427, 1979

Error 131

More vincristine errors

Since medication errors involving vincristine (Oncovin) were first published in error #71, we have received reports of four more errors. All cases, thus far, are overdoses that led to severe toxicity or death. There is no known antidote of value.

In my opinion, a contributing factor to these errors is the availability of a 5 mg vial of vincristine, even though the maximum single adult dose of vincristine is no greater than 2 mg. The problem is that many of the doses incorrectly ordered have been in the 5-20 mg range because of prescriber miscalculation of dose, confusion with vinblastine (Velban), or a decimal point that was not seen.

With the availability of a 5 mg vial, which is really meant to be used for multiple dose preparation in cancer centers, one may substantiate the erroneous higher doses ("why would 5 mg vials be available if not for these higher doses?"). We have previously suggested that only 1 mg vials be stocked in non-cancer center hospitals. However, we are now finding that even some of the largest cancer centers in the United States will not stock the 5 mg vials because of the error potential. This has been called to the attention of the manufacturer, but they plan to continue manufacturing the larger vials. We urge all hospital pharmacists to delete the 5 mg vial from their inventories immediately. It is just too dangerous to have around.

Something else has come out of the most recent overdose reports mailed to us. In three of the four cases, pharmacists were intimidated into dispensing the overdoses. The pharmacists knew that the doses were high. The ordering physician each time was a resident of a staff oncologist. The resident insisted that the dose was correct (after all, an expert, the staff oncologist, had ordered it) and insisted on obtaining the dose. You are less than a pharmacist if you bow to such pressures. If you are not positive of a drug or dose, you owe it to your patient, and to yourself, to check it out completely.

I would be interested in learning about other vincristine errors and the circumstances in which they occurred.

14:427, 1979

Error 132

Use ml/h or units/h for heparin infusions

An order was received for "heparin 30,000 units in 1000 ml D5/W — run at 24 drops/min." Pharmacy made the infusion and labeled it with the ordered rate. The bottle was hung by a nurse who maintained the rate throughout her shift. When an ordered APTT was reported as greater than 100 seconds on the next shift, a second nurse checked the bottle and realized that the infusion was running at 24 drops/min as ordered — not at the usual *micro*drops per minute. When informed, the physician said, "She should have known what I meant," but the nurse confessed that she was too unfamiliar with heparin infusions to question the order.

Obviously, had the physician correctly written microdrops/min, the error would not have occurred. But an even better way to list the rate of a heparin infusion is in ml/h or units/h. It is easier to think in ml/h for constant infusions and allows easy time taping of bottles. A nurse would realize that a microdrop set would be necessary, since a macrodrop set would be nearly impossible to regulate at such a slow rate. Infusion pumps used for constant infusion are set at rates in ml/h. In fact, a pump or rate controller should be used for constant heparin infusion, as a gravity flow delivery is too risky. Many hospi-

Table 2. Heparin 20,000 units per 1000 ml D5/W solution*

Flow rate (ml/h)	Units/hour delivered
15	300
20	400
25	500
30	600
35	700
40	800
45	900
50	1000
55	1100
60	1200
65	1300
70	1400

*At Temple University Hospital, a continuous heparin infusion flow-rate chart is taped to the side of the infusion pump. Rate changes ordered in ml/h or units/h are made by consulting the chart.

tals have established standard solution concentrations so that infusion rate changes are more easily and accurately accomplished (see Table 2).

14:428, 1979

Error 133

Heparin overdose due to injection of wrong concentration

A patient suffering from phlebitis was being maintained on anticoagulant therapy of heparin, 5000 units intravenously every four hours. The concentration on the medication vial dispensed routinely by pharmacy for intravenous heparin read 1000 units per ml, so the patient was receiving 5 ml (5000 units) intravenously per dose. Eventually, the patient was changed to subcutaneous injections of heparin, 5000 units every four hours. The dosage on the medication vial used routinely for subcutaneous heparin read 10,000 units per ml, indicating the patient should receive 0.5 ml of heparin subcutaneously. Unfor-

tunately, the medication nurse hurriedly rewrote the medication sheet, neglecting to change the volume, and gave the patient 5 ml of the concentration used for subcutaneous heparin instead of 0.5 ml. Therefore, the patient received 50,000 units instead of 5000 units. The patient survived, but developed a subdural hemorrhage that necessitated further surgery and a more prolonged hospitalization. Obviously, the nurse should have read the order more carefully and the concentration on the vials more accurately.

Everyone knows the importance of reading labels, but unfortunately there are those among us who do not always take the time to do so. After these people get burned badly enough, they change their methods.

To make errors such as this one less likely to occur, the unit dose drug distribution system, with its inherent checks and double checks, has been developed. Had prefilled syringes of heparin been dispensed by pharmacy, this error would probably not have occurred. Alternatively, pharmacy might consider dispensing only one strength of heparin to be used systemically; 5000 units/ml can easily be used by either I.V. or S.C. routes.

14:477, 1979

Error 134

Nurses should know about treatment of acetaminophen overdose

A patient with an acetaminophen overdose was admitted to an emergency department and therapy begun with the antidote, acetylcysteine. She was then transferred to a special care unit where therapy was continued. The physician's original order read "Mucomyst Solution 20%, 3.5 g p.o. q

4 h." Because the nurse was familiar with the use of Mucomyst only in respiratory therapy as a mucolytic, the nurse questioned the oral use of the drug and the dose. She tried unsuccessfully to get further information on this from her supervisor, two other nurses, and a physician. The package insert mentioned only its mucolytic activity. Finally, after considerable delay, she changed the 3.5 g to 3.5 ml (3.5 g would be 17.5 ml) and administered it orally.

The incident occurred on a Sunday night. On Monday morning, pharmacy dispensed the balance of the order, properly labeled as 3.5 g = 17.5 ml. However, four days later, a pharmacist noted that the majority of the Mucomyst dispensed was being returned. After floor personnel were questioned, the original error was discovered and it was determined that the patient had not received the proper dose at any time during the four-day period. Fortunately, the patient survived the error. The error could have been prevented if one of the nurses had contacted the pharmacist on call or if a pharmacist had been on duty at the time the drug was ordered.

Now that acetylcysteine is being used as a safe and effective antidote for acetaminophen overdose,[1] we should expect to see orders for this drug. Nurses should be prepared for this, just as we should be. Pharmacists should consider providing inservice education on this topic, as well as including an article on the subject in their pharmacy bulletin.

14:447, 1979

---

[1]Gates, T.N.: Management of acetaminophen overdose with N-acetylcysteine. 1979, McNeil Consumer Products Co., Fort Washington, Pa. 19034.

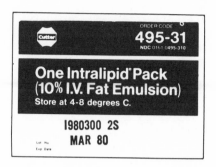

Figure 42. Intralipid package label. Note the word "fat."

Error 135

An interesting cause of patient refusal

An interesting incident occurred with the use of intravenous fat emulsion that should be brought to the attention of readers. A patient suffering from anorexia nervosa had been receiving parenteral alimentation and was to be started on Intralipid. A nurse started the infusion peripherally. Before the nurse left the patient's room, the patient screamed and began crying about the fluid being administered. She refused to allow the infusion to continue. The reason for this was that she did not want to receive *fat*, as indicated on the label (see Fig. 42).

It is understandable that this patient became upset. The last thing a patient with anorexia nervosa wants to do is gain weight. A good deal of psychotherapy goes along with alimentation attempts before the patient's condition can be corrected. In this case, reassurance from the nurse and psychiatrist were necessary to get the patient to cooperate.

As with any type of therapy being dispensed, pharmacists should first have a record of patient diagnosis. When a patient with anorexia nervosa is to receive intravenous fat emulsion, it is advisable that the manufacturer's label be covered with an auxiliary I.V. additive label listing the brand name. The new Abbott product, Liposyn, also lists "fat" in the labeling.

14:545, 1979

Error 136

Remind others of teaspoon volume variance

A pediatrician ordered ampicillin suspension (125 mg/5 ml), one teaspoonful q.i.d. for 10 days. A 125 mg/5 ml concentration in a 200 ml bottle was supplied by pharmacy. Eight days after the antibiotic was begun, an instructor supervising nursing students on a pediatric rotation discovered that only 50% of the solution had thus far been administered. Yet all doses were signed for on the medication administration record. The medication nurses were asked about the discrepancy and were asked how the suspension was being administered. They showed the colorful plastic teaspoons that they obtain from the dietary department to administer oral liquids to children (they assumed they were 5 ml). The capacity of the spoons was measured and found to be less than 3 ml.

Pharmacists are made aware of the variance in volumes of different teaspoons sometimes as early as freshman orientation in pharmacy school. Yet how many of us take the time to remind our nursing colleagues of this? Do we make available accurate measuring devices to be dispensed along with liquid prescriptions to families of pediatric outpatients? Some of the liquid medication doses are extremely critical and fraught with dosing inaccuracies (e.g., phenytoin suspension).

Pharmacists should really make an effort to stay on top of institutional drug administration practices if they are going to prevent such happenings. We are, after all, responsible for the entire drug distribution cycle — including the safety of drug administration practices.

Incidentally, the person who sent me this report stated that they had "corrected" the problem. From now on, they will be using 5 ml syringes to administer a teaspoon of medication. Of course, this practice may be more hazardous than an inaccurate teaspoon since the potential exists for a needle to be attached and the suspension injected. Pharmacists must never allow such a practice. Oral syringe devices that will not accommodate a needle should be used. Unfortunately, even these devices have been used successfully to inject, so be careful with these, too. It must be noted that the ordering physician, by writing for a "teaspoon" dose, might have contributed to this inpatient error.

14:545, 1979

Error 137

Problems with pharmacy-prepared Kayexalate suspension

As hospital pharmacists know, Kayexalate (sodium polystyrene sulfonate) is a powder that must first be made into a suspension before administration. The package insert states that 15 g is "equal to approximately 4 level teaspoons."

A physician wrote an order for "Kayexalate 15 g (4 level teaspoons) q.i.d."

The pharmacy prepared and dispensed the drug as a suspension with sorbitol and water. The bottle label read:

Kayexalate	15 g
Sorbitol 70%	30 ml
Water	30 ml
For oral use	
SHAKE WELL BEFORE USING	

Soon after the drug was dispensed (in unit dose containers as above) it was discovered that only 20 ml of the suspension was being administered four times a day. Apparently, the "4 level teaspoons" was transcribed onto the nursing medication administration record.

To prevent this error, pharmacists should label the container so that it is clear what volume contains the requested dose. For unit dose containers, state that the entire bottle contains the dose. For bottles dispensed in bulk sizes, list the volume specifically.

The author of this report mentioned that in-service education on the use of Kayexalate also proved valuable.

14:628, 1979

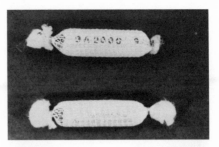

Figure 43. An amyl nitrate capsule looks almost identical to an aromatic ammonia capsule.

Some hospitals have removed amyl nitrate capsules from floor stock and have added them to their list of controlled drugs because of their potential for abuse. This would also decrease the chance for error.

14:682, 1979

Error 138

Mixup of amyl nitrate and aromatic ammonia crushable capsules

If you maintain stocks of crushable capsules of amyl nitrate and aromatic ammonia (Burroughs Wellcome), it might pay to keep watch on any area in which they might be stored. A reader reports to us that she recently witnessed an amyl nitrate capsule used mistakenly in place of the ammonia. She discovered this when she noticed the lack of the characteristic ammonia odor. Upon checking, she found the drugs mixed in the same stock box. Although the amyl nitrate capsule netting is yellow and the ammonia white, it is nearly impossible to read the labeling underneath (Fig. 43). One could foresee a newly assigned employe using one for the other and not recognizing a difference at first. The incident occurred in a delivery room with a newly delivered mother who had become faint. Perhaps the last thing she needed was a lower blood pressure.

Error 139

Platinol (cisplatin) must be refrigerated until reconstitution

There has been some confusion recently over the storage of Platinol (cisplatin). The shelf package, the vial box, and the vial itself all mention that the drug should be refrigerated at 2-8° C. However, on one of the box flaps there appears the statement: "Do not refrigerate," followed on a second line by "Reconstituted Solution . . ." (Fig. 44). We know of two incidents in which pharmacy technical personnel only read the "Do not refrigerate" line and were misguided into storing this important product at room temperature.

The company has begun placing a red warning label on the shelf package (10 vials), but the individual vial boxes remain the same.

Storeroom personnel must be supervised.

14:682, 1979

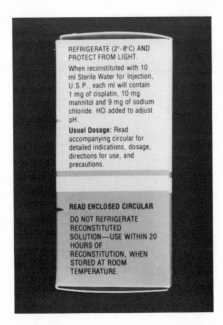

REFRIGERATE (2°-8°C) AND
PROTECT FROM LIGHT.
When reconstituted with 10
ml Sterile Water for Injection,
U.S.P., each ml will contain
1 mg of cisplatin, 10 mg
mannitol and 9 mg of sodium
chloride. HCl added to adjust
pH.
Usual Dosage: Read
accompanying circular for
detailed indications, dosage,
directions for use, and
precautions.

READ ENCLOSED CIRCULAR
DO NOT REFRIGERATE
RECONSTITUTED
SOLUTION—USE WITHIN 20
HOURS OF
RECONSTITUTION, WHEN
STORED AT ROOM
TEMPERATURE.

Figure 44. The statement that appears on the vial box of Platinol can be confusing. Notice the phrase, "Do not refrigerate."

Error 140

Nurses should hang only those I.V. bags that they have prepared themselves or that have been prepared and labeled by pharmacy

During a cardiac-arrest procedure, a nurse removed the outer wrap of a 5% D/W plastic I.V. bag and added 4 ampuls of dopamine HCl (Intropin). She put the bag on the crash cart next to the empty wrapper, but did not label the bag to show that the drug had been added. As it turned out, the patient never needed a dopamine drip.

After the "code," another nurse saw the unused, unlabeled bag. Assuming it had just been taken from the nearby wrapper, she put it back into the wrapper and returned it to I.V. floor stock.

Later, a third nurse went to the stock to pick up a 5% D/W bag for one of her patients. When she saw the opened package on the shelf, she assumed it had been opened by mistake and that it contained a fresh bag. She used it to start her patient's I.V. Fortunately, the first nurse, after completing her report on the "code," went to clean up. She remembered the bag that she had prepared but could not locate it. After questioning the other nurses, the bag was traced and the infusion stopped just after it had started.

In this case the patient escaped harm, but the consequences could have been serious. Of course, the error would have been prevented if the bag had not been left unlabeled. But a good rule to follow is never to use I.V. bags from stock when they are found out of the outer package. The same could be said for glass bottles from which the aluminum pull tabs and seals have been removed. The only exception would be when the solution is prepared and properly labeled by a pharmacy I.V. admixture service and still within the expiration date.

14:738, 1979

Error 141

Misidentification of a patient

One of the most common causes of medication error stems from misidentification of patients at the time of drug administration. Errors 53-56 discussed in detail the problem of not checking armbands to assure identity at all times. One of the errors occurred when a nurse asked the patient her name. She answered "Johnson" and the nurse gave Mrs. Johnson her medications. Later, the nurse discovered that another patient in the same room had the same surname and that she had given the medications to the wrong Mrs. Johnson.

A nurse has sent me a similar error report, but with a different twist. She was relieving the regular medication nurse on a ward for tuberculosis patients. The men were all alert and she identified them by asking their names. All went fine until she asked a patient, "Are you Mr. Thomas?" "Wright," he answered. Mr. Wright was given Mr. Thomas' drugs.

As much of a bother as it may be, there is no substitution for checking armbands prior to drug administration to identify patients properly.

14:738, 1979

Error 142

Use caution and sense when clinical information about patient is written on prescription

A revolting and very unfortunate incident occurred recently in a hospital outpatient pharmacy that should serve as a lesson to all physicians and pharmacists.

Two prescriptions, one for 120 Dilaudid 4-mg tablets, the other for 120 Valium 2-mg tablets, were written upon discharge for a cancer patient who had severe pain. Although aware of the disease, the patient, a 50-year-old woman, was unaware that she was considered "terminal." She had not been informed because the physician and family thought that knowledge of the gravity of her disease at that time would be detrimental to the patient.

The physician was concerned that the patient might have trouble getting the Dilaudid prescription filled because it was well known that several fraudulent Dilaudid prescriptions had been presented to the hospital pharmacy and community pharmacies in recent months. As a matter of fact, many area pharmacies were

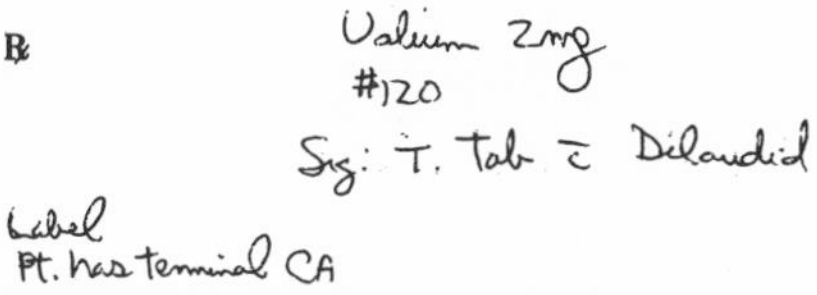

℞   Valium 2mg
    #120
    Sig: T. Tab c̅ Dilaudid
Label
Pt. has terminal CA

Figure 45

refusing to fill Dilaudid prescriptions. Because of this concern, the physician included the statement "Pt. has terminal Ca" on both the Valium and Dilaudid prescriptions. He placed both prescriptions in an envelope and handed this to the patient. He then accompanied the patient to the pharmacy to make sure that she could obtain the prescriptions without delay. The physician explained the need for the quantity and drugs ordered and then left. The pharmacist then dispensed the prescriptions, placed them in a bag, and handed them to the patient with brief instructions.

When the patient arrived at home, she opened the bag and read the labels on the containers. The statement "Pt. has terminal Ca" appeared on the label. Needless to say, the patient was shocked. She was quite distressed that her family and physician had kept this from her and she became severely depressed. Immediate medical attention was necessary.

On examination of the prescription, it is easy to see how this tragic error occurred (see Fig. 45). This physician placed the note just under his direction to "label" the prescription. The pharmacist assumed that the physician meant for him to include this on the label. No information was communicated to indicate that the patient had not been told about her condition. The pharmacist actually rationalized that the patient might be going on an overseas trip and that such information might be necessary to get through customs. Still, the pharma-

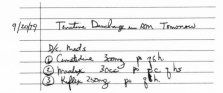

Figure 46

cist did not use much sense. He should have checked with the physician before placing the statement on the label.

The physician could have prevented the error by simply telephoning the information to the pharmacist. If it could not be determined what pharmacy would be used, the physician could have had the patient ask her pharmacist to phone him. If for some reason it is necessary to write clinical information about the patient, then it should be placed in parentheses, away from the main directions of the prescription or, better yet, on a separate note.

In the state in which this prescription was written, it is law that all prescriptions must be labeled with drug name. Therefore, the statement "label" was unnecessary and should not have been included.

Finally, health professionals should never use the term "terminal" when referring to patients.

15:27, 1980

Error 143

D/C: a potentially misunderstood abbreviation

In hospitals, the abbreviation D/C is widely used to mean "discontinue" (D/C meds). However, the abbreviation has also been used to mean "discharge" (D/C pt. in AM). As with all abbreviations that have more than one meaning, users normally under-stand the intended meaning of the abbreviation when taken in context with other information provided at the time. However, this is not always the case. The abbreviation D/C, when taken in the wrong context, has led to medication error. An example of misunderstood meaning of D/C appears in Fig. 46. The person noting these orders erroneously discontinued the medications 24 hours prior to the time of discharge. The patient received no doses until the discharging physician gave a nurse the patient's prescriptions at discharge time. The error was then discovered. The physician intended "D/C meds" to mean "discharge meds." A nurse thought he meant for them to be discontinued.

The abbreviation D/C should not be used to mean "discharge" when referring to medication orders to be taken by discharged patients. Pharmacists and nurses should be on the lookout for misuse of this abbreviation and should check on its meaning when necessary.

15:28, 1980

Error 144

Ambiguous drug orders

For oral solid dosage forms and most liquids, the specific weight of each dose should be used in medication orders. Orders expressing the dose in number of tablets, milliliters, and so forth, are ambiguous and misleading when more than one tablet strength or liquid concentration exists (see Error #33, December 1975). For example, how would you fill an order for "Lasix, one tablet?"

When both strength *and* number of tablets appear in an order, the meaning is as ambiguous as if no strength were mentioned. For example, what is the meaning of "Inderal ½ tablet 40 mg q.i.d.?" It is unclear whether the intended dose here is 20 mg (one-half of 40 mg tablet) or 40 mg (one-half of 80 mg tablet). Physicians should always specify the dose of medication desired in terms of strength.

15:28, 1980

Error 145
Confusion of "similar" oral theophylline products

An ambulatory asthmatic patient was stabilized on Slo-phyllin Gyrocaps (sustained release anhydrous theophylline) 250 mg twice daily. A refill prescription labeled Slow-Phyllin 250 mg (SIC) was dispensed. The patient, who happened to be a pharmacist, noticed that the capsules dispensed were different in appearance from those he had been taking. He questioned the dispensing pharmacist about this difference and learned that what was dispensed was Somophyllin-T 250 mg capsules (anhydrous theophylline, but *not* sustained release). The dispensing pharmacist had substituted this product. Although substitution was legal in the state in which this occurred, there was a lack of recognition on the part of the pharmacist of the difference in dosage form. Depending upon the patient's body clearance of theophylline, the error may have led to transiently toxic peak levels and subtherapeutic trough levels.

The names of these two products are quite similar. It is important that labels be read completely and that pharmacists differentiate them.

Even more confusing is the situation that exists with the various dosage forms of Slo-Phyllin. Mentioned above was the sustained release product Slo-Phyllin Gyrocap. It is available in 60 mg, 125 mg, and 250 mg

capsules. Slo-Phyllin is also available in non-sustained release tablets of 100 mg and 200 mg and a syrup of 80 mg per 15 ml. The capsule and non-sustained release forms are obviously not interchangeable. The name *Slo*-phyllin implies slow release, but this is not the case with the tablets or syrup. The physician, pharmacist, and nurse must be aware of the differences. When the sustained release is prescribed, "Gyrocap" or "sustained release" should be included as part of the order. Otherwise, confusion will exist. Inclusion of the dose required is a necessity and should also help to prevent confusion since the doses are different with the various dosage forms.

15:109, 1980

Error 146
Dispensing errors: Estratab for Ethatab*

In Memphis, Tennessee, an adult male presented a pharmacist with a prescription for Ethatab. The pharmacist dispensed Estratab.

Ethatab is the smooth muscle relaxant, ethaverine, made by Meyer Laboratories. Estratab is a female hormone made by Reid-Provident Labs, Inc. The patient sued the pharmacist for malpractice after taking the drug for 1 year. The plaintiff claimed breast enlargement, nausea, physical and mental fatigue, loss of memory, impotence, and psychological changes.

Not having seen the prescription, I cannot comment on its legibility. One could speculate that the prescription was illegible and looked like Estratab,

*Abstracted from the Newsletter of the American Society of Pharmacy Law, RX Ipsa Loquitur, October 1979.

that the pharmacist was not familiar with Ethatab and focused in on what he was familiar with, Estratab, or that the pharmacist just reached for the wrong bottle. The last possibility is unlikely since the prescription was used for 1 year.

If the pharmacist had effectively communicated with the patient initially, this error could have been prevented. The pharmacist should have satisfied himself that the female hormone he or she was dispensing was indicated for the condition being treated. Estrogens are used in the treatment of prostatic cancer.

At the trial, the plaintiff was awarded $135,000 for damages suffered due to the pharmacist's negligence.

This error points out the value of experienced, well-trained pharmacists who are given time (or take the time) to do the things they should do.

15:109, 1980

Error 147

Enteral alimentation fluids must have special labels and solution administration sets

A 60-year-old man, unconscious as a result of a cardiopulmonary arrest with resuscitation, was receiving enteral alimentation through a Silastic nasogastric tube. The 24-hour supply of 3000 ml of nutrient (Vivonex) was being divided into three bottles daily, each administered over eight hours by infusion pump. Powdered nutrient was dissolved in sterile water for irrigation contained in liter bottles with screw caps. The screw cap was modified to accept an I.V. solution administration set with a pump chamber and the luer tip of the set connected directly to the nasogastric tube. The solution set and screw cap were to be changed every 24 hours. On the second day, the person placing the fresh set and cap on the first bottle that day connected the line to a central venous catheter instead of to the nasogastric tube. The patient received approximately 400 ml of solution before the error was recognized. Although the patient experienced seizures, it could not be determined with certainty whether these were due to inadvertent I.V. infusion or to the patient's previous cerebral anoxia. The patient was placed on prophylactic antibiotic therapy. He experienced no fevers after the incident. Since the patient was also already on a ventilator, respiratory difficulty, if it occurred, was not readily recognizable.

Obviously, the person who connected the solution to the I.V. catheter did not think about what he or she was doing. The container was not an I.V. bottle; it had a special screw cap. The solution was not a clear liquid. The individual should have been aware of what type of therapy the patient was receiving and of the difference between enteral and parenteral alimentation (some are confused by the term "hyperalimentation" and do not differentiate).

There are other considerations. A pharmacist prepared the final solutions and labeled the bottles with labels normally used for intravenous therapy. If enteral alimentation is to be used, off-color labels should be utilized. They should prominently warn that the solution is "for enteral use — not for injection." Manufacturers can be of assistance by providing such labels (with space for listing other additives) with their products. These labels would help greatly to prevent errors in administration.

Tubing used with enteral alimentation should have connections that cannot fit I.V. catheters. At least one company (Abbott) manufactures an infusion pump set for use specifically with enteral alimentation. It has a screw cap already attached, and the set tip will not accommodate an I.V. catheter. Other companies should make such sets available. Alternatively, special administration bags are available from some manufacturers of enteral alimentation products, but these are not easily used with infusion pumps.

Lastly, if enteral and parenteral alimentation are being used in your institution, make sure that hospital personnel receive the educational support necessary to understand and utilize this type of therapy properly.

15:158, 1980

Error 148

More on cisplatin storage

Cisplatin (Platinol) requires special storage conditions depending upon the physical state of the product. Each unopened vial contains 10 mg of the drug as a dry powder which must be stored in the refrigerator (2-8°C). If stored in this manner, the drug remains stable for two years. Cisplatin powder may be stable for at least several days if unrefrigerated, although this change in labeling has not yet been approved by the FDA.[1]

When the powder is reconstituted with 10 ml of sterile water for injection, the resulting solution contains cisplatin in a concentration of 1 mg/ml. Such reconstituted solutions are stable for 20 hours at room temperature (27°C).[2] Although reconstituted solutions for parenteral use are often refrigerated to inhibit bacterial growth, vials containing reconstituted solutions of cisplatin must *not* be refrigerated, as this will lead to precipitation of the drug. The man-

ufacturer currently cannot guarantee stability of cisplatin when vials containing solutions have been refrigerated for variable lengths of time, and it is recommended that such solutions be discarded.

It has been shown that precipitation can be avoided for 48 hours if the concentration of cisplatin in refrigerated solutions is less than 0.6 mg/ml but that precipitation may occur within one hour if solutions are refrigerated in concentrations of 1 mg/ml.[3] The drug goes back into solution very slowly when rewarmed, but because of possible instability, rewarming of precipitated solutions is not currently recommended. The solution should be discarded if there is a haze or any other evidence of precipitation.

Pharmacists have encountered such precipitation, as well as several other instances in which improper storage of cisplatin has necessitated destruction of large quantities of the drug. In one instance, the pharmacy sent eight of the 10 mg vials of the dry powder to the nursing station, where they were properly refrigerated. The I.V. team reconstituted them later but then incorrectly placed the reconstituted vials back into the refrigerator. The drug precipitated, and the vials had to be discarded.

The pharmacy department subsequently instructed appropriate personnel about proper storage conditions for the product. However, eight

1. Personal communication. Syracuse: Bristol Laboratories, Division of Bristol-Myers Company, November 16, 1979.

2. Platinol: cisplatin for injection. Package insert. Syracuse: Bristol Laboratories, Division of Bristol-Myers Company, August 1978.

3. Greene RF, Chatterji DC, Hiranaka PK, Gallelli JF. Stability of cisplatin in aqueous solution. Am J Hosp Pharm 1979; 36:38-43.

vials of the dry powder sent up after this incident were later found on the same nursing station stored at room temperature. Because the length of time these vials had been improperly stored could not be determined, these vials were also discarded.

Cisplatin is supplied in a carton of ten vials that is clearly marked with a red label that states: "Perishable drug. Must refrigerate. Store at (2-8°C). Protect from light." This carton must *not* be used to deliver multiple reconstituted solutions to nursing station, oncology nurses, I.V. teams, or others. It is recommended that the pharmacy clearly label reconstituted vials *"Do not refrigerate"* or *"Not to be refrigerated."* Even this precaution may not be enough, as a third incident of improper storage occurred when a pharmacy technician placed in the refrigerator several vials containing reconstituted solutions that were clearly marked with such a label. For this reason, nurses, technicians, and all other personnel who handle cisplatin should be carefully instructed about the proper storage conditions for the drug. To further avoid confusion, the drug should be reconstituted immediately before administration whenever feasible.

Also see Error #139, November 1979.

15:158, 1978

Error 149

Neutra-Phos capsules should not be swallowed

A patient experienced severe gastrointestinal upset after swallowing a Neutra-Phos capsule. Neutra-Phos capsules, a product for oral phosphorus supplementation, contain powder *concentrate. The capsule is not* *meant to be swallowed.* Rather, its contents are to be emptied and dissolved in water (⅓ glass of water per capsule).

Unfortunately, previous labeling of the manufacturer's (Willen Drug Company, Baltimore, Maryland) container did not make the above information clear. However, they claim that their new label in use since October 1979, does. It is important that pharmacists communicate to nurses the need for dissolving the capsule before administering it. The MAR sheet should carry a notation of this.

One might want to recommend packaging each capsule in unit dose form with appropriate labeling, but the company warned us that the product is extremely hygroscopic and does not lend itself to packaging in other than "tight containers" (i.e., no glassine envelopes or c-cups). Probably the best way for pharmacists to dispense Neutra-Phos capsules is in bulk with an auxiliary label or in unit dose form with each capsule placed in a plastic vial with sealer cap and appropriate labeling.

15:213, 1980

Error 150

Cytarabine dispensed and administered instead of vidarabine

A physician's order for Ara-A was received by a pharmacy late in the day. A dose of 487 mg of Ara-A was ordered to be infused over 12 hours. This was to be repeated after the first dose was administered. The pharmacist processing the order was unsure of the identity of the product and asked another pharmacist to clarify the identity of the drug. The second pharmacist responded that he thought that Ara-A was an abbreviation for Cytosar-U, but recommended that a reference source be checked. The *American Drug Index* was then consulted. Although no listing for Ara-A was found, the listing for Cytosar-U was checked, "ara" was noticed as part of many names listed, and the pharmacist believed identification was confirmed. Five 100-mg vials of Cytosar-U were dispensed.

Later, the nurse who received the drug called the pharmacy to verify that Cytosar-U and Ara-A were the same drug. The pharmacist assured the nurse that they were. The I.V. solution was prepared and administration begun. Several hours later, the mistake was discovered; however, 275 mg of Cytosar-U had already been infused.

The pre-marketing research nomenclature that the physician used in writing this order led to this serious error. The abbreviation Ara-A was used rather than the generic or trade name. The intended product, vidarabine, has also been referred to as adeniol arabinoside and by its brand name, Vira-A. The product that it was confused with, Cytosar-U (cytarabine), was formerly known as cytosine arabinoside and abbreviated as Ara C. Only the generic or brand name should be used when referring to these drugs.

The error was further preventable by the pharmacists if they had clarified the order to the extent necessary. If a pharmacist is ever unfamiliar with the drug name written on a prescription or with the use and dose of an ordered drug, dispensing must not occur until this is clarified with certainty. The same can be said for a nurse required to administer a drug.

The error demonstrates once again the need for pharmacists to maintain patient profiles with information about patient diagnosis. Cytosar-U is used primarily for the treatment of

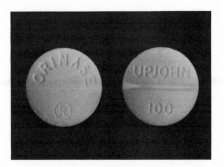

Figure 47. Upjohn's Orinase.

leukemias. Vira-A is used as an antiviral agent.

This error indicates the need for researchers, government, industry, publishers, and practitioners to stop using and referring to chemical names and their abbreviations as soon as a substance is given a United States Adopted Name (USAN). The full USAN (generic name) should be the only name used.

Of related interest is the brand name change of Cytosar to Cytosar-U. This was done by Upjohn because handwritten orders for Cytosar were being incorrectly interpreted as Cytoxan. The likelihood of Cytosar-U being mistaken for Cytoxan is more remote.

15:213, 1980

HAZARD WARNING #1

Code number hazard

Upjohn's system for identifying their drug products may lead to misidentification of the dose of their Orinase 500 mg tablet. The tablets now include the drug name as well as a code number to identify drug and dose. In the case of their Orinase 500 mg tablet the code number is 100 (Fig. 47). This may lead to misidentification by health professionals or pa-

228

tients as 100 mg. It should be noted that Upjohn has never manufactured such a strength. I can foresee a situation in which a patient may take five tablets to equal a 500 mg dose. Even more likely is the chance that an inexperienced physician or nurse may identify a supply of tablets brought to the hospital or office as 100 mg and prescribe this dose for a patient, or "five tablets." Upjohn should reassign the tablet another code number or else print in the dose and leave the code number off.

12:44, 1977

HAZARD WARNING #2

Preventing errors in prescriptions for travelers

A plea for physicians to use generic names of drugs when prescribing for travelers has been made by Eisenberg et al. in the *Journal of the American Medical Association* 233: 277, 1975. The authors caution that trade names for drugs in different countries may not always be for the same agents. Their letter bears repeating and publication in your pharmacy newsletter or communication sheet:

To the Editor: In our world of rapid transport, patients can find themselves in a foreign country where the loss of baggage can mean the loss of their drug supply. Obtaining the correct drug may be made more complex not only by the biological availability variation of the foreign product but by its trade name, made evident by the following two examples.
First, the trade name Cardoxin is used in Israel for dipyridamole, the coronary dilater; the same name is used in Australia for digoxin. Second, the trade name Didion, used in Europe to indicate the antiepileptic ethadione, is used in Israel for the indandione anticoagulant diphenadione.
These two examples only emphasize the care that must be taken in writing that "safety" prescription for the traveler. The generic or chemical name must always be included with the trade name to prevent this type of inadvertent and potentially dangerous error.

HAZARD WARNING #3

Poor labeling of prefilled syringes of emergency drugs may lead to error

The labeling on prefilled disposable syringes of emergency drugs manufactured by Bristol Laboratories can lead to dangerous error (Fig. 48). The dose contained in the syringe (see lower left of package) is difficult to see because of the small size of the numbers in relation to other lettering and numbering on the package. Especially since these drugs are used during medical emergencies, the dose should be listed more prominently so that people do not have to waste time looking for the dose (in tense situations such as cardiac arrest this can be very frustrating, can add to the confusion and delay therapy).

Another problem is in the way the dose is printed as 100.0 mg in 5 ml, (20.0 mg per ml) for lidocaine. Syringes for epinephrine, calcium and atropine are similarly labeled. Since the printing is so small, this can be taken for 1000 mg per 5 ml and 200 mg per ml (lidocaine). There is no reason ever to use a zero after a decimal point when drug doses are listed. There is also no reason for a decimal point to be present.

Yet another drawback with Bristol's labeling is the fact that the box containing the syringes also has one end on which only the drug name appears — no dose. Since these drugs are often stored in emergency drug supplies with only the end visible, the problem here is obvious.

Bristol Laboratories has since improved the labeling of their prefilled disposable syringes.

11:487, 1976

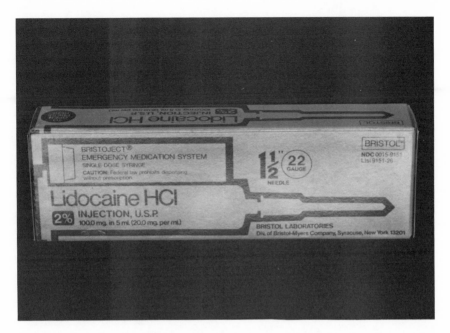

Figure 48. Hazardous labeling of prefilled syringe. Notice small size of numbers used to label dose in comparison to size of numbers for less important needle size. The 100.0 mg and 20.0 mg in the lower left corner can easily be misinterpreted as 1000 mg and 200 mg.

HAZARD WARNING #4

A recent issue of APhA Weekly contained the following item.

Firm's Name May Confuse Pharmacists and Patients

The April issue of the Duquesne University's toxicology newsletter reports that the name "Purepac"—a major generic drug manufacturer—is often confused with Ipecac.

According to the newsletter, the poison control director at the Nassau County Medical Center in East Meadow, N.Y., reports several cases in which Syrup of Ipecac has been confused with the Purepac brand of methyl salicylate or tincture of benzoin.

The newsletter suggested that one means of avoiding the possible confusion would be for the manufacturer to change its label design to place the brand name in smaller letters at the bottom of the label.

11:436, 1976

HAZARD WARNING # 5

Inadvertent I.V. Injection

A hazard of intravascular injection of benzathine penicillin G (Bicillin) exists when the 2,400,000 unit syringe manufactured by Wyeth Laboratories is used.

When an intramuscular injection is administered, it is standard practice to aspirate the syringe to see if the needle level has been inadvertently positioned in an artery or vein. If this is the case, blood will appear at the needle junction.

The Wyeth Bicillin syringe does not allow for this. If one withdraws in the space available, sufficient suction is not accomplished to move the drug suspension away from the needle junction for blood detection. Also a blue rubber apparatus located within

230

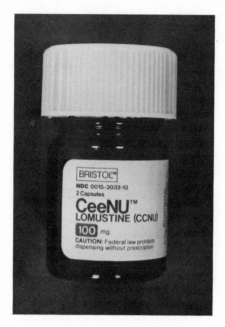

Figure 49. CeeNU label.

an anticonvulsant. The drug is available as a 0.5 mg, 1 mg or 2 mg tablet. Clonidine (Catapres—Boehringer-Ingelheim) is an antihypertensive available as 0.1 mg and 0.2 mg tablets. Both drugs have the prefix clon-. Since there were no drugs available in the United States with this prefix, the confusion is magnified.

Clonazepam dosage ranges from 0.5 mg to 20 mg per day. Clonidine doses range from 0.1 to 2.4 mg per day.

Publicity should be given to this situation within your institution. Inadvertent name switching may occur at any point along the drug distribution cycle. To avoid problems, close attention should be paid to the patient's diagnosis to learn of the condition for which the drug is to be used.

11:207, 1976

the syringe neck obscures visibility of aspirated blood.

Editor's note: Experimenting with methylene blue, I was unable to detect the dye at the needle junction. The syringe does not allow for visible blood aspiration.—MRC

Editors' Update: Wyeth has redesigned this Bicillin Syringe to correct this problem. Aspirated blood is now visible.

11:282, 1976

HAZARD WARNING #6

Clonazepam and Clonidine

A potentially hazardous situation exists because two recently released drugs with very different indications have names that are easily confused. Their dosage ranges also overlap.

Clonazepam (Clonapin—Roche) is

HAZARD WARNING #7

CeeNU capsule package labeling

The recently marketed CeeNU (lomustine) capsules from Bristol Laboratories are packaged with hazardous labeling. The following error report illustrates the problem.

An order was received for "CeeNU 100 mg PO." The labeling on the manufacturer's bottle reads (Fig. 49) "2 capsules, CeeNU, 100 mg." The bottle had been dispensed as packaged and the capsules subsequently administered to the patient. The capsules each contain 100 mg; the patient received both capsules. The error was discovered a few minutes after the dose was administered and lavage was immediately begun.

Hospital personnel are becoming used to unit dose packaging and the person administering the drug thought the bottle with two capsules contained 100 mg total. More precise labeling on the immediate container would have prevented this error. A package insert (labeled "important information") is contained in a box with three bottles of CeeNU, each of different strengths. Although the insert gives more complete information about capsule strength, it was not consulted in this case and did not help to prevent the error. The label should state "100 mg per capsule."

Bristol Laboratories and the USP have been informed of this problem. You should consider dispensing the drug in unit dose form until a label change occurs.

12:191, 1977

HAZARD WARNING #8

Elixophyllin Pediatric Suspension is four times as strong as Elixophyllin

A 14 kg boy, an asthmatic, was hospitalized for status asthmaticus. After successful treatment with intravenous aminophylline and steroids for three days, the child was converted to an oral theophylline product at a dose of 80 mg QID. After two days of this therapy, it was decided to discharge the patient.

In preparing discharge medication orders, the house officer was informed by the parent that they had a full bottle of Elixophyllin at home. The house officer, therefore, told the parent to administer one tablespoonful QID. The next morning during a conference the physician learned of a new product called Elixophyllin Pediatric Suspension. The physician called the parent and learned that they did, indeed, have Elixophyllin Pediatric Suspension, which has a concentration of 100 mg/5 ml, not regular Elixophyllin (27 mg/5 ml).

Therefore, the child was receiving 300 mg QID instead of 80 mg QID. Fortunately, the child had received only two doses separated by 12 hours and serious toxicity was avoided.

An incomplete drug history here played a major role in causing this error. Because of the similarity of the name assigned the new product, it is easy to see how the mix-up occurred. Although termed "Pediatric Suspension," the new product is much more concentrated. It is also free of dye, sugar and alcohol.

Note: The name Elixophyllin Pediatric Suspension has been changed to Elixicon.

12:427, 1977

HAZARD WARNING #9

The name "Percocet-5"

Attention is called to a hazardous situation that exists because of the brand name given by Endo Laboratories, Inc. to its tablets of oxycodone HCl, 5 mg with acetaminophen 325 mg in combination. The name of the product is Percocet-5. For some reason the fact that the product contains 5 mg of oxycodone HCl was deemed so important that it needed to be highlighted as part of the drug name.

The danger is that some physicians erroneously do not use the full name or number of tablets per dose when prescribing on a physician's order form of the patient's chart. Commonly, I have seen orders for "Percocet q 6 h prn pain." If a nurse becomes familiar with this type of order and is not familiar with the actual name of the product, the following might occur:

Another physician, using the correct name when prescribing but again not stating the number of tablets per dose writes "Percocet-5 q 6 h prn pain" with possible serious consequences to the patient.

Whenever a number is used as part of a drug name there is a potential for error. Errors have been reported in the "Medication Error Reports" with 6-Mercaptopurine, Tylenol No. 3 and 6-Thioguanine (Errors #13, #27, #104). Some have resulted in death.

I believe it is already too late for Endo to change the name of the product. By dropping the "5," physicians who continue to write "Percocet-5" might then cause an error because nurses will see labeling and become familiar with only "Percocet." But manufacturers really ought to consider this problem when giving names to their products. A number should never appear as part of a drug name.

In the meantime, hospital personnel should have the problem called to their attention immediately. In-service departments should mention this during orientation of new personnel. I strongly recommend that only unit dose packaging be used in inpatient areas. This will reduce the potential for error, as each tablet is labeled Percocet-5. Any repackaging by pharmacists must clearly be labeled as Percocet-5, never just "Percocet."

14:278, 1979

HAZARD WARNING #10

Metoprolol-metaproterenol

Metoprolol (Lopressor) is a recently released beta blocker indicated for the treatment of hypertension. Metaproterenol is a beta stimulant indicated for the treatment of bronchospastic diseases. Since the available tablet strengths of metoprolol (50 and 100 mg) are relatively close in strength to those of metaproterenol (10 and 20 mg) and because of the similarity of generic names and pharmacologic involvement (both affecting beta adrenergic system of autonomic nervous system) we should be concerned that these drugs may inadvertently be confused for one another. It is suggested that appropriate publicity be given to this situation via your pharmacy newsletter or other communication system. Perhaps it would be safer to utilize brand names when referring to these drugs. When receiving orders for these drugs, you should make sure of the patient's diagnosis.

14:367, 1979

HAZARD WARNING #11

Lopress-Lopressor

Until 1976, Tutag Pharmaceuticals of Broomfield, Colorado manufactured hydralazine under the trade name Lopress. Although they relinquished rights to the name and no longer market the product, some reference books still list this brand name. At least one error has occurred because of the similarity of this name and the recently marketed Lopressor (metoprolol). The doses also overlap.

A nurse, in transcribing a physician's order for Lopressor 50 mg, realized that she was unfamiliar with this drug. She went to a reference book kept on the nursing unit (*The Nurse's Drug Handbook*, New York, John Wiley & Sons, 1977) and found Lopress listed as the brand name for hydralazine. Without considering that the small difference in spelling was of any significance, she called the pharmacy and asked for a dose of "hydralazine 50 mg." Unfortunately, the first dose was dispensed without the original order first being reviewed by a pharmacist (a break in procedure for this pharmacy department). Subsequently, after the original order was seen, the pharmacist recognized that metoprolol was being requested, not hydralazine, and the error was not repeated.

Lopress is also listed in American Drug Index, 1977 edition.

It would be a good idea to update the aforementioned texts if they are available anywhere in your hospital or library. You should be aware of the potential for confusion, but the error also points out the need for a pharmacist's reviewing a copy of the original order before dispensing doses other than in an emergency.

14:428, 1979

HAZARD WARNING #12

Danger in "similar" color-coded labels

A potentially dangerous labeling problem has been identified by the University of Kansas Medical Center, Department of Pharmacy. The 50 ml single dose vial of 50% dextrose and the 50 ml multiple-dose vial of 1% lidocaine hydrochloride packaged by Cutter Laboratories have "almost" identical color-coded labels. One product is labeled with an orange and white label and is sealed with a similarly colored cap, and the other has a tan label and cap.

A near mishap occurred when 50 ml of 1% lidocaine was drawn up in place of 50 ml of 50% dextrose for a patient undergoing renal dialysis. For patient convenience the room light was dim, making the distinction between orange and tan labels difficult. The labels were accurate, but the personnel were relying upon the color code rather than the label.

Pharmacists are advised to double check the label on all products that are dispensed and to be especially watchful of products that are the same size, shape, and color.

14:553, 1979

HAZARD WARNING # 13

Color Coding

In Hazard Warning #12 an error was reported that described a near mishap when 1% lidocaine was drawn up instead of 50% dextrose. In addition to not reading the label, the problem was traced to similar coloring of the individual containers manufactured by Cutter Laboratories. One is orange while the other is tan. In a dimly lit room they appeared to be the same color and the user did not read the label.

Since this went to press, I have received two error reports also involving Cutter color-coded containers. In each case, bacteriostatic sodium chloride injection 30 ml was confused with concentrated sodium chloride injection (120 mEq/30 ml). Both have yellow labels and caps. In addition, on the bacteriostatic sodium chloride label, the only indication of strength is the lettering in the upper right hand corner and the list of ingredients on the back. This lettering, "0.9%," is 1 mm in height. The manufacturer's name and the NDC are twice that size. There is a definite lack of easily and quickly identifiable markings to create a clear distinction between the different vials.

Both of the reports came from hospital pharmacists with TPN services, which is where the problems occurred. In one of the cases, the problem-causing vials were emptied into the sink. In the words of the author,

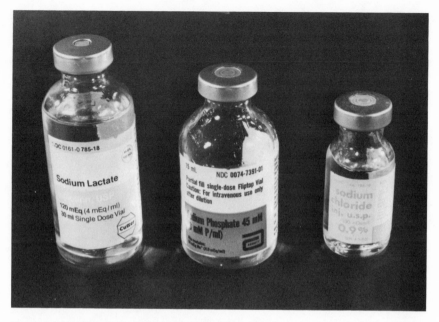

Figure 50. Small-volume parenterals intended for single-dose use have nonremovable caps and vial stoppers that are meant for multi-dose use.

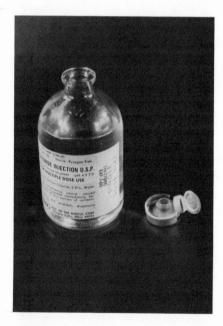

Figure 51. Some small-volume parenterals have completely removable ("peel-off") caps.

". . . These measures are less costly in time and money than the waste created by the destruction of the questionable I.V. admixtures, replacement of those bags with the proper ones, and the filing of medication error reports when necessary."

It has been recommended that Cutter take a hard look at their labeling practices and especially the way color coding is used.

14:628, 1979

HAZARD WARNING #14

Misuse of single-dose vials with multi-dose caps

Small-volume parenterals packed in glass vials are convenient to use and eliminate the problem of glass particles being drawn up in a syringe when preparing a dose. Several companies market small-volume parenterals intended for single use only (these contain no preservative and are marked "single-dose vial"). Some of these have nonremovable caps and vial stoppers meant for multi-dose use (Fig. 50). Such vials should never be dispensed as floor stock. The reason is that users, unaware of the vials' single-use limit, may use them as multi-dose vials and risk contamination of the solution. They are meant for single use only and are best utilized in conjunction with pharmacy I.V. admixture programs.

Because completely removable vial caps are also available (Fig. 51) for solutions packaged in vials ("peel-off caps"), these should be used whenever it is necessary to dispense vials as floor stock. Some users will complain that this type of cap and stopper, when removed, makes it more difficult to draw up medication, because when tilted, it may spill. For those users, the tab can be partially removed, exposing a target area (Fig. 52) that still allows for the vial's use in multi-dose fashion.

It should be pointed out that the "peel off caps" can also be misused as multi-dose containers when the cap is not completely removed. In fact, even glass ampuls have been discovered used as multi-dose containers by the uninformed (Fig. 53). To prevent those problems, nothing will take the place of the pharmacist making routine checks of the patient care area. Be on the lookout for misuse of small-volume parenteral containers and incorporate this point in your nursing in-service programs.

14:682, 1979

HAZARD WARNING #15

Pavulon and Pancuronium

The Food and Drug Administration (FDA) has recently received a report that two products having similar proprietary names were confused during dispensing. These products are

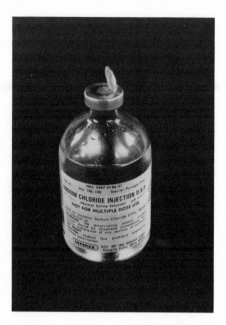

Figure 52. On this vial, the tab of the peel-off cap has been partially removed to expose a target area, permitting medication to be dispensed easily without spilling.

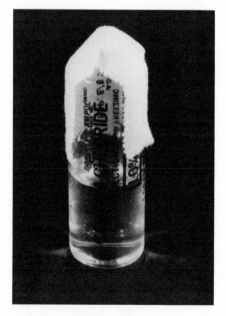

Figure 53. Glass ampul being misused as a multi-dose container.

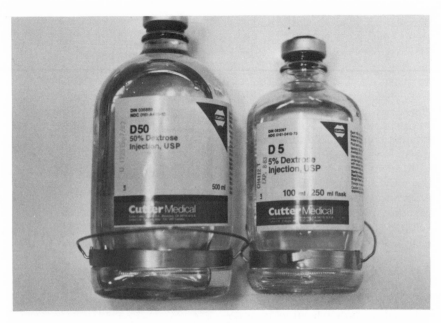

Figure 54. Label of Cutter 50% dextrose injection contains no warning of high concentration. Its color coding is the same as that of 5% dextrose injection partial fill.

Pavulon (Organon; pancuronium bromide; ampul) and Peptavlon (Ayerst; pentagastrin; ampul). Because these drugs are frequently requested by departmental requisition, it would be a good idea to inform both pharmacists and technical personnel of the potential for mix-up.

14:738, 1979

HAZARD WARNING #16

Cutter LVP of 50% dextrose injection

The labeling of 50% dextrose injection manufactured by Cutter Medical is hazardous (Fig. 54). No warning statement of its high concentration (other than the word "hypertonic") appears. In addition, the label is color-coded brown, the same as their 5% dextrose injection partial fills.

Danger exists because the appearance of the labels of 5% and 50% concentrations are so similar. Inad-

vertent administration of 50% dextrose has had disastrous consequences (see Error #9). For safety's sake, a vivid warning should appear on the face of the label. It should state that the product should be administered only after dilution and through a central venous catheter.

Since the product is mainly used in preparing TPN solutions and since TPN products should be prepared by a pharmacist, these containers must not be permitted in patient-care areas.

Other parenteral manufacturers include warning statements on their labels of 50% dextrose in LVP containers. Cutter Medical has been contacted and has stated that they will look into the matter.

This potential type of error emphasizes the need for the pharmacist to check drugs and supplies throughout the hospital.

15:109, 1980

Appendix 2

ASHP Guidelines on Hospital Drug Distribution and Control (with References)

Drug control (of which drug distribution is an important part) is among the pharmacist's most important responsibilities. Therefore, adequate methods to assure that these responsibilities are met must be developed and implemented. These guidelines will assist the pharmacist in preparing drug control procedures for all medication-related activities. The guidelines are based on the premise that the pharmacy is responsible for the procurement, distribution, and control of *all* drugs used within the institution. In a sense, the entire hospital is the pharmacy, and the pharmacy service is simply a functional service extending throughout the institution's physical and organizational structures.

It should be noted that, although this document is directed toward hospitals, much of it is relevant to other types of health care facilities.

Pharmacy Policies, Procedures, and Communications

Policy and Procedure Manuals. [1] The effectiveness of the drug control system depends upon adherence to policies (broad, general statements of philosophy) and procedures (detailed

guidelines for implementing policy). The importance of an up-to-date policy and procedure manual for drug control cannot be overestimated. All pharmacy staff must be familiar with the manual; it is an important part of orientation for new staff and crucial to the pharmacy's internal communication mechanism. In addition, preparing written policies and procedures requires a thorough analysis of control operations; this review might go undone otherwise.

Drug control begins with the setting of policy. The authority to enforce

Developed by the ASHP Council on Professional Affairs. Approved by the ASHP Board of Directors on March 20, 1980.

This document contains numerous references to various official ASHP documents and other publications. Inclusion of the latter does not constitute endorsement of their content by the Society; they are, however, considered to be useful elaborations on certain subjects contained herein. To avoid redundancy with other ASHP documents, relevant references are cited in many sections of these Guidelines. Most may be obtained from ASHP through its publications catalog. (American Society of Hospital Pharmacists, 4630 Montgomery Ave., Washington, D.C. 20014) drug control policy and procedures must come from the administration of the institution, with the endorsement of the medical staff, via the pharmacy and therapeutics (P&T) committee and/or other appropriate committee(s). Because the drug control system interfaces with numerous departments and professions, the P&T committee should be the focal point for communications relating to drug control in the institution. The pharmacist, with the cooperation of the P&T committee, should develop media such as newsletters, bulletins, and seminars to communicate with persons functioning within the framework of the control system.

In-service Training and Education. Intra- and inter-departmental education and training programs are important to the effective implementation of policies and procedures and the institution's drug control system in general. They are part of effective communication and help establish and maintain professional relationships among the pharmacy staff and between it and other hospital departments. Drug control policies and procedures should be included in the pharmacy's educational programs.

Standards, Laws, and Regulations

The pharmacist must be aware of and comply with the laws, regulations, and standards governing the profession. Many of these standards and regulations deal with aspects of drug control. Among the agencies and organizations affecting institutional pharmacy practice are those described below.

Regulatory Agencies and Organizations. The U.S. government, through its Food and Drug Administration (FDA), is responsible for implementing and enforcing the federal Food, Drug and Cosmetic Act. The FDA is responsible for the control and prevention of misbranding and of adulteration of food, drugs, and cosmetics moving in interstate commerce. The FDA also sets label requirements for food, drugs, and cosmetics; sets standards for investigational drug studies and for marketing of new drug products; and compiles data on adverse drug reactions.

The U.S. Department of the Treasury influences pharmacy operation by regulating the use of tax-free alcohol through the Bureau of Alcohol, Tobacco and Firearms. The U.S. Department of Justice affects pharmacy practice through its Drug Enforcement Agency (DEA) by enforcing the Controlled Substances Act of 1970 and other federal laws and regulations for controlled drugs.

Another federal agency, the Health Care Financing Administration, has established Conditions of Participation for hospitals and skilled nursing facilities to assist these institutions to qualify for reimbursement under the health insurance program for the aged (Medicare) and for Medicaid.

The state board of pharmacy is the agency of state government responsible for regulating pharmacy practice within the state. Practitioners, institutions, and community pharmacies must obtain licenses from the board to practice pharmacy or provide pharmacy services in the state. State boards of pharmacy promulgate numerous regulations pertaining to drug dispensing and control. (In some states, the state board of health licenses the hospital pharmacy separately or through a license that includes all departments of the hospital.)

Standards and guidelines for pharmaceutical services have been established by the Joint Commission on Accreditation of Hospitals (JCAH)[2] and the American Society of Hospital Pharmacists (ASHP).[3] The United States Pharmacopeial Convention also promulgates certain pharmacy practice procedures as well as official standards for drugs and drug testing. Professional practice guidelines and standards generally do not have the force of law, but rather, are intended to assist pharmacists in achieving the highest level of practice. They may, however, be employed in legal proceedings as evidence of what constitutes acceptable practice as determined by the profession itself.

In some instances, both federal and state laws may deal with a specific activity; in such cases, the more stringent law will apply.

The Medication System

Procurement: Drug Selection, Purchasing Authority, Responsibility and Control.[4-6] The selection of pharmaceuticals is a basic and extremely important professional function of the hospital pharmacist, who is charged with making decisions regarding products, quantities, product specifications and sources of supply. It is the pharmacist's obligation to establish and maintain standards assuring the quality, proper storage, control, and safe use of all pharmaceuticals and related supplies (e.g., fluid administration sets); this responsibility must not be delegated to another individual. Although the actual purchasing of drugs and supplies may be performed by a nonpharmacist, the setting of quality standards and specifications requires professional knowledge and judgment and must be performed by the pharmacist.

Economic and therapeutic consid-erations make it necessary for hospitals to have a well-controlled, continuously updated formulary. It is the pharmacist's responsibility to develop and maintain adequate product specifications to aid in the purchase of drugs and related supplies under the formulary system. The *USP-NF* is a good base for drug product specifications; there also should be criteria to evaluate the acceptability of manufacturers and distributors. In establishing the formulary, the pharmacy and therapeutics committee recommends guidelines for drug selection. However, when his knowledge indicates, the pharmacist must have the authority to reject a particular drug product or supplier.

Though the pharmacist has the authority to select a brand or source of supply, he must make economic considerations subordinate to those of quality. Competitive-bid purchasing is an important method for achieving a proper balance between quality and cost when two or more acceptable suppliers market a particular product meeting the pharmacist's specifications. In selecting a vendor, the pharmacist must consider price, terms, shipping times, dependability, quality of service, returned goods policy, and packaging; however, prime importance always must be placed on drug quality and the manufacturer's reputation. It should be noted that the pharmacist is responsible for the quality of all drugs dispensed by the pharmacy.

Records. The pharmacist must establish and maintain adequate record-keeping systems. Various records must be retained (and be retrievable) by the pharmacy because of governmental regulations; some are advisable for legal protection; others are needed for JCAH accreditation, and still others are necessary for sound management (evaluation of productivity, workloads and expenses, and assessment of departmental growth and progress) of the pharmacy department. Records must be retained for at least the length of time prescribed by law (where such requirements apply).

It is important the pharmacist study federal, state, and local laws to become familiar with their requirements for permits, tax stamps, storage of alcohol and controlled substances, records, and reports.

Among the records needed in the drug distribution and control system are:

• Controlled substances inventory and dispensing records.
• Records of medication orders and their processing.
• Manufacturing and packaging production records.
• Pharmacy workload records.
• Purchase and inventory records.
• Records of equipment maintenance.
• Records of results and actions taken in quality assurance and drug audit programs.

Receiving Drugs. Receiving control should be under the auspices of a responsible individual, and the pharmacist must ensure that records and forms provide proper control upon receipt of drugs. Complete accountability from purchase order initiation to drug administration must be provided.

Personnel involved in the purchase, receipt, and control of drugs should be well-trained in their responsibilities and duties and must understand the serious nature of drugs. All nonprofessional personnel employed by the pharmacy should be selected and supervised by the pharmacist.

Delivery of drugs directly to the pharmacy or other pharmacy receiving area is highly desirable; it should be considered mandatory for controlled drugs. Orders for controlled substances must be checked against the official order blank (when applicable) and against hospital purchase order forms. All drugs should be placed into stock promptly upon receipt, and controlled substances must be directly transferred to safes or other secure areas.

Drug Storage and Inventory Control. Storage is an important aspect of the total drug control system. Proper environmental control (i.e., proper temperature, light, humidity, conditions of sanitation, ventilation, and segregation) must be maintained wherever drugs and supplies are stored in the institution. Storage areas must be secure; fixtures and equipment used to store drugs should be constructed so that drugs are accessible only to designated and authorized personnel. Such personnel must be carefully selected and supervised. Safety also is an important factor, and proper consideration should be given to the safe storage of poisons and flammable compounds. Externals should be stored separately from internal medications. Medications stored in a refrigerator containing items other than drugs should be kept in a secured, separate compartment.

Proper control is important wherever medications are kept, whether in general storage in the institution or the pharmacy or patient care areas (including satellite pharmacies, nursing units, clinics, emergency rooms, operating rooms, recovery rooms, and treatment rooms). Expiration dates of perishable drugs must be considered in all of these locations and stock rotated as required. A method to detect and properly dispose of outdated, deteriorated, recalled, or obsolete drugs and supplies should be established. This should include monthly audits of all medication storage areas in the institution. (The results of these audits should be documented in writing.)

Since the pharmacist must justify and account for the expenditure of pharmacy funds, he must maintain an adequate inventory management system. Such a system should enable the pharmacist to analyze and interpret prescribing trends and their economic impacts, and appropriately minimize inventory levels. It is essential that a system to indicate subminimum inventory levels be developed to avoid "outages," along with procedures to procure emergency supplies of drugs when necessary.

In-house Manufacturing, Bulk Compounding, Packaging and Labeling. [7,8] As with commercially marketed drug products, those produced by the pharmacy must be accurate in identity, strength, purity, and quality. Therefore, there must be adequate process and finished-product controls for all manufacturing/bulk compounding and packaging operations. Written master formulas and batch records (including product test results) must be maintained. All technical personnel must be adequately trained and supervised.

Packaging and labeling operations must have controls sufficient to prevent product/package/label mixups. A lot number to identify each finished product with its production and control history must be assigned to each batch.

The Good Manufacturing Practices of the Food and Drug Administration is a useful model for developing a comprehensive control system.

The pharmacist is encouraged to prepare those drug dosage forms, strengths, and packagings which are needed for optimal drug therapy, but which are commercially unavailable. Adequate attention must be given to the stability, palatability, packaging, and labeling requirements of these products.

Medication Distribution (The Unit Dose System). [9-11] Medication distribution is the responsibility of the pharmacy. The pharmacist, with the assistance of the pharmacy and therapeutics committee and the department of nursing, must develop comprehensive policies and procedures that provide for the safe distribution of all medications and related supplies to inpatients and outpatients.

For reasons of safety and economy, the preferred method to distribute drugs in institutions is the *unit dose system.* Though the unit dose system may differ in form depending on the specific needs, resources, and characteristics of each institution, four elements are common to all: (1) medications are contained in, and administered from, single-unit or unit-dose packages; (2) medications are dispensed in ready-to-administer form, to the extent possible; (3) for most medications, not more than a 24-hour supply of doses is provided to or available at the patient care area at any time, and (4) a patient medication profile is concurrently maintained in the pharmacy for each patient. Floor stocks of drugs are minimized and limited to drugs for emergency use and routinely used "safe" items such as mouthwash and antiseptic solutions.

(1) Physician's Drug Order: Writing the Order. Medications should be given (with certain specified exceptions) only on the *written* order of a qualified physician or other authorized prescriber. Allowable exceptions to this rule (i.e., telephoned or verbal orders) should be put in writ-

ten form immediately and the prescriber should countersign the nurse's or pharmacist's signed record of these orders within 48 (preferably 24) hours. Only a pharmacist or registered nurse should accept such orders. Provision should be made to place physician's orders in the patient's chart, and a method for sending this information to the pharmacy should be developed.

Prescribers should specify the date and time medication orders are written.

Medication orders should be written legibly in ink and should include:

- Patient's name and location (unless clearly indicated on the order sheet).
- Name (generic) of medication.
- Dosage expressed in the metric system, except in instances where dosage must be expressed otherwise (i.e., units, etc.).
- Frequency of administration.
- Route of administration.
- Signature of the physician.
- Date and hour the order was written.

Any abbreviations used in medication orders should be agreed to and jointly adopted by the medical, nursing, pharmacy, and medical records staff of the institution.

Any questions arising from a medication order, including the interpretation of an illegible order, should be referred to the ordering physician by the pharmacist. It is desirable for the pharmacist to make (appropriate) entries in the patient's medical chart pertinent to the patient's drug therapy. (Proper authorization for this must be obtained.[12]) Also, a duplicate record of the entry can be maintained in the pharmacy profile.

In computerized patient data systems, each prescriber should be assigned a unique identifier; this number should be included in all medication orders. Unauthorized personnel should not be able to gain access to the system.

(2) Physician's Drug Order: Medication Order Sheets. The pharmacist (except in emergency situations) must receive the physician's original order or a direct copy of the order before the drug is dispensed. This permits the pharmacist to resolve questions or problems with drug orders before the drug is dispensed and administered. It also eliminates errors which may arise when drug orders are transcribed onto another form for use by the pharmacy. Several methods by which the pharmacy may receive physicians' original orders or direct copies are:

1. Self-copying order forms. The physician's order form is designed to make a direct copy (carbon or NCR) which is sent to the pharmacy. This method provides the pharmacist with a duplicate copy of the order and does not require special equipment. There are two basic formats:
   a. Orders for medications included among treatment orders. Use of this form allows the physician to continue writing his orders on the chart as he has been accustomed in the past, leaving all other details to hospital personnel.
   b. Medication orders separated from other treatment orders on the order form. The separation of drug orders makes it easier for the pharmacist to review the order sheet.
2. Electromechanical. Copying machines or similar devices may be used to produce an exact copy of the physician's order. Provision should be made to transmit physi-

cians' orders to the pharmacy in the event of mechanical failure.

3. Computerized. Computer systems, in which the physician enters orders into a computer which then stores and prints out the order in the pharmacy or elsewhere, are used in some institutions. Any such system should provide for the pharmacist's verification of any drug orders entered into the system by anyone other than an authorized prescriber.

(3) Physician's Drug Order: Time Limits and Changes. Medication orders should be reviewed automatically when the patient goes to the delivery room, operating room, or a different service. In addition, a method to protect patients from indefinite, open-ended drug orders must be provided. This may be accomplished through one or more of the following: (1) routine monitoring of patients' drug therapy by a pharmacist; (2) drug class-specific, automatic stop-order policies covering those drug orders not specifying a number of doses or duration of therapy; (3) automatic cancellation of all drug orders after a predetermined (by the pharmacy and therapeutics committee) time interval unless rewritten by the prescriber. Whatever the method used, it must protect the patient, as well as provide for a timely notification to the prescriber that the order will be stopped *before* such action takes place.

(4) Physician's Drug Order: Receipt of Order and Drug Profiles. A pharmacist must review and interpret every medication order, and resolve any problems or uncertainties with it, before the drug is entered into the dispensing system. This means that he must be satisfied that each questionable medication order is, in fact, acceptable. This may occur through study of the patient's medical record, research of the professional literature or discussion with the prescriber or other medical, nursing, or pharmacy staff. Procedures to handle a drug order the pharmacist still believes is unacceptable (e.g., very high dose or a use beyond that contained in the package insert) should be prepared (and reviewed by the hospital's legal counsel). In general, the physician must be able to support the use of the drug in these situations. It is generally advisable for the pharmacist to document actions (e.g., verbal notice to the physician that a less toxic drug was available and should be used) relative to a questionable medication order on the pharmacy's patient medication profile form or other pharmacy document (not in the medical record).

Once the order has been approved, it is entered into the *patient's medication profile.* A medication profile must be maintained in the pharmacy for all inpatients and those outpatients routinely receiving care at the institution. (Note: equivalent records also should be available at the patient care unit.) This essential item, which is continuously updated, may be a written copy or computer-maintained. It serves two purposes. First, it enables the pharmacist to become familiar with the patient's total drug regimen, enabling him to detect quickly potential interactions, unintended dosage changes, drug duplications and overlapping therapies, and drugs contraindicated because of patient allergies or other reasons. Second, it is required in unit dose systems in order for the individual medication doses to be scheduled, prepared, distributed, and administered on a timely basis. The profile information must be reviewed by the pharmacist *before* dispensing the patient's drug(s). (It also may be useful in retrospective review of drug use.)

Patient profile information should include:

- Patient's full name, date hospitalized, age, sex, weight, hospital I.D. number, and provisional diagnosis or reason for admission (the format for this information will vary from one hospital to another).
- Laboratory test results.
- Other medical data relevant to the patient's drug therapy (e.g., information from drug history interviews).
- Sensitivities, allergies, and other significant contraindications.
- Drug products dispensed, dates of original order, strengths, dosage forms, quantities, dosage frequency or directions, and automatic stop dates.
- Intravenous therapy data (this information may be kept on a separate profile form but there should be a method for the pharmacist to review both concomitantly).
- Blood products administered.
- Pharmacist's or technician's initials.
- Number of doses or amounts dispensed.
- Items relevant or related to the patient's drug therapy (e.g., blood products) not provided by the pharmacy.

(5) Physician's Drug Order: Records. Appropriate records of each medication order and its processing in the pharmacy must be maintained. Such records must be retained in accordance with applicable state laws and regulations. Any changes or clarifications in the order should be written in the chart. The signature(s) or initials of the person(s) verifying the transcription of medication orders into the medication profile should be noted. A way should be provided to determine, for all doses dispensed, who prepared the dose, its date of dispensing, the source of the drug, and the person who checked it. Other information, such as the time of receipt of the order and management data (number of orders per patient day, and the like) should be kept as desired. Medication profiles also may be useful for retrospective drug use review studies.

(6) Physician's Drug Order: Special Orders. [5,6,13,14] Special orders (i.e., "stat" and emergency orders, and those for nonformulary drugs, investigational drugs, restricted-use drugs or controlled substances) should be processed according to specific written procedures meeting all applicable regulations and requirements.

(7) Physician's Drug Order: Other Considerations. The pharmacy, nursing, and medical staffs, through the pharmacy and therapeutics committee, should develop a schedule of standard drug administration times. The nurse should notify the pharmacist whenever it is necessary to deviate from the standard medication schedule.

A mechanism to continually inform the pharmacy of patient admissions, discharges, and transfers should be established.

(8) Intravenous Admixture Services. [15] The preparation of sterile products (e.g., i.v. admixtures, "piggybacks," irrigations) is an important part of the drug control system. The pharmacy is responsible for assuring that all such products used in the institution are: (1) therapeutically and pharmaceutically appropriate (i.e., are rational and free of incompatibilities or similar problems) to the patient; (2) free from microbial and pyrogenic contaminants; (3) free

from unacceptable levels of particulate and other toxic contaminants; (4) correctly prepared (i.e., contain the correct amounts of the correct drugs), and (5) properly labeled, stored, and distributed. Centralizing all sterile compounding procedures within the pharmacy department is the best way to achieve these goals.

Parenteral admixtures and related solutions are subject to the same considerations presented in the preceding sections "Physician's Drug Order." However, their special characteristics (e.g., complex preparation or need for sterility assurance) also mandate certain additional requirements concerning their preparation, labeling, handling, and quality control. These are described in Reference 15.

It is important that the pharmacy is notified of any problems that arise within the institution pertaining to the use of intravenous drugs and fluids (infections, phlebitis, product defects).

(9) Medication Containers, Labeling and Dispensing: Stock Containers. The pharmacist is responsible for labeling medication containers. Medication labels should be typed or machine-printed. Labeling with pen or pencil and the use of adhesive tape or china marking pencils should be prohibited. A label should not be superimposed on another label. The label should be legible and free from erasures and strikeovers. It should be firmly affixed to the container. The labels for stock containers should be protected from chemical action or abrasion and bear the name, address, and telephone number of the hospital. Medication containers and labels should not be altered by anyone other than pharmacy personnel. Prescription labels should not be distributed outside the pharmacy. Accessory labels and statements (shake well, may

not be refilled, and the like) should be used as required. Any container to be used outside the institution should bear its name, address, and phone number.

Important labeling considerations are:

1. The metric system should be given prominence on all labels when both metric and apothecary measurement units are given.
2. The names of all therapeutically active ingredients should be indicated in compound mixtures.
3. Labels for medications should indicate the amount of drug or drugs in each dosage unit (e.g., per 5 ml, per capsule).
4. Drugs and chemicals in forms intended for dilution or reconstitution should carry appropriate directions.
5. The expiration date of the contents, as well as proper storage conditions, should be clearly indicated.
6. The acceptable route(s) of administration should be indicated for parenteral medications.
7. Labels for large-volume sterile solutions should permit visual inspection of the container contents.
8. Numbers, letters, coined names, unofficial synonyms, and abbreviations should not be used to identify medications, with the exception of approved letter or number codes for investigational drugs (or drugs being used in blinded clinical studies).
9. Containers presenting difficulty in labeling, such as small tubes, should be labeled with no less than the prescription serial number, name of drug, strength, and name of the patient. The container should then be placed in a

larger carton bearing a label with all necessary information.

10. The label should conform to all applicable federal, state, and local laws and regulations.

11. Medication labels of stock containers and repackaged or prepackaged drugs should carry codes to identify the source and lot number of medication.

12. Nonproprietary name(s) should be given prominence over proprietary names.

13. Amount dispensed (e.g., number of tablets) should be indicated.

14. Drug strengths, volumes, and amounts should be given as recommended in References 11 and 16.

(10) Medication Containers, Labeling and Dispensing: Inpatient Medications. [11,16] Drug products should be as ready for administration to the patient as the current status of pharmaceutical technology permits. Inpatient medication containers and packages should conform to applicable USP requirements and the guidelines in References 11 and 16.

Inpatient self-care and "discharge" medications should be labeled as outpatient prescriptions (see below).

(11) Medication Containers, Labeling and Dispensing: Outpatient Medications. [17] Outpatient medications must be labeled in accordance with state board of pharmacy and federal regulations. As noted, medications given to patients as "discharge medication" must be labeled in the pharmacy (not by nursing personnel) as outpatient prescriptions.

The source of the medication and initials of the dispenser should be noted on the prescription form at the time of dispensing. If feasible, the lot number also should be recorded.

An identifying check system to ensure proper identification of outpatients should be established.

Outpatient prescriptions should be packaged in accordance with the provisions of the Poison Prevention Packaging Act of 1970 and any regulations thereunder. They must also meet any applicable requirements of the USP.

Any special instructions to or procedures required of the patient relative to the drug's preparation, storage, and administration should be either a part of the label or accompany the medication container received by the patient. Counseling of the patient sufficient to ensure understanding and compliance (to the extent possible) with his medication regimen must be conducted. Nonprescription drugs, if used in the institution, should be labeled as any other medication.

(12) Delivery of Medications. Couriers used to deliver medications should be reliable and carefully chosen.

Pneumatic tubes, dumbwaiters, medication carts, and the like, should protect drug products from breakage and theft. In those institutions having automatic delivery equipment, such as a pneumatic tube system, provision must be made for an alternate delivery method in case of breakdown.

All parts of the transportation system must protect medications from pilferage. Locks and other security devices should be used where necessary. Procedures for the orderly transfer of medications to the nurse should be instituted, i.e., drug carts or pneumatic tube carriers should not arrive at the patient care area without the nurse or her designee acknowledging their arrival.

Medications must always be properly secured. Storage areas and equipment should meet the requirements presented in other sections of these guidelines.

(13) Administration of Medications. The institution should develop detailed written procedures governing

medication administration. In doing so, the following guidelines should be considered:

1. All medications should be administered by appropriately trained and authorized personnel in accordance with the laws, regulations, and institutional policies governing drug administration. It is particularly important that there are written policies and procedures defining responsibility for starting parenteral infusions, administering all intravenous medications, and adding medications to flowing parenteral fluids. Procedures for drug administration by respiratory therapists and during emergency situations also should be established. Exceptions to any of these policies should be provided in writing.

2. All medications should be administered directly from the medication cart (or equivalent) at the patient's room. The use of unit-dose packaged drugs eliminates the need for medication cups and cards (and their associated trays), and they should not be used. A medication should not be removed from the unit-dose package until it is to be administered.

3. Medications prepared for administration but not used must be returned to the pharmacy.

4. Medications should be given as near the specified time as possible.

5. The patient for whom the medication is intended should be positively identified by checking the patient's identification band or hospital number, or by other means as specified by hospital policy.

6. The person administering the medication should stay with the patient until the dose has been taken. Exceptions to this rule are specific medications which may be left at the patient's bedside, upon the physician's written order for self-administration.

7. Parenteral medications that are not to be mixed together in a syringe should be given in different injection sites on the patient or separately injected into the administration site of the administration set of a compatible intravenous fluid.

8. The pharmacy should receive copies of all medication error reports or other medication-related incidents.

9. A system to assure that patients permitted to self-medicate do so correctly should be established.

(14) Return of Unused Medication. All medications that have not been administered to the patient must remain in the medication cart and be returned to the pharmacy. Only those medications returned in unopened sealed packages may be reissued. Medications returned by outpatients should not be reused. Procedures for crediting and returning drugs to stock should be instituted. A mechanism to reconcile doses not given with nursing and pharmacy records should be provided.

(15) Recording of Medication Administration. All administered, refused, or omitted medication doses should be recorded in the patient's medical record according to an established procedure. Disposition of doses should occur immediately after administering medications to each patient and before proceeding to the next patient. Information to be recorded should include the drug name, dose and route of administration, the date and time of administration, and the initials of the person administering the dose.

Drug Samples and Medical Sales Representatives. [18] The use of drug samples within the institution is strongly discouraged and should be eliminated to the extent possible. They should never be used for inpatients (unless, for some reason, no other source of supply is available to the pharmacy). Any samples used must be controlled and dispensed through the pharmacy.

Written regulations governing the activities of medical sales representatives within the institution should be established. Sales representatives should receive a copy of these rules and their activities monitored.

Investigational Drugs. [13] Policies and procedures governing the use and control of investigational drugs within the institution are necessary. Detailed procedural guidelines are given in Reference 13.

Radiopharmaceuticals. The basic principles of compounding, packaging, sterilizing, testing, and controlling drugs in institutions apply to radiopharmaceuticals. Therefore, even if the pharmacy department is not directly involved with the preparation and dispensing of these agents, the pharmacist must ensure that their use conforms to the drug control principles set forth in this document.

"Bring-in" Medications. The use of a patient's own medications within the hospital should be avoided to the extent possible. They should be used only if the drugs are not obtainable by the pharmacy. If they are used, the physician must write an appropriate order in the patient's medical chart. The drugs should be sent to the pharmacy for verification of their identity; if not identifiable, they must not be used. They should be dispensed as part of the unit dose system, not separate from it.

Drug Control in Operating and Recovery Rooms. [19] The institution's drug control system must extend to its operating room complex. The pharmacist should ensure that all drugs used within this area are properly ordered, stored, prepared, and accounted for.

Emergency Medication Supplies. A policy to supply emergency drugs when the pharmacist is off the premises or when there is insufficient time to get to the pharmacy should exist. Emergency drugs should be limited in number to include only those whose prompt use and immediate availability are generally regarded by physicians as essential in the proper treatment of sudden and unforeseen patient emergencies. The emergency drug supply should not be a source for normal "stat" or "p.r.n." drug orders. The medications included should be primarily for the treatment of cardiac arrest, circulatory collapse, allergic reactions, convulsions, and bronchospasm. The pharmacy and therapeutics committee should specify the drugs and supplies to be included in emergency stocks.

Emergency drug supplies should be inspected by pharmacy personnel on a routine basis to determine if contents have become outdated and are maintained at adequate levels. Emergency kits should have a seal which visually indicates when they have been opened. The expiration date of the kit should be clearly indicated.

Pharmacy Service When the Pharmacy is Closed. Hospitals provide services to patients 24 hours a day. Pharmaceutical services are an integral part of the total care provided by the hospital, and the services of a pharmacist should be available at all times. Where around-the-clock operation of the pharmacy is not feasible, a pharmacist should be available on an "on-call" basis. The use of "night cabinets" and drug dispensing by nonpharmacists should be minimized, and eliminated wherever possible.

Drugs must not be dispensed to outpatients or hospital staff by anyone other than a pharmacist while the pharmacy is open. If it is necessary for nurses to obtain drugs when the pharmacy is closed and the pharmacist is unavailable, written procedures covering this practice should be developed. They generally should provide for a limited supply of the drugs most commonly needed in these situations; the drugs should be in proper single-dose packages and a log should be kept of all doses removed. This log must contain the date and time the drugs were removed, a complete description of the drug product(s), name of the (authorized) nurse involved, and the patient's name.

Drugs should not be dispensed to emergency room patients by nonpharmacist personnel if the pharmacy is open. When no pharmacist is available, emergency room patients should receive drugs packaged, to the extent possible, in single unit packages; no more than a day's supply of doses should be dispensed. The use of an emergency room "formulary" is recommended.[20]

Adverse Drug Reactions. The medical, nursing, and pharmacy staffs must always be alert to the potential for, or presence of, adverse drug reactions. A written procedure to record clinically significant adverse drug reactions should be established. These should be reported to the Food and Drug Administration, the involved drug manufacturer, and the institution's pharmacy and therapeutics committee (or its equivalent). Adverse drug reaction reports should contain:

- Patient's age, sex, and race.
- Description of the drug reaction and suspected cause.
- Name of drug(s) suspected of causing the reaction.
- Administration route and dose.
- Name(s) of other drugs received by patient.
- Treatment of the reaction, if any.

These reports, along with other significant reports from the literature, should be reviewed and evaluated by the pharmacy and therapeutics committee. Steps necessary to minimize the incidence of adverse drug reactions in the facility should be taken.

Medication Errors. If a medication error is detected, the patient's physician must be informed immediately. A written report should be prepared describing any medication errors of clinical import observed in the prescribing, dispensing, or administration of a medication. This report, in accordance with hospital policy, should be prepared and sent to the appropriate hospital officials (including the pharmacy) within 24 hours. These reports should be analyzed, and any necessary action taken, to minimize the possibility of recurrence of such errors. Properly utilized, these incident reports will help to assure optimum drug use control. Medication error reports should be reviewed periodically by the pharmacy and therapeutics committee. (It should be kept in mind that, in the absence of an organized, independent error detection system, most medication errors will go unnoticed.)

Special Considerations Contributing to Drug Control

Pharmacy Personnel and Management.[21-24] Adequate numbers of competent personnel and a well-managed pharmacy are the keys to an effective drug control system. References 21-24 provide guidance on the competencies required of the pharmacy staff and on administrative requirements of a well-run pharmacy department.

Assuring Rational Drug Therapy: Clinical Services.[21,25] Maximizing rational drug use is an important part of the drug control system. Although all pharmacy services contribute to this goal in a sense, the provision of drug information to the institution's patients and staff and the pharmacy's clinical services are those that most directly contribute to rational drug therapy. They are, in fact, institutional pharmacists' most important contribution to patient care.

Facilities. Space and equipment requirements relative to drug storage have been discussed previously. In addition to these considerations, space and equipment must be sufficient to provide for safe and efficient drug preparation and distribution, patient education and consultation, drug information services, and proper management of the department.

Hospital Committees Important to Drug Control.[26,27] Several hospital committees deal with matters of drug control, and the pharmacist must actively participate in their activities. Among these committees (whose names may vary among institutions) are the pharmacy and therapeutics committee, infection control committee, use review committee, product evaluation committee, patient care committee, and the committee for protection of human subjects. Of particular importance to the drug control system are the formulary and drug use review (DUR) functions of the pharmacy and therapeutics committee (though DUR in many institutions may be under a use review or quality assurance committee).

Drug Use Review.[28] Review of how drugs are prescribed and used is an important part of institutional quality assurance and drug control systems. DUR programs may be performed retrospectively or, preferably, concurrently or prospectively. They may utilize patient outcomes or therapeutic processes as the basis for judgments about the appropriateness of drug prescribing and use. Depending on the review methodology, the pharmacist should be involved in:

1. Preparing, in cooperation with the medical staff, drug use criteria and standards.
2. Obtaining quantitative data on drug use, i.e., information on the amounts and types of drugs used, prescribing patterns by medical service, type of patient, and so forth. These data will be useful in setting priorities for the review program. They also may serve as a measure of the effectiveness of DUR programs, assist in analyzing nosocomial infection and culture and sensitivity data, and help in preparing drug budgets.
3. Reviewing medication orders against the drug use criteria and standards.
4. Consulting with prescribers concerning the results of (3) above.
5. Participating in the follow-up activities of the review program, i.e., educational programs directed at prescribers; development of recommendations for the formulary, and changes in drug control procedures in response to the results of the review process.

It should be noted that the overall drug use review program is a joint responsibility of the pharmacy and the organized medical staff; it is not unilaterally a pharmacy or medical staff function.

Quality Assurance for Pharmaceutical Services.[29] In order to ensure that the drug control system is functioning as intended, there should be a formalized method to: (1) set precise objectives (in terms of outcome and process criteria and standards) for the system; (2) measure and verify the degree of compliance with these standards, i.e, the extent to which the objectives have been realized; and (3) eliminate any noncompliance situations. Such a *quality assurance program* will be distinct from, though related to, the drug use review activities of the department.

Drug Recalls. A written procedure to handle drug product recalls should be developed. Any such system should have the following elements:

1. Whenever feasible, notation of the drug manufacturer's name and drug lot number should appear on outpatient prescriptions, inpatient drug orders or profiles, packaging control records, and stock requisitions and their associated labels.
2. Review of these documents (prescriptions, drug orders, and so forth) to determine the recipients (patients, nursing stations) of the recalled lots. Optimally, this would be done by automated means.
3. In the case of product recalls of substantial clinical significance, a notice should go to the recipients that they have a recalled product. The course of action they should take should be included. In the case of outpatients, caution should be exercised not to cause undue alarm. The uninterrupted therapy of the patients must be assured, i.e., replacement of the recalled drugs generally will be required. The hospital's administration and nursing and medical staffs should be informed of any recalls having significant therapeutic implications. Some situations also may require notifying the physicians of patients receiving drugs that have been recalled.
4. Personal inspection of all patient care areas should be made to deter-

mine if any of the recalled products are present.
5. Quarantine of all recalled products obtained (marked: Quarantined — Do Not Use") until they are picked up by or returned to the manufacturer.
6. Maintenance of a written log of all recalls, the actions taken, and their results.

Computerization. [30] Many information-handling tasks in the drug control system (e.g., collecting, recording, storing, retrieving, summarizing, transmitting and displaying drug use information) may be done more efficiently by computers than by manual systems. Before the drug control system can be computerized, however, a comprehensive, thorough study of the existing manual system must be conducted. This study should identify the data flow within the system and define the functions to be done and their interrelationships. This information is then used as the basis to design or prospectively evaluate a computer system; any other considerations, such as those of the hospital accounting department, are subordinate.

The computer system must include adequate safeguards to maintain the confidentiality of patient records.

A backup system must be available to continue the computerized functions during equipment failure. All transactions occurring while the computer system is inoperable should be entered into the system as soon as possible.

Data on controlled substances must be readily retrievable in written form from the system.

Defective Drug Products, Equipment, and Supplies. The pharmacist should be notified of any defective drug products (or related supplies and equipment) encountered by the nursing or medical staffs. All drug product defects should be reported to the USP-FDA-ASHP Drug Product Defect Reporting Program.

Disposal of Hazardous Substances. Hazardous substances (e.g., toxic or flammable solvents, carcinogenic agents) must be disposed of properly in accordance with the requirements of the Environmental Protection Agency or other applicable regulations. The substances should not be poured indiscriminately down the drain or mixed in with the usual trash.

Unreconstituted vials or ampuls and unopened bottles of oral medications supplied by the National Cancer Institute (NCI) should be returned to the NCI's contract storage and distribution facility.

Other intact products should be returned to the original source for disposition.

Units of anticancer drugs no longer intact, such as reconstituted vials, opened ampuls, and bottles of oral medications, and any equipment (e.g., needles and syringes) used in their preparation, require a degree of caution greater than with less toxic compounds to safeguard personnel from accidental exposure. The National Institutes of Health recommends that all such materials be segregated for special destruction procedures. The items should be kept in special containers marked *"Danger–Chemical Carcinogens."* Needles and syringes first should be rendered unusable, then placed in specially marked plastic bags. Care should be taken to prevent penetration and leakage of the bags. Excess liquids should be placed in sealed containers; the original vial is satisfactory. Disposal of all of the above materials should be by incineration to destroy organic material.

Alternate disposal for BCG vaccine products has been recommended by the Bureau of Biologics (BOB). The BOB suggests all containers and equipment used with BCG vaccines be sterilized prior to disposal. Autoclaving at 121°C for 30 minutes will sterilize the equipment.

At all steps in the handling of anticancer drugs and other hazardous substances, care should be taken to safeguard professional and support services personnel from accidental exposure to these agents.

References

1. Ginnow WK, King CM Jr. Revision and reorganization of a hospital pharmacy policy and procedure manual. *Am J Hosp Pharm.* 1978; 35:698-704.
2. Accreditation manual for hospitals, 1980 ed. Chicago: Joint Commission on Accreditation of Hospitals; 1979.
3. Publications, reprints and services. Washington, DC: American Society of Hospital Pharmacists; current edition.
4. ASHP guidelines for selecting pharmaceutical manufacturers and distributors. *Am J Hosp Pharm.* 1976; 33-645-6.
5. ASHP guidelines for hospital formularies. *Am J Hosp Pharm.* 1978; 35:326-8.
6. ASHP statement of guiding principles on the operation of the hospital formulary system. *Am J Hosp Pharm.* 1964; 21:40-1.
7. ASHP guidelines for repackaging oral solids and liquids in single unit and unit dose packages. *Am J Hosp Pharm.* 1979; 36:223-4.
8. 21 CFR Parts 210 and 211. Current good manufacturing practices in manufacturing, processing, packing or holding of drugs. April 1979.

9. Sourcebook on unit dose drug distribution systems. Washington, DC: American Society of Hospital Pharmacists; 1978.

10. ASHP statement on unit dose drug distribution. *Am J Hosp Pharm.* 1975; 32:835.

11. ASHP guidelines for single unit and unit dose packages of drugs. *Am J Hosp Pharm.* 1977; 34:613-4.

12. ASHP guidelines for obtaining authorization for pharmacists' notations in the patient medical record. *Am J Hosp Pharm.* 1979; 36:222-3.

13. ASHP guidelines for the use of investigational drugs in institutions. *Am J Hosp Pharm.* 1979; 36:221-2.

14. ASHP guidelines for institutional use of controlled substances. *Am J Hosp Pharm.* 1974; 31:582-8.

15. Recommendations of the National Coordinating Committee on Large Volume Parenterals. Washington, DC: American Society of Hospital Pharmacists; 1980.

16. National Coordinating Committee on Large Volume Parenterals. Recommendations for the labeling of large volume parenterals. *Am J Hosp Pharm.* 1978; 35:49-51.

17. ASHP guidelines on pharmacist-conducted patient counseling. *Am J Hosp Pharm.* 1976; 33:644-5.

18. Lipman AG, Mullen HF. Quality control of medical service representative activities in the hospital. *Am J Hosp Pharm.* 1974; 31:167-70.

19. Evans DM, Guenther AM, Keith TD et al. Pharmacy practice in an operating room complex. *Am J Hosp Pharm.* 1979; 36:1342-7.

20. Mar DD, Hanan ZI, LaFontaine R. Improved emergency room medication distribution. *Am J Hosp Pharm.* 1978; 35:70-3.

21. ASHP minimum standard for pharmacies in institutions. *Am J Hosp Pharm.* 1977; 34:1356-8.

22. ASHP guidelines on the competencies required in institutional pharmacy practice. *Am J Hosp Pharm.* 1975; 32:917-9.

23. ASHP training guidelines for hospital pharmacy supportive personnel. *Am J Hosp Pharm.* 1976; 33:646-8.

24. ASHP competency standard for pharmacy supportive personnel in organized health care settings. *Am J Hosp Pharm.* 1978; 35:449-51.

25. ASHP statement on clinical functions in institutional pharmacy practice. *Am J Hosp Pharm.* 1978; 35:813.

26. ASHP statement on the pharmacy and therapeutics committee. *Am J Hosp Pharm.* 1978; 35:813-4.

27. ASHP statement on the hospital pharmacist's role in infection control. *Am J Hosp Pharm.* 1978; 35:814-5.

28. Antibiotic use review and infection control: evaluating drug use through patient care audit. Chicago: InterQual, Inc.; 1978. (Available through ASHP).

29. Model quality assurance program for hospital pharmacies, revised. Washington, DC: American Society of Hospital Pharmacists; 1980.

30. Sourcebook on computers in pharmacy. Washington, DC: American Society of Hospital Pharmacists; 1978.

Accreditation Manual for Hospitals 1980 Edition

Pharmaceutical Services

Principle

The hospital shall maintain a pharmaceutical department/service that is conducted in accordance with accepted ethical and professional practices and all legal requirements.

Standard I

The pharmaceutical department/service shall be directed by a professionally competent and legally qualified pharmacist. It shall be staffed by a sufficient number of competent personnel, in keeping with the size and scope of services of the hospital.

Interpretation

The pharmaceutical department/service shall be directed by a competent pharmacist who is appropriately licensed and who is responsible to the chief executive officer of the hospital or his designee. The director should either be a graduate of a college of pharmacy accredited by the American Council on Pharmaceutical Education and oriented and knowledge-able in the specialized functions of hospital pharmacies, or have completed a hospital pharmacy residency program accredited by the American Society of Hospital Pharmacists. Consideration may be given to graduates of foreign colleges of pharmacy who are appropriately licensed and otherwise qualified to perform the responsibilities of the job. The director may be employed full-time or part-time.

The pharmaceutical services provided shall be sufficient to meet the needs of the patients as determined by the medical staff. It is recommended that a pharmacist be available at all times. Whether this is on an on duty, on call, or consultative basis should be determined by the pharmacy work load.

When the hospital pharmaceutical department/service is decentralized, a licensed pharmacist, responsible to the director of the pharmaceutical department/service, shall supervise each satellite pharmacy or separate organizational element involved with the preparation and dispensing of drugs and with the provision of drug information and other pharmaceutical services.

The director of the pharmaceutical department/service should be assisted by additional qualified pharmacists and pharmacy supportive personnel commensurate with the scope of services provided. Nonpharmacist personnel shall work under the direct supervision of a licensed pharmacist and in such a relationship that the supervising pharmacist is fully aware of all activities involved in the preparation and dispensing of medications, including the maintenance of appropriate records. The duties and responsibilities of nonpharmacist personnel must be consistent with their training and experience, and they shall not be assigned duties that by law or regulation must be performed only by a licensed pharmacist. Clerical and stenographic assistance should be provided as needed to assist with records, reports, and correspondence.

The organizational structure of the pharmaceutical department/service will vary with the size and complexity of the hospital and the scope of services provided. The pharmacy shall be licensed as required.

If the hospital does not have an organized pharmacy, pharmaceutical services shall be obtained from another hospital having such services or from a community pharmacy. Prepackaged drugs then shall be stored in, and distributed from, the hospital drug storage area, under the supervision of the director of the pharmaceutical department/service. Prepackaged drugs obtained from pharmacies outside the hospital shall be identified and labeled so that recalls can be effected as necessary and the proper controls established. There shall be an approved written procedure for obtaining drugs from another hospital or community pharmacy on a routine basis and in emergencies.

Standard II

Space, equipment, and supplies shall be provided for the professional and administrative functions of the pharmaceutical department/service as required, to promote patient safety through the proper storage, preparation, dispensing, and administration of drugs.

Interpretation

Hospitals with an organized pharmaceutical department/service shall have the necessary space, equipment, and supplies for the storage, preparation (compounding, packaging labeling), and dispensing of drugs. As appropriate, this shall include the preparation and dispensing of parenteral products and radiopharmaceuticals.

Drug storage and preparation areas within the pharmacy and throughout the hospital must be under the supervision of the director of the pharmaceutical department/service or his pharmacist-designee. Drugs must be stored under proper conditions of sanitation, temperature, light, moisture, ventilation, segregation, and security. Properly controlled drug preparation areas should be designated, and locked storage areas or locked medication carts provided, for each nursing unit as required. Drug preparation areas should be well-lighted and should be located where personnel preparing drugs for dispensing or administration will not be interrupted. The director of the pharmaceutical department/service or his qualified designee must conduct at least monthly inspections of all nursing care units or other areas of the hospital where medications are dispensed, administered, or stored.

A record of all such monthly inspections shall be maintained to verify that:

- antiseptics, other drugs for external use, and disinfectants are stored separately from internal and injectable medications.
- drugs requiring special conditions for storage to assure stability are properly stored. For example, biologicals and other thermolabile medications shall be stored in a separate compartment within a refrigerator that is capable of maintaining the necessary temperature. All drugs must be stored in accordance with current established standards (United States Pharmacopeia). Drugs not listed in the official compendia must be stored so that their integrity, stability, and effectiveness are maintained.
- outdated or otherwise unusable drugs have been identified and their distribution and administration prevented. The director of the pharmaceutical department/service, with the approval of the chief executive officer, shall designate one or more areas for the authorized storage of such drugs prior to their proper disposition.
- distribution and administration of controlled drugs are adequately documented by the pharmacy, nursing service, and other involved services or personnel, and are in accordance with federal and state law.
- any investigational drugs in use are properly stored, distributed, and controlled.
- emergency drugs, as approved by the medical staff, are in adequate and proper supply within the pharmacy and in designated hospital areas. The pharmacist should be responsible both for the contents of emergency medication carts, kits, and so forth, and for the inspection procedure to be used.
- the metric system is in use for all medications. Metric-apothecaries' weight and measure conversion charts should be available to those professional individuals who may require them.

There should be a suitable area for the manipulation of parenteral medications. When laminar airflow hoods are used, quality control requirements shall include cleaning of the equipment used on each shift, microbiological monitoring as required by the infection control committee, and periodic checks for operational efficiency at least every 12 months by a qualified inspector. Appropriate records shall be maintained.

Materials and equipment necessary for the administration of the pharmaceutical department/service should be provided. Effective messenger and delivery service, when appropriate, should be provided for the pharmacy.

Up-to-date pharmaceutical reference materials shall be provided in order to furnish the pharmaceutical, medical, and nursing staffs with adequate information concerning drugs. These should include official pharmaceutical compendia and periodicals, as well as current editions of text and reference books covering the following: theoretical and practical pharmacy; general, organic, pharmaceutical, and biological chemistry; toxicology; pharmacology; therapeutics; bacteriology; sterilization and disinfection; compatibility and drug interaction references; and other related matters important to good pharmaceutical practice in its relation to patient care. Authoritative, current antidote information and the telephone number of the regional poison control information center should be readily available in the pharmacy for emergency reference. Current federal and state drug law information should be readily available to the pharmaceutical department/service.

Standard III

The scope of the pharmaceutical department/service shall be consistent with the medication needs of the patients as determined by the medical staff.

Interpretation

All drugs, chemicals, and biologicals shall meet national standards of quality or shall be clearly and accurately labeled as to contents, and such information shall be disclosed to the medical staff. All drugs should be obtained and used in accordance with written policies and procedures that have been approved by the medical staff. Such policies and procedures should relate to the selection, the distribution, and the safe and effective use of drugs in the hospital, and should be established by the combined effort of the director of the pharmaceutical department/service, the medical staff, the nursing service, and the administration.

Within this framework, the director of the pharmaceutical department/service should be responsible for at least the following:

- Maintaining an adequate drug supply.
- Establishing specifications for the procurement of all approved drugs, and those chemicals and biologicals related to the practice of pharmacy.
- Preparing and dispensing drugs and chemicals.
- Preparing, sterilizing, and labeling parenteral medications and solutions that are manufactured in the hospital. There shall be an associated quality control program to monitor personnel qualifications, training and performance, and equipment and facilities. The end product should be examined on a sampling basis, as determined by the director of the pharmaceutical department/service, to assure that it meets the required specifications. Appropriate records shall be maintained. The compounding and admixture of large volume parenterals should ordinarily be the responsibility of a qualified pharmacist. Individuals who prepare or administer large volume parenterals should have special training to do so. When any part of the above functions (preparing, sterilizing, and labeling parenteral medications and solutions) is performed within the hospital but not under direct pharmacy supervision, the director of the pharmaceutical department/service shall be responsible for providing written guidelines and for approving the procedure to assure that all pharmaceutical requirements are met. In the interest of safety of preparation and administration, and effective nutritional content, overall direction shall be provided by a qualified physician when total parenteral nutrition products (hyperalimentation) are required.
- Participating in the initial orientation and subsequent in-service education, including the provision of appropriate incompatibility information, of all personnel involved in the preparation or administration of sterile parenteral medications and solutions.
- Any in-hospital manufacturing of pharmaceuticals, with proper control procedures.

- Maintaining and keeping available the medical staff-approved stock of antidotes and other emergency drugs, both in the pharmacy and in patient care areas. Authoritative, current antidote information, as well as the phone number of the regional poison control information center, should also be readily available in areas outside the pharmacy where these drugs are stored.
- Filling and labeling all drug containers issued to the departments/services from which medications are to be administered.
- Maintaining records of the transactions of the pharmacy as required by federal, state, and local laws, and as necessary to maintain adequate control and accountability of all drugs. This should include a system of controls and records for the requisitioning and dispensing of pharmaceutical supplies to nursing care units and to other departments/services of the hospital.
- Participating in the development and subsequent updating of a hospital formulary or drug list. The medical staff, through its pharmacy and therapeutics function, shall determine the hospital formulary to be used. When properly annotated, a formulary developed outside the hospital will suffice if it is maintained as a current document and if it has been approved by the medical staff. Any hospital formulary or drug list should be readily available to the professional staff who use it, and the staff should be kept informed of any changes. The formulary or drug list should also include the availability of non-legend medications. The existence of a formulary does not preclude the use of unlisted drugs, and there should be a written policy and procedure for their procurement.

- Requiring and documenting the participation of pharmacy personnel in relevant education programs, including orientation of new employees, as well as in-service and outside continuing education programs. Frequency of programs and participation shall be related to the scope of the pharmaceutical services offered and shall be established with the approval of the chief executive officer.
- Participating in those aspects of the overall hospital quality assurance program that relate to drug utilization and effectiveness. This may include determining usage patterns for each drug according to clinical department/service or individual prescribers, and assisting in the setting of drug use criteria. Refer also to the Quality Assurance section of this *Manual*.
- Participating in all meetings of the pharmacy and therapeutics committee and implementing the decisions of that committee throughout the hospital.
- Communicating new product information to nursing service and other hospital personnel, as required.
- Performing an annual review of all pharmaceutical policies and procedures for the purpose of establishing their consistency with current practices within the hospital.
- Maintaining confidentiality of patient/medical staff information.
- Maintaining a means of identifying the signature of all practitioners authorized to use the pharmaceutical services for ambulatory care patient prescriptions, as well as a listing of their Drug Enforcement Administration numbers.
- Cooperating in the teaching and research programs of the hospital.

Within the limits of available resources, the pharmaceutical department/service should provide drug monitoring services in keeping with each patient's needs. These may include, but are not necessarily limited to, the following:

* The maintenance of a medication record or drug profile for each patient, which is based on available drug history and current therapy and includes the name, age, and weight of the patient, the current diagnosis(es), the current drug therapy, any drug allergies or sensitivities, and other pertinent information relating to the patient's drug regimen. This information should be available to the responsible practitioners at all times.
* A review of the patient's drug regimen for any potential interactions, interferences, or incompatibilities, prior to dispensing drugs to the patient. Such irregularities must be resolved promptly with the prescribing practitioner, and when appropriate, with notification of the nursing service and administration.
* The instruction of the patient or of the appropriate nursing department/service personnel who advise the patient, verbally or in writing, on the importance and correct use of medication to be taken following discharge, in the interest of assuring safe and correct self-administration, when such instruction is requested by the responsible practitioner or as provided by written medical staff policy.

The director of the pharmaceutical department/service and staff pharmacists should be invited to participate on a regular basis in the education of medical staff and nursing service personnel in regard to drugs and biologicals in use in the hospital. This may include information on drug incompatibilities and sensitivities, on

the monitoring of end-points for initial signs of toxicity or optimum drug effect, and on new drugs. Individuals who have responsibility for drug storage or administration should be instructed in the recognition of signs of drug deterioration. Greatest benefit occurs when qualified pharmaceutical department/service staffing permits the establishment of a drug information center in the hospital, which is available at all times to professional staff members.

Standard IV

Written policies and procedures that pertain to the intrahospital drug distribution system shall be developed by the director of the pharmaceutical department/service in concert with the medical staff and, as appropriate, with representatives of other disciplines.

Interpretation

Drug preparation and dispensing shall be restricted to a licensed pharmacist, or to his designee under the direct supervision of the pharmacist. A pharmacist should review the prescriber's order, or a direct copy thereof, before the initial dose of medication is dispensed (with the exception of emergency orders when time does not permit). In cases when the medication order is written when the pharmacy is "closed" or the pharmacist is otherwise unavailable, the medication order should be reviewed by the pharmacist as soon thereafter as possible, preferably within 24 hours.

The use of floor stock medications should be minimized; the unit dose drug distribution system, which permits identification of the drug up to the point of administration, is recommended for use throughout the hospital.

Written policies and procedures that are essential for patient safety and for the control, accountability, and intrahospital distribution of drugs shall be reviewed annually, revised as necessary, and enforced. Such policies and procedures shall include, but not be limited to, the following:

- All drugs shall be labeled adequately, including the addition of appropriate accessory or cautionary statements, as well as the expiration date when applicable.
- Discontinued and outdated drugs, and containers with worn, illegible, or missing labels, shall be returned to the pharmacy for proper disposition.
- Only a pharmacist, or authorized pharmacy personnel under the direction and supervision of a pharmacist, shall dispense medications, make labeling changes, or transfer medications to different containers.
- Only prepackaged drugs shall be removed from the pharmacy when a pharmacist is not available. These drugs shall be removed only by a designated registered nurse or a physician, and only in amounts sufficient for immediate therapeutic needs. Such drugs should be kept in a separate cabinet, closet, or other designated area and shall be properly labeled. A record of such withdrawals shall be made by the authorized individual removing such drugs and shall be verified by a pharmacist.
- There shall be a written drug recall procedure that can be implemented readily and the results documented. This requirement shall apply to both inpatient and ambulatory care patient medications.
- Drug product defects should be reported in accordance with the ASHP-USP-FDA Drug Product Problem Reporting Program.
- Medications to be dispensed to inpatients at the time of discharge from the hospital shall be labeled as for ambulatory care patient prescriptions.
- A system designed to assure accurate identification of ambulatory care patients at the time they receive prescribed medications should be established.
- Unless otherwise provided by law, ambulatory care patient prescription labels should bear the following information:
  - Name, address, and telephone number of the hospital pharmacy;
  - Date and pharmacy's identifying serial number for the prescription;
  - Full name of the patient;
  - Name of the drug, strength, and amount dispensed;
  - Directions to the patient for use;
  - Name of the prescribing practitioner;
  - Name or initials of the dispensing individual; and
  - Any required Drug Enforcement Administration cautionary label on controlled substance drugs, and any other pertinent accessory cautionary labels.
- In the interest of effective control, the distribution of drug samples within the hospital should be eliminated if possible. Sample drugs brought into the hospital shall be controlled through the pharmaceutical department/service.

Standard V

Written policies and procedures governing the safe administration of drugs and biologicals shall be developed by the medical staff in cooperation with the pharmaceutical department/service, the nursing service, and, as necessary, representatives of other disciplines.

Interpretation

Written policies and procedures governing the safe administration of drugs shall be reviewed at least annually, revised as necessary, and enforced. Such policies and procedures shall include, but not necessarily be limited to, the following:

- Drugs shall be administered only upon the order of a member of the medical staff, an authorized member of the house staff, or other individual who has been granted clinical privileges to write such orders. Verbal orders for drugs may be accepted only by personnel so designated in the medical staff rules and regulations and must be authenticated by the prescribing practitioner within the stated period of time.
- All medications shall be administered by, or under the supervision of, appropriately licensed personnel in accordance with laws and governmental rules and regulations governing such acts and in accordance with the approved medical staff rules and regulations.
- There shall be an automatic cancellation of standing drug orders when a patient undergoes surgery. Automatic drug stop orders shall otherwise be determined by the medical staff and stated in medical staff rules and regulations. There shall be a system to notify the responsible practitioner of the impending expiration of a drug order, so that the practitioner may determine whether the drug administration is to be continued or altered.
- Cautionary measures for the safe admixture of parenteral products

shall be developed. Whenever drugs are added to intravenous solutions, a distinctive supplementary label shall be affixed to the container. The label shall indicate the patient's name and location; the name and amount of the drug(s) added; the name of the basic parenteral solution; the date and time of the addition; the date, time, and rate of administration; the name or identifying code of the individual who prepared the admixture; supplemental instructions; and the expiration date of the compounded solution.

- Drugs to be administered shall be verified with the prescribing practitioner's orders and properly prepared for administration. The patient shall be identified prior to drug administration, and each dose of medication administered shall be recorded properly in the patient's medical record.
- Medication errors and adverse drug reactions shall be reported immediately in accordance with written procedures. This requirement shall include notification of the practitioner who ordered the drug. An entry of the medication administered and/or the drug reaction shall be properly recorded in the patient's medical record. Hospitals are encouraged to report any unexpected or significant adverse reactions promptly to the Food and Drug Administration and to the manufacturer.
- Drugs brought into the hospital by patients shall not be administered unless the drugs have been identified and there is a written order from the responsible practitioner to administer the drugs. If the drugs are not to be used during the patient's hospitalization, they should

be packaged and sealed, and either given to the patient's family or stored and returned to the patient at the time of discharge, provided such action is approved by the responsible practitioner.

- Self-administration of medications by patients shall be permitted on a specific written order by the authorized prescribing practitioner and in accordance with established hospital policy.
- Investigational drugs shall be properly labeled and stored, and shall be used only under the direct supervision of the authorized principal investigator. Such drugs should be approved by an appropriate medical staff committee. Investigational drugs should be administered in accordance with an approved protocol that includes any requirements for a patient's appropriate informed consent. On approval of the principal investigator, registered nurses may administer these drugs after they have been given, and have demonstrated an understanding of, basic pharmacologic information about the drugs. In the absence of an organized pharmaceutical department/service, a central unit should be established where essential information on such drugs is maintained.
- Orders involving abbreviations and chemical symbols should be carried out only if the abbreviations/symbols appear on an explanatory legend approved by the medical staff. In the interest of minimizing errors, the use of abbreviations is discouraged, and the use of the leading decimal point should be avoided. Each practitioner who prescribes medication must clearly state the administration times or the time interval between doses. The use of "prn" and "on call" with medication orders should be qualified.

- Drugs prescribed for ambulatory care patient use in continuity with hospital care shall be released to patients upon discharge only after they are labeled for such use under the supervision of the pharmacist and only on written order of the authorized prescribing practitioner. Each drug released to a patient on discharge should be recorded in the medical record.
- Individual drugs should be administered as soon as possible after the dose has been prepared, particularly medications prepared for parenteral administration, and, to the maximum extent possible, by the individual who prepared the dose, except where unit dose drug distribution systems are used.

Unless otherwise provided by the medical staff bylaws, rules and regulations or by legal requirements, prescribing practitioners may, within their discretion at the time of prescribing, approve or disapprove the dispensing of a nonproprietary drug or the dispensing of a different proprietary brand to their patients by the pharmacist.

Refer also to the Anesthesia Services, Emergency Services, Functional Safety and Sanitation, Home Care Services, Hospital-Sponsored Ambulatory Care Services, Infection Control, Medical Record Services, Medical Staff, Nuclear Medicine Services, Nursing Services, Respiratory Care Services, and Special Care Units sections of this *Manual.*

INDEX

Numerals in *italics* indicate figures, "t" indicates tabular matter.